Innovations in Healthcare and Outcome Measurement

Philipp Plugmann • Dorothea Portius
Editors

Innovations in Healthcare and Outcome Measurement

New Approaches for a Healthy Lifestyle

Springer

Editors
Philipp Plugmann
SRH University of Applied Sciences
Cologne, Germany

Dorothea Portius
Institute for Agriculture and Nutritional Sciences
Martin-Luther-University Halle-Wittenberg
Halle (Saale), Germany

ISBN 978-3-031-77301-3 ISBN 978-3-031-77302-0 (eBook)
https://doi.org/10.1007/978-3-031-77302-0

This Springer imprint is published by the registered company Springer Nature Switzerland AG
The registered company address is: Gewerbestrasse 11, 6330 Cham, Switzerland

Foreword

In recent years, the healthcare landscape has been dynamically transformed by a confluence of groundbreaking innovations. With the integration of digital technologies, advanced molecular profiling, and artificial intelligence, the realm of healthcare and outcome measurement has been elevated to unprecedented heights. This edited volume, *Innovations in Healthcare and Outcome Measurement*: *New Approaches for a Healthy Lifestyle*, seeks to encapsulate the myriad advancements and their profound impact on modern medicine.

The chapters within this volume are a testament to the interdisciplinary efforts and the relentless pursuit of excellence in healthcare. From precision medicine, which tailors treatment to individual genetic profiles, to the revolutionary use of AI in diagnostics and treatment planning, each contribution offers a deep dive into the cutting-edge technologies and methodologies that are reshaping patient care. The authors, both from industry and academia, are esteemed experts in their respective fields. They provide a comprehensive overview of the current state of healthcare innovations and their future potential.

The editors, Dr. Dorothea Portius and Prof. Dr. Dr. Philipp Plugmann, have meticulously curated this volume to ensure it encompasses a broad spectrum of topics relevant to modern healthcare challenges and solutions. Each chapter not only presents state-of-the-art research and developments but also provides critical insights into the practical applications and future directions of these innovations.

As you embark on this journey through the pages of *Innovations in Healthcare and Outcome Measurement*, I hope you find inspiration and valuable knowledge that will contribute to your understanding and the furthering of healthcare excellence. This compilation is not just a reflection of current advancements but a beacon guiding future explorations in the quest for a healthier world. I am sure that this volume will be a valuable resource for anyone interested in advances in healthcare, from students and researchers to industry professionals and policymakers. I wish you every success in reading this work and implementing the recommendations for action contained therein.

Deggendorf Institute of Technology
Deggendorf, Germany
July 2024

Patrick Glauner

Preface

In the ever-evolving landscape of healthcare, the pursuit of a healthier lifestyle through innovation has become a driving force for remarkable advancements. We are honored to present this book, *Innovations in Healthcare and Outcome Measurement*: *New Approaches for a Healthy Lifestyle*, which brings together pioneering ideas and critical developments from a diverse array of experts.

The past decade has witnessed transformative changes in healthcare, spurred by breakthroughs in digitalization, personalized medicine, advanced cell and tissue engineering, and artificial intelligence (AI). These innovations are not merely incremental improvements but revolutionary strides that are redefining how we approach the prevention and treatment of diseases, particularly noncommunicable diseases that pose significant challenges to global health and our healthcare systems.

One of the cornerstones of this revolution is precision medicine. By understanding the unique genetic, environmental, and lifestyle factors that influence an individual's health, precision medicine offers the promise of highly tailored interventions. The integration of genomics, proteomics, and other molecular profiling techniques has equipped healthcare providers with unprecedented insights into patients' molecular blueprints. These insights enable the development of targeted therapies that maximize efficacy while minimizing adverse effects, thereby enhancing patient outcomes and the quality of life.

Moreover, the advent of advanced diagnostic tools has significantly improved the accuracy and efficiency of disease detection and monitoring. High-resolution imaging technologies, wearable sensors, and liquid biopsies are revolutionizing the diagnostic landscape. When combined with the power of AI and machine learning, these innovations are augmenting the capabilities of healthcare management and precision medicine, paving the way for more precise and effective treatments.

This book is a comprehensive guide to the latest advancements, opinions, and critical issues in healthcare and personalized medicine. It covers a wide range of topics, including advances in medical devices, digitalization and data-driven technologies, AI in drug development, diagnostic imaging, personalized medicine, nutrition, the microbiome, oral healthcare, and more. Each chapter delves into these subjects with depth and clarity, offering valuable insights for researchers, clinicians, and policymakers.

Among the compelling topics covered, we explore the transformative potential of cloud computing in healthcare and the profound insights derived from data analytics and AI. We also examine the integration of nature and technology in biohacking, the future of human disease diagnosis through saliva, and the revolutionary use of 3D technology in orthopedics. Each chapter is a testament to the relentless pursuit of innovation and its potential to reshape healthcare from diverse perspectives.

As guest editors, we are thrilled to bring together this collection of cutting-edge research and thought leadership. We hope this book will serve as a valuable resource for those dedicated to advancing healthcare and improving patient outcomes. We extend our deepest gratitude to all the contributors for their invaluable work and to our readers for their commitment to fostering a healthier, more innovative future.

Cologne, Germany — Philipp Plugmann
Halle (Saale), Germany — Dorothea Portius

Contents

Part I

Pioneering Technological Healthcare Innovations

1 Unlocking the Code of Innovation: TRIZ Theory's Blueprint for Precision Medicine Breakthroughs

Rudi Schmidt

Is there a fundamental "grand unified theory" that can systematically explain and predict innovations and inventions in precision medicine? An approach that is more than 70 years old may be able to answer this question in the affirmative. The Theory of Inventive Problem Solving (TRIZ) with its innovation patterns has revolutionized the space of innovation and problem-solving since its inception in the mid-twentieth century [1]. Based on the analysis of hundreds of thousands of inventions in many fields it extrapolated a 39 × 39 matrix of contradictory patterns (problems) and 40 generalizable innovation principles to solve these problems. Research on TRIZ culminates in three findings:

1. Problems and solutions are repeated across industries and sciences.
2. Patterns of technical evolution are replicated in industries and sciences.
3. The innovations have scientific effects outside the field in which they were developed [2, 3].

This chapter suggests that large parts of Precision Medicine (PM) could be interpreted as an application of the TRIZ innovation principles. Basically, precision medicine can be seen as an implementation of the first TRIZ innovation principle, segmentation.

For example, one of the most important applications of precision medicine, targeted cancer therapy, is based on segmentation of tumors or tumor genetics analogous to the first TRIZ innovation principle (segmentation). Another example beyond genetics is the multi-omics subtyping (patient, disease segmentation) for directing state-of-the-art therapeutics in oncology and other medical fields [4–10] that is now evolving into single-cell multi-omics [11, 12]. Artificial intelligence and machine learning are playing an increasing role in this segmentation process [13–16].

R. Schmidt (✉)
COO IHLAD Abu Dhabi, Abu Dhabi, United Arab Emirates
e-mail: rudi.schmidt@rudischmidt.eu

P. Plugmann, D. Portius (eds.), *Innovations in Healthcare and Outcome Measurement*, https://doi.org/10.1007/978-3-031-77302-0_1

An important question is whether further TRIZ principles point the way, for example, to get the side effects of targeted therapies under control. Number 9 "Preliminary anti-action" could be considered for immune-related adverse events in ICI-Therapy of cancer. Apart from approaches known from treating auto-immune diseases, modulating the gut microbiota by probiotics, prebiotics, postbiotics, and fecal microbiota transplantation as an emerging trend in cancer or Parkinson's disease patient [17–22] could be seen as such a preliminary anti-action.

It makes sense to consider the TRIZ approach for an additional systematic taxonomy in PM and for hypothesis generation of innovations and inventions.

1.1 Introduction

1.1.1 Theories of Innovation, Other Scientific Theories and Perspectives in Innovation Failure

One of the fundamental problems in science is the understanding of discovery and innovation process to explain scientific and technological change in society. Recent research suggests that the likelihood of discoveries may be consistent across various fields. However, other studies indicate that the occurrence of inventions and innovations varies between research fields, influenced by the ecosystem and nature of each discipline. So-called market-oriented sciences tend to have a higher probability of generating inventions and innovations. In particular, the field of medicine sees a significant number of inventions, driven by the opportunistic behavior of its practitioners [23].

From the view of a philosophy of science, theories of innovations seem to be at the intersections of science and technology [24]. Scientific theories about innovation tend to differ from scientific theories dealing with other areas in their focus and application. Theories of innovation seemed to be concerned with the process of introducing new ideas, processes, or products and their diffusion within a population or system. They often emphasize the practical application of these innovations to improve performance, such as enhancing quality, safety, outcomes, or reducing costs, especially in fields like healthcare [25]. On the other hand, typical scientific theories in other fields focus more on explaining natural phenomena, understanding underlying mechanisms, or predicting outcomes based on empirical evidence. These theories are more about understanding the "why" and "how" of things, rather than the practical application or implementation of new solutions [26–28].

Moreover, innovation theories often involve a multi-stakeholder approach and consider the social context, whereas other scientific theories might be more focused on isolated, individual components or elements within a system. Theories of innovation also tend to be more interdisciplinary, integrating knowledge from various fields to foster the creation and adoption of new solutions [29, 30].

A recent paper suggested that while journals in the life sciences disciplines publish a greater number of articles without funding compared to those with funding, the proportion of citations for funded articles surpasses their overall publication count. In every field of life science examined, articles with funding are cited more frequently than those without [31]. So far it remains elusive if medical innovations based on more cited papers are more successful on their way from bench to bedside than other innovations or if biomedical inventions based on industrial (and thus funded) systematic approaches such as TRIZ have a lower failure rate when it comes to implementation. In general, major causes of innovation failure seemed to be located in planning and design, execution, and market orientation and are associated with goal difficulty, environmental complexity, and uncertainty [32, 33].

1.1.2 Precision Medicine

Precision Medicine (PM) has triggered unparalleled increases in scientific research across the pathophysiology of basic disease processes. The exponentially growing number of scientific insights beyond genomics (based on multi-omics such as immunology, proteomics, metabolomics, metagenomics within the microbiota/microbiomes—of the gut, the oral cavity, the skin, tumors, and their microenvironment, etc., epigenetics, virology, and other omics in parallel with big data science and artificial intelligence) promise a more individualized medicine. However, despite all these advances, the translation from bench to bedside turned out to be a disappointment as drug development and clinical trials come with an extremely high failure rate. This development was coined into the "valley of death" between bench and bedside [34].

If we take precision medicine (PM) to its logical extreme, it results in what isknown as n-of-1 clinical trials or real-world evidence of only one individual participant - some literature considers this as the epitome of individualized healthcare. *N*-of-1 trials target differences in treatment response and adverse events between individual patients [35] while underreporting of adverse events in healthcare systems is already a global concern. Those trials come with several challenges, and they demonstrate the dilemma of many individualized approaches in general—to name only one example, with precision nutrition and weight loss interventions for patients with obesity [36]. Implementing *N*-of-1 trials in clinical settings presents considerable logistical, temporal, and acceptance hurdles. However, monitoring with medical device wearables or the implementation of a TRIZ-based model to increase the reporting of adverse events [37] could promote the adoption of *N*-of-1 methodologies in everyday clinical practice [38].

Nevertheless, PM aims to tailor patient treatment plans based on their individual biological characteristics, environment, and lifestyle. It often utilizes biomarkers, indicators of biological or pathogenic processes, or responses to treatments, to guide therapy choices. This approach is moving healthcare from a general to a more targeted treatment model.

The difference between PM and typical or traditional medicine in clinical routine lies in the approach to treatment decisions, therapies, and care. So far, clinical routine follows a more generalized approach, where treatments are designed for large groups of people with the same condition, not always considering factors like sex, age, or weight ("one size fits all").

Clinical routine utilizes standard diagnostic tools and treatments that are broadly applicable, while PM propagates more sophisticated diagnostic tools and big data analytics to understand a person's unique biological makeup and predict which treatments will work best for an individual, reducing trial and error. In essence, precision medicine is more targeted and personalized.

1.1.3 TRIZ

TRIZ originated in the mid-twentieth century Soviet Union. It was developed by Genrich Altshuller who analyzed over 200,000 patents to find patterns of innovation. Despite initial back draws, including Altshuller's imprisonment in a Gulag, TRIZ gained recognition for its effectiveness in various fields. Post-Soviet Union, TRIZ spread globally and has been integrated with other methodologies. It is now used worldwide for problem-solving and innovation, supported by many organizations like, to name only one example, the Association of German Engineers, which created the TRIZ guideline VDI4521 to facilitate access to its methods and tools.

TRIZ identifies recurring patterns in technical evolution and inventive solutions. Similarly, in medical innovation, certain challenges and solutions tend to repeat across different healthcare contexts—for example, drug delivery methods or immune-related adverse events (oncology, autoimmune diseases). TRIZ emphasizes resolving contradictions—problems, where improving one aspect of a system negatively impacts another. In medicine, such trade-offs can be found between drug efficacy, safety, cost, and patient comfort.

The TRIZ contradiction matrix is the main tool designed to help innovators identify and overcome contradictions in engineering and design problems. It consists of 39 parameters that describe common features of physical and engineering systems. By analyzing the most inventive patents, it was possible to map contradictions between these parameters and identify the most frequently used inventive principles that resolved these contradictions [39, 40].

The matrix works by selecting the parameters that need to be improved and then identifying the parameters that worsen as a result. At the intersection of these two parameters in the matrix, references to the inventive principles most commonly used to resolve the contradiction are noted. This approach has been refined over time, with the latest iteration known as Matrix 2022, which serves as the fourth generation of this contradiction-solving tool. The analysis of contradictions and the strategies used to resolve them has in many ways now been automated to an extent that offers innovators in real time a list of ranked inventive principles used by others to challenge a given pair of conflicting parameters [41].

The so-called innovative principles, on the other hand, are a set of 40 principles derived from the study of patterns in inventive solutions that have successfully overcome specific problems. These principles serve as a heuristic guide for problem-solving and innovation. They are used in conjunction with the contradiction matrix to provide systematic solutions to complex problems [42].

TRIZ differs from other innovation theories in several ways:

1. Transversal Problem-Solving Approach.

   Unlike some other theories that focus on specific industries or contexts, TRIZ aims to uncover universal patterns in innovation. TRIZ posits the existence of universal problem-solving mechanisms and principles. These mechanisms serve as the foundation for innovation. Essentially, no matter the problem, it is highly likely that someone, somewhere, has already devised a solution mechanism—even if it was originally applied to a different problem. Creative problem-solving in TRIZ involves identifying these universal principles or solution mechanisms and adapting them to address the specific problem at hand. TRIZ's successful application extends across various fields [43]. Thus, TRIZ is not limited to specific domains; it provides a transversal problem-solving methodology applicable across various disciplines [44].
2. Structured Rules and Patterns

   TRIZ assumes that innovation is governed by certain rules that can be studied and extracted. It offers a systematic approach to solving problems, emphasizing structured patterns rather than randomness [22].
3. Application Beyond Technical Systems

   While TRIZ originated as a tool for technical problem-solving, it has been widely applied beyond engineering. TRIZ has found use in fields such as science, business, and even politics [45] or healthcare.

1.1.3.1 TRIZ in Healthcare

Recently, a study developed a healthcare-specific TRIZ framework with an adapted 16 × 16 solution matrix for health service providers derived from the original 39 × 39 TRIZ conflict matrix [46]. Another work used TRIZ theory and bibliometrics to deduce new ideas about cancer treatments and identified eight promising innovation principles [47]:

1. Principle 21: Skipping.
2. Principle 23: Feedback.
3. Principle 33: Homogeneity.
4. Principle 1: Segmentation.
5. Principle 34: Discarding and Recovering.
6. Principle 40: Composite Materials.
7. Principle 11: Beforehand Cushioning.
8. Principle 12: Equipotentiality.

Another study tried to develop a lean healthcare contradiction matrix with eight new parameters [48]:

1. Informatization.
2. Securitization.
3. Specialization.
4. Funds control.
5. Timeliness.

6. Streamlined.
7. Employees growth.

Total quality and innovation management in healthcare (TQIM-H) [49] and critical service failures in medical and care services (hospitals, nursing homes) [50, 51], seem to be an obvious domain for the applications of TRIZ methods. Various publications describe the use of TRIZ in other fields:

- Analyze and improve healthcare quality in general.
- Discover and develop new drugs and vaccines.
- Design medical devices.
- Design medical equipment.
- Develop smart product-service system that combines digital health and artificial intelligence within the Internet of (Medical) Things (IoT, IoMT) [52–59].

A remarkable article of experts in the TRIZ methods analyzed problems associated with the impossibility of effectively using artificial intelligence, especially existing neural networks, for the analysis of medical information [60].

1.2 TRIZ in Precision Medicine

In certain areas of medicine, PM has transitioned from an academic promise to innovations close to clinical routine. Genetic testing, for example, has improved treatment of numerous inherited disorders, including cystic fibrosis, which has notably increased the survival rates of affected children. Within oncology, the introduction of specialized treatments has extended the life expectancy of individuals with cancers such as breast, NSCLC, colorectal, melanoma, and various blood-related malignancies. While achievements in other medical fields may not be as widely recognized, they are equally significant [61]. In general, in PM the challenge is to determine if patients can be grouped based on shared factors, similar responses to treatments or other feature to classify them into the right subgroups [62]. The convergence of artificial intelligence (AI) and PM promises to boost innovations by deep phenotyping of patient cohorts [63].

Table 1.1 gives several medical examples that can be systematically classified with the help of TRIZ principles (contradiction matrix) and explain their transferability

Segmentation (divide an object into independent parts) is the primus inter pares of TRIZ principles in PM where patients are segmented based on criteria such as genomics and other omics, deep clinical phenotyping, environmental, lifestyle, or other factors. Based on segmentation, treatments are tailored to specific patient subgroups, aiming to optimize patient outcomes.

The TRIZ principle Local Quality and its solution (transition from homogeneous to heterogeneous structure of an object or outside environment) finds applications in PM where local quality refers to tailoring treatments to

Table 1.1 Innovations in precision medicine

Examples for innovations in precision medicine	Somatic	Psychiatry/mental health	Oral health, dentistry	Prevention/lifestyle/aging
Data classes (examples)				
Gene-related, including gene-regulation, epigenetics	CDx in oncology, hereditary diseases, pharmacogenomics	Major depressive disorder, autism spectrum disorder (ASD)	Taste receptors, Wolf-Hirschhorn, saliva biomarkers	Genetic risk exposure, taste receptors and behaviour/diet, aging clocks, nutrigenomics
Multi-omics (including spatial, single cell)	Drug repurposing, coronary artery diseases, bioavailability (e.g. gut microbiome)	Drug repurposing, schizophrenia	Bi-directional interplay with systemic health, periodontitis, diabetes, CRC	Strategies for personalized and predictive medicine, saliva biomarkers, microbiota of social groups, buildings
Systemic (immunology)	Antibodies in autoimmune diseases, biologics in inflammatory bowel disease	Psychoneuroimmunology: PANS/PANDAS, dementia, Alzheimer's	Autoimmunity, gum infections	Regenerative medicine, infections, mucosal immunity, aging clocks, longevity biomarkers
Methods				
AI, ML, DL, Big Data, bioinformatics	Insilico approaches for drug discovery, toxicology, deep clinical phenotyping	Predictive models for Alzheimer's, Parkinson, molecular profiling, speech patterns	Image analysis, AI-supported preventive teledentistry, oral and maxillofacial surgical planning	Public health, coaching (chatbots etc.), prognosis of lifestyle diseases, deep clinical phenotyping, aging clocks

(continued)

Table 1.1 (continued)

Examples for innovations in precision medicine	Somatic	Psychiatry/mental health	Oral health, dentistry	Prevention/lifestyle/aging
Imaging, video, audio (pathology, radiology, retina, skin, oral, gait pattern)	Radiogenomics, retinal diseases, pathology expert systems, melanoma	Neuroimaging, motor neuron diseases, traumatic brain injury, Parkinson	3D imaging, AI-based image analysis	Aging clocks, (high) performance athletes, retina imaging, diet identification
Technologies				
Virtual Reality, Augmented Reality, Metaverse	Aging, visualization of high dimensional data models	Exposure therapy (anxiety, PTSD, ICD…), organizational health/leadership skills (empathy)	Teledentistry	Public health, population health, aging, health apps, telemedicine
Devices, wearables, smartphones incl. 5G/6G	Seamless monitoring, (saliva) biomarkers, location, time-based clustering, patient adherence	Context-triggered assessment for schizophrenia. Depression, panic attacks, aggressive behavior prediction (e.g. autism), patient adherence	Intraoral cams for teledentistry, orofacial wearables, saliva biomarkers	Telemedicine, new sensors for wearables, environmental surveillance

Several medical examples can be systematically classified with the help of TRIZ principles (contradiction matrix) and explain their transferability. Examples for innovations in precision medicine can be found across all medical areas such as somatic, psychiatry/mental health, oral health/dentistry and lifestyle/prevention/aging

The innovations and inventions can be classified within data classes (genomic, multi-omics, systemic/immunology), clinical phenotypes), methods (AI/ML, deep learning, big data, bioinformatics, imaging) and technologies (virtual reality, augmented reality, metaverse, wearables, medical devices, consumer devices, smartphones, apps including 5G/6G technology) individual patient needs. Precision medicine aims to optimize treatment efficacy while minimizing side effects by considering patient-specific factors. Drug delivery is prominent example of applying this TRIZ principle. The application of numerous promising therapeutic agents has been impeded by pharmacological challenges such as toxicity and resistance to drugs. However, advancements in drug delivery materials and methods have reached a stage where they can adjust the pharmacological attributes of a drug without affecting its intended impact on molecular targets. In particular, these advancements can regulate a drug's absorption, stability, pharmacokinetics, and distribution to both tumors and normal tissues, as well as support the use of combined drugs that work in synergy [64].

The TRIZ principles addressing inherent contradictions and ideality can be linked with typical contradictions and challenges in PM like balancing ideal efficacy (ideality) and minimizing side effects. In cancer therapy, for example, patients often receive a chemotherapy. Applying TRIZ principles could lead this interpretation:

- Segmentation: Divide the treatment plan into phases (induction, maintenance, etc.) based on tumor type and patient response.
- Local Quality: Tailor drug dosages and schedules to minimize toxicity while maximizing tumor suppression.
- Contradiction Resolution: Develop targeted therapies that selectively attack cancer cells without harming healthy tissues.
- Ideality: Strive for a treatment plan that maximizes cancer control while minimizing adverse effects.

1.2.1 Patient Segmentation Via Biomarker and Companion Diagnostic (CDx) Tests

The effectiveness of PM relies on accurate biomarker identification through companion diagnostic (CDx) tests, which inform therapeutic decisions [65]. Companion diagnostics (CDx) are changing treatment decisions by enabling the segmentation of patients for more personalized therapies. CDx tests determine which patients are likely to benefit from a particular drug and who may have adverse reactions, ensuring treatments are both safe and effective. However, the predictive value of treatment based on CDx results is compromised if the test lacks proper diagnostic performance or validation.

Challenges may arise when new clinical performance tests are required to comply with updated standards or clinical data requirements, such as obtaining clinical samples, institutional support, funding, and time constraints. Consequently, a streamlined clinical regulatory process is vital to adhere to rigorous regulatory demands. This study advocates for reinforcing the existing clinical regulatory structure for CDx by comparing the approaches of various regulatory agencies, including the FDA, EMA, and MFDS.

The critical role of CDx in clinical biomarker application necessitates stringent regulatory oversight. Regulatory bodies are tightening rules and updating guidelines to reflect this. The EU's In Vitro Diagnostic Regulation, for instance, has formally recognized CDx, highlighting its significance [66].

Targeted drug-eluting stents (DES) for localized treatment of coronary artery disease could be seen as another example of TRIZ principles in PM [67]:

- Contradiction Resolution: DES were developed to overcome the contradiction between the effectiveness of stents in keeping arteries open and the problem of in-stent restenosis, where arteries become blocked again. This aligns with the TRIZ principle of resolving contradictions without compromise.
- Ideality: The TRIZ concept of ideality, where the ideal system performs its function without existing, is reflected in the design of DES. They aim to restore blood flow and then gradually release medication to prevent restenosis, effectively treating the condition with minimal intervention.
- Use of Resources: TRIZ encourages the use of available resources to solve problems. In the case of DES, the stent itself serves as a delivery system for medication, utilizing its physical presence as a resource.
- Local Quality: The medication is only released at the site of the stent, targeting the specific area that needs treatment.
- Dynamics: The stent adapts to the changing environment inside the artery as it releases medication over time.
- Nested Doll: The stent has multiple layers, with the outer structure supporting the artery and the inner layer containing the drug.

1.2.2 Outlook: Artificial Intelligence and Machine Learning at the Intersection of PM and TRIZ

Advocates for precision medicine argue that conventional methods of innovations in health sciences have been overly focused on assessing the average effectiveness rather than addressing the specific needs of individuals. That resonates with the current zeitgeist [1] where (in theory) the wealth of detailed, accessible individual longitudinal data, coupled with the implementation of adaptable machine learning techniques, presents a thrilling opportunity for a paradigm shift. At the forefront is the vision of new innovations in precision medicine shaped by machine learning.

However, the validity of these assertions is up for debate as currently they fall short of the hype and expectation that has grown around them [68]. Several systematic challenges are roadblocks to the integration of digital health products [69], automated evolutionary discovery of product design improvements [70], PM, and TRIZ. These challenges stem from data limitations, such as biases, and research incentives, like optimizing data and interpretation for publication.

The accuracy on diagnostic tasks is promising only in academic cohorts, while the algorithms often fail in real-life settings. Cohorts and bioinformatic approaches are often guided by the availability of data rather than clinical relevance [71]. In precision psychiatry [72], for example, the challenges range from the distance to clinical practice, over the lack of valid real-world databases (to feed data-intensive algorithms), models that are disconnected from the core principles of clinical utility and ethical acceptability [73].

The crux of modern machine learning is its failure to meet the transparency that clinicians and patients require "to buy in." To roll out medical AI successfully in future, doctors and patients should have reason to trust a model. This requires a change in how medical AI and precision medicine are designed and validated to meet the transparency requirements that are standard for all other serious medical interventions [74]. Without a doubt, the combination of big data, medical AI, and TROZ will offer exciting opportunities for disruptive innovations and inventions—but disruption in medicine demands greater scrutiny, not less when it comes to transparency and benefit assessments in health technology assessments (HTA).

Once this is given, artificial intelligence and machine learning will play an important role at the intersection of PM and TRIZ. Because developing innovations in precision medicine requires a very deep understanding of disease biology and the ability to dissect the relationship between molecular, multi-omics factors and their phenotypic consequences.

Obviously, biomedical knowledge explodes every year with tens of thousands of publications and uncounted terabytes of new raw data in nonstandardized repositories, in nonstandardized ontologies and taxonomies—with some taxonomies that tend to **change** more often than other—especially in some data classes such as metagenomics. That makes it difficult to connect the biomolecular foundation of PM and its innovations with clinical phenotypes and clinical routine.

AI-based approaches are ideal to create multimodal knowledge graphs for PM and TRIZ analyses. Some publications suggest that these knowledge graphs have to connect more than 17,000 diseases with more than four million relationships representing ten major biological scales, including disease-associated protein perturbations, biological processes and pathways, anatomical and phenotypic scales, and the entire range of approved drugs with their therapeutic action [75].

AI may also help to overcome a joint issue of TRIZ and PM: finding discrete groups and subgroups and divide patients into the right segments and applicable TRIZ-principles [76]. Academic research often missed that assigning a patient to a particular group is anything but trivial. Clinical routine is full of diagnostic challenges, differential diagnoses, and vague syndromic presentations [77]. That leads to ambiguous clinical phenotyping and real-world data. However, both are necessary to define the adequate contradictions in the TRIZ matrix as well as in the diagnostic process. AI will help to personalize the clinical phenotyping of each patient especially in the challenging fields of autoimmune diseases (rheumatology), brain disorders, cardiovascular and gastroenterological diseases—where different pathophysiological mechanisms underlie the same manifestation [78]. Thus, dAI will remove many roadblocks of PM and TRIZ at the same time.

References

1. Brad S. Mapping the evolutionary journey of TRIZ and pioneering its next S-curve in the age of AI-aided invention. In: Cavallucci D, Livotov P, Brad S, editors. Towards AI-aided invention and innovation. TFC 2023. IFIP advances in information and communication technology, vol. 682. Cham: Springer; 2023. https://doi.org/10.1007/978-3-031-42532-5_1.
2. Vidal R, et al. Fuzzy cognitive map-based selection of TRIZ (theory of inventive problem solving) trends for eco-innovation of ceramic industry products. J Clean Prod. 2015;107:202–14. https://doi.org/10.1016/j.jclepro.2015.04.131.
3. Chechurin L, Borgianni Y. Understanding TRIZ through the review of top cited publications. Comput Ind. 2016;82:119–34. https://doi.org/10.1016/j.compind.2016.06.002.
4. Ayton SG, et al. Multiomics subtyping for clinically prognostic cancer subtypes and personalized therapy: a systematic review and meta-analysis. Genet Med. 2022;24(1):15–25. https://doi.org/10.1016/j.gim.2021.09.006.
5. Duan R, et al. Evaluation and comparison of multi-omics data integration methods for cancer subtyping. PLoS Comput Biol. 2021;17(8):e1009224. https://journals.plos.org/ploscompbiol/article?id=10.1371/journal.pcbi.1009224.
6. Lee W, Huang DS, Han K. Constructing cancer patient-specific and group-specific gene networks with multi-omics data. BMC Med Genet. 2020;13(Suppl 6):81. https://doi.org/10.1186/s12920-020-00736-7.
7. Gillenwater LA, et al. Multi-omics subtyping pipeline for chronic obstructive pulmonary disease. PLoS One. 2021;16(8):e0255337. https://journals.plos.org/plosone/article?id=10.1371/journal.pone.0255337.
8. Maiorino E, Loscalzo J. Phenomics and robust multiomics data for cardiovascular disease subtyping. Arterioscler Thromb Vasc Biol. 2023;43(7):1111–23. https://www.ahajournals.org/doi/abs/10.1161/ATVBAHA.122.318892.
9. Brière G, Darbo É, Thébault P, et al. Consensus clustering applied to multi-omics disease subtyping. BMC Bioinform. 2021;22:361. https://doi.org/10.1186/s12859-021-04279-1.
10. Manganaro L, Bianco S, Bironzo P, et al. Consensus clustering methodology to improve molecular stratification of non-small cell lung cancer. Sci Rep. 2023;13:7759. https://doi.org/10.1038/s41598-023-33954-x.
11. Cui H, Wang C, Maan H, et al. scGPT: toward building a foundation model for single-cell multi-omics using generative AI. Nat Methods. 2024;21(8):1470–80. https://doi.org/10.1038/s41592-024-02201-0.
12. Schäfer PSL, Dimitrov D, Villablanca EJ, et al. Integrating single-cell multi-omics and prior biological knowledge for a functional characterization of the immune system. Nat Immunol. 2024;25:405–17. https://doi.org/10.1038/s41590-024-01768-2.
13. Piroozkhah M, et al. Computational methods for multi-omics data analysis in cancer precision medicine. Front Genet. 2023;14:1226975. https://www.frontiersin.org/journals/genetics/articles/10.3389/fgene.2023.1226975.
14. Wang L, Zhang Y, Yao R, et al. Identification of distinct clinical phenotypes of cardiogenic shock using machine learning consensus clustering approach. BMC Cardiovasc Disord. 2023;23:426. https://doi.org/10.1186/s12872-023-03380-y.
15. Acosta JN, Falcone GJ, Rajpurkar P, et al. Multimodal biomedical AI. Nat Med. 2022;28:1773–84. https://doi.org/10.1038/s41591-022-01981-2.
16. Wang H, Fu T, Du Y, et al. Scientific discovery in the age of artificial intelligence. Nature. 2023;620:47–60. https://doi.org/10.1038/s41586-023-06221-2.
17. Ciernikova S, et al. Modulating the gut microbiota by probiotics, prebiotics, postbiotics, and fecal microbiota transplantation: an emerging trend in cancer patient care. Biochim Biophys Acta Rev Cancer. 2023;1878(6):188990. https://doi.org/10.1016/j.bbcan.2023.188990.
18. Esfahani K, Elkrief A, Calabrese C, et al. Moving towards personalized treatments of immune-related adverse events. Nat Rev Clin Oncol. 2020;17:504–15. https://doi.org/10.1038/s41571-020-0352-8.

19. Bruggeman A, et al. Safety and efficacy of faecal microbiota transplantation in patients with mild to moderate Parkinson's disease (GUT-PARFECT): a double-blind, placebo-controlled, randomised, phase 2 trial. EClinicalMedicine. 2024;71:102563. https://doi.org/10.1016/j.eclinm.2024.102563.
20. Vongsavath T, et al. The potential role of fecal microbiota transplantation in Parkinson's disease: a systematic literature review. Appl Microbiol. 2023;3(3):993–1002.
21. DuPont HL, et al. Fecal microbiota transplantation in Parkinson's disease—a randomized repeat-dose, placebo-controlled clinical pilot study. Front Neurol. 2023;14:1104759.
22. Cheng Y, et al. Efficacy of fecal microbiota transplantation in patients with Parkinson's disease: clinical trial results from a randomized, placebo-controlled design. Gut Microbes. 2023;15(2):2284247.
23. Coccia M. Probability of discoveries between research fields to explain scientific and technological change. Technol Soc. 2022;68:101874. https://www.sciencedirect.com/science/article/abs/pii/S0160791X2200015X.
24. Clark N. Similarities and differences between scientific and technological paradigms. Futures. 1987;19(1):26–42. https://doi.org/10.1016/0016-3287(87)90037-1.
25. Kechagioglou P. What we know from existing theories of innovation. In: Healthcare innovation success. Cham: Springer; 2023. https://doi.org/10.1007/978-3-031-28353-6_2.
26. Li K, Wijaya TT, Chen X, et al. Exploring the factors affecting elementary mathematics teachers' innovative behavior: an integration of social cognitive theory. Sci Rep. 2024;14:2108. https://doi.org/10.1038/s41598-024-52604-4.
27. Frietsch R, Reiß T, Schmoch U. Development of innovation monitoring and innovation indicators in the past 50 years. Systems and innovation research in transition: research questions and trends in historical perspective. Cham: Springer Nature Switzerland; 2024. p. 39–72.
28. Yan WY, Loang OK. Building a research model for the relationship between enterprise innovation values and employees' innovation behavior: with innovation self-efficacy as a mediator. In: El Khoury R, editor. Technology-driven business innovation. Studies in systems, decision and control, vol. 223. Cham: Springer; 2024. https://doi.org/10.1007/978-3-031-51997-0_5.
29. Greenacre P, Gross R, Speirs J. Innovation theory: a review of the literature. London: Imperial College Centre for Energy Policy and Technology. 2012. https://www.imperial.ac.uk/media/imperial-college/research-centres-and-groups/icept/Innovation-review%2D%2D-ICEPT-working-paper-version-(16.05.12).pdf.
30. Salonen J. Realizing strategic value from digital innovation initiatives-digital innovation theory-driven portfolio and transformation management; 2024.
31. Mosleh M, Roshani S, Coccia M. Scientific laws of research funding to support citations and diffusion of knowledge in life science. Scientometrics. 2022;127:1931–51. https://doi.org/10.1007/s11192-022-04300-1.
32. Coccia M. New perspectives in innovation failure analysis: a taxonomy of general errors and strategic management for reducing risks. Technol Soc. 2023;75:102384. https://doi.org/10.1016/j.techsoc.2023.102384.
33. Coccia M. Theory of innovation failure and strategic management implications. Technology analysis & strategic management, in press (Forthcoming) (2024). https://papers.ssrn.com/sol3/papers.cfm?abstract_id=4902697.
34. Subbiah V. The next generation of evidence-based medicine. Nat Med. 2023;29:49–58. https://doi.org/10.1038/s41591-022-02160-z.
35. Grammatikopoulou MG, Gkouskou KK, Gkiouras K, et al. The niche of n-of-1 trials in precision medicine for weight loss and obesity treatment: back to the future. Curr Nutr Rep. 2022;11:133–45. https://doi.org/10.1007/s13668-022-00404-5.
36. Allman-Farinelli M, et al. Nutrition-related N-of-1 studies warrant further research to provide evidence for dietitians to practice personalized (precision) medical nutrition therapy: a systematic review. Nutrients. 2023;15(7):1756. https://doi.org/10.3390/nu15071756.
37. Lee JY, Lee PS, Chiang CH, et al. Implementation of a novel TRIZ-based model to increase the reporting of adverse events in the healthcare center. Sci Rep. 2024;14:26905. https://doi.org/10.1038/s41598-024-78661-3.

38. Wilmont I, Loeffen M, Hoogeboom T. A qualitative study on the facilitators and barriers to adopting the N-of-1 trial methodology as part of clinical practice: potential versus implementation challenges. Int J Qual Stud Health Well Being. 2024;19(1):2318810. https://doi.org/10.1080/17482631.2024.2318810.
39. Lux S. Application of the TRIZ contradictory matrix to foster innovation for sustainable chemical engineering. Chemie Ingenieur Technik. 2022;94(8):1071–9. https://onlinelibrary.wiley.com/doi/abs/10.1002/cite.202100205.
40. Hipple J. The TRIZ contradiction table. In: The ideal result. New York, NY: Springer; 2012. https://doi.org/10.1007/978-1-4614-3707-9_10.
41. Mann D. Matrix 2022: re-imagining the contradiction matrix. In: Borgianni Y, Brad S, Cavallucci D, Livotov P, editors. Creative solutions for a sustainable development. TFC 2021. IFIP advances in information and communication technology, vol. 635. Cham: Springer; 2021. https://doi.org/10.1007/978-3-030-86614-3_16.
42. Borgianni Y, et al. The process for individuating TRIZ inventive principles: deterministic, stochastic or domain-oriented? Des Sci. 2021;7:e12. https://www.cambridge.org/core/journals/design-science/article/process-for-individuating-triz-inventive-principles-deterministic-stochastic-or-domainoriented/81CEAB2A6483D6A7D42010A22F5B9839.
43. Sala AJ, Felez J, Cano-Moreno JD. Efficient railway turnout design: leveraging TRIZ-based approaches. Appl Sci. 2023;13(17):9531. https://doi.org/10.3390/app13179531.
44. Bolaños-Ruiz EA. Technology roadmapping and TRIZ: a practical approach for inventive problem-solving and product innovation. In: Cortes Robles G, editor. TRIZ in Latin America. Cham: Springer; 2023. https://doi.org/10.1007/978-3-031-20561-3_7.
45. Bersano G, Fayemi PE. Application of TRIZ and innovation management theory on decision support for transport infrastructure. In: Benmoussa R, De Guio R, Dubois S, Koziołek S, editors. New opportunities for innovation breakthroughs for developing countries and emerging economies. TFC 2019. IFIP advances in information and communication technology, vol. 572. Cham: Springer; 2019. https://doi.org/10.1007/978-3-030-32497-1_38.
46. Guner S, Ilker KOSE. A new approach that proposes TRIZ as a creative problem solving technique in health services. Res J Bus Manag. 2020;7(2):67–79. https://www.researchgate.net/profile/Seyma-Guener-3/publication/342503897_A_new_approach_that_proposes_TRIZ_as_a_creative_problem_solving_technique_in_health_services/links/5ef7b6be299bf18816edd3a0/A-new-approach-that-proposes-TRIZ-as-a-creative-problem-solving-technique-in-health-services.pdf.
47. Huiquan Y, et al. Triz theory and the method of cancer document selection for chemical complexes and innovation schemes of meta-analysis with lymphomas as an example. J Chem. 2020;2020:1–12. https://www.hindawi.com/journals/jchem/2020/6294613/.
48. Wang J, Zhao D, Han Z. Two-stage construction of lean healthcare contradiction matrix based on LDA topic model and TRIZ theory. In: Proceedings of the 2nd international conference on public management, digital economy and internet technology, ICPDI 2023, September 1–3, 2023, Chongqing, China, 2023. https://eudl.eu/doi/10.4108/eai.1-9-2023.2338802.
49. Tonjang S, Thawesaengskulthai N. TRIZ inventive principle in healthcare quality and innovation development. Int J Qual Reliab Manag. 2023;40(10):2664–721. https://doi.org/10.1108/IJQRM-11-2021-0389.
50. Shie A-J, et al. Design and process optimization of combined medical and elderly care services: an integrated service blueprint–TRIZ model. Front Public Health. 2022;10:965443. https://www.frontiersin.org/journals/public-health/articles/10.3389/fpubh.2022.965443.
51. Chen C-K, et al. An ageing-in-place service innovation model by using TRIZ methodology. Hum Factors Ergonomics Manuf Serv Ind. 2015;25(2):166–82. https://doi.org/10.1002/hfm.20536.
52. Hemeng B, Aoming X, Fang Z. Literature review on the development of new drugs based on TRIZ. Asian J Soc Pharm. 2021;16(1):60–7. http://asianjsp.syphu.edu.cn/CN/abstract/abstract599.shtml.

53. Mansootian AR, Naini FH. 40 inventive principles and biological models. TRIZ J. 2004;9(6):129–32.
54. Chang D, et al. A TRIZ-inspired knowledge-driven approach for user-centric smart product-service system: a case study on intelligent test tube rack design. Adv Eng Inform. 2023;56:101901. https://doi.org/10.1016/j.aei.2023.101901.
55. Degland A, Jean C, Gazo C. Using TRIZ in the healthcare environment: first proposition of a new design method. In: Benmoussa R, De Guio R, Dubois S, Koziołek S, editors. New opportunities for innovation breakthroughs for developing countries and emerging economies. TFC 2019. IFIP advances in information and communication technology, vol. 572. Cham: Springer; 2019. https://doi.org/10.1007/978-3-030-32497-1_34.
56. Gao C, et al. Innovation design of medical equipment based on TRIZ. Technol Health Care. 2015;23(Suppl 2):S269–76. https://content.iospress.com/articles/technology-and-health-care/thc962.
57. Ramírez-Rios LY, et al. Design of a modular plantar orthosis system through the application of TRIZ methodology tools. Appl Sci. 2021;11(5):2051. https://doi.org/10.3390/app11052051.
58. Mawale MB, Kuthe A, Mawale A. Rapid prototyping assisted fabrication of a device for medical infusion therapy using TRIZ. Health Technol. 2019;9:167–73. https://doi.org/10.1007/s12553-018-0259-x.
59. Motyl B, Filippi S. Integration of creativity enhancement tools in medical device design process. Procedia Eng. 2014;69:1316–25.
60. Farber B, et al. Progressive artificial neural network for medical applications. Ann Mechnikovs Inst. 2021;4:91–100. https://journals.uran.ua/ami/article/view/246527.
61. García-Foncillas J, Argente J, Bujanda L, et al. Milestones of precision medicine: an innovative, multidisciplinary overview. Mol Diagn Ther. 2021;25:563–76. https://doi.org/10.1007/s40291-021-00544-4.
62. Mori M, Krumholz HM, Allore HG. Using latent class analysis to identify hidden clinical phenotypes. JAMA. 2020;324(7):700–1. https://jamanetwork.com/journals/jama/article-abstract/2769454.
63. Johnson KB, et al. Precision medicine, AI, and the future of personalized health care. Clin Transl Sci. 2021;14(1):86–93. https://doi.org/10.1111/cts.12884.
64. Manzari MT, Shamay Y, Kiguchi H, et al. Targeted drug delivery strategies for precision medicines. Nat Rev Mater. 2021;6:351–70. https://doi.org/10.1038/s41578-020-00269-6.
65. Keeling P, Clark J, Finucane S. Challenges in the clinical implementation of precision medicine companion diagnostics. Expert Rev Mol Diagn. 2020;20(6):593–9. https://doi.org/10.1080/14737159.2020.1757436.
66. Kang SL, et al. Necessity of strengthening the current clinical regulatory framework for companion diagnostics: a institutional comparison of the FDA, EMA, and MFDS. Mol Ther Methods Clin Dev. 2023;30:447–58. https://doi.org/10.1016/j.omtm.2023.08.008.
67. Mendiola J, Manuel J. Design of a bioabsorbable stent as preventive treatment of complication in bariatric surgery RYGBP; 2017. https://repositorio.tec.mx/handle/11285/629758.
68. Wilkinson J, et al. Time to reality check the promises of machine learning-powered precision medicine. Lancet Digit Health. 2020;2(12):e677–80. https://www.thelancet.com/journals/landig/article/PIIS2589-7500(20)30200-4/fulltext#seccestitle60.
69. Kaliteevskii V, Bryksin M, Chechurin L. Integration of TRIZ methodologies into the digital product development process. In: Nowak R, Chrząszcz J, Brad S, editors. Systematic innovation partnerships with artificial intelligence and information technology. TFC 2022. IFIP advances in information and communication technology, vol. 655. Cham: Springer; 2022. https://doi.org/10.1007/978-3-031-17288-5_24.
70. Iuga M, Brad S. Integrating generative AI with TRIZ for evolutionary product design. In: Cavallucci D, Brad S, Livotov P, editors. World conference of AI-powered innovation and inventive design. TFC 2024. IFIP advances in information and communication technology, vol. 735. Cham: Springer; 2025. https://doi.org/10.1007/978-3-031-75919-2_3.

71. Varoquaux G, Cheplygina V. Machine learning for medical imaging: methodological failures and recommendations for the future. npj Digit Med. 2022;5:48. https://doi.org/10.1038/s41746-022-00592-y.
72. Manchia M, et al. Challenges and future prospects of precision medicine in psychiatry. Pharmacogenomics Pers Med. 2020;13:127–40. https://www.tandfonline.com/doi/abs/10.2147/PGPM.S198225.
73. Koutsouleris N, et al. From promise to practice: towards the realisation of AI-informed mental health care. Lancet Digit Health. 2022;4(11):e829–40. https://www.thelancet.com/journals/landig/article/PIIS2589-7500(22)00153-4/fulltext.
74. Quinn TP, et al. The three ghosts of medical AI: can the black-box present deliver? Artif Intell Med. 2022;124:102158. https://www.sciencedirect.com/science/article/pii/S0933365721001512.
75. Chandak P, Huang K, Zitnik M. Building a knowledge graph to enable precision medicine. Sci Data. 2023;10:67. https://doi.org/10.1038/s41597-023-01960-3.
76. Wu K, Duan Y. DIKWP-TRIZ: a revolution on traditional TRIZ towards invention for artificial consciousness. Appl Sci. 2024;14(23):10865. https://www.preprints.org/manuscript/202410.0751.
77. Seymour CW, Gomez H, Chang CCH, et al. Precision medicine for all? Challenges and opportunities for a precision medicine approach to critical illness. Crit Care. 2017;21:257. https://doi.org/10.1186/s13054-017-1836-5.
78. Cesario A, et al. Personalized clinical phenotyping through systems medicine and artificial intelligence. J Pers Med. 2021;11(4):265. https://doi.org/10.3390/jpm11040265.

Innovations and Solutions in Precision and Systems Medicine Using Artificial Intelligence

2

Tatsiana Akhrymenka

2.1 Introduction

Precision medicine, or more commonly known as personalised medicine, another widely used term is stratified or P4 medicine, is medicine based on the 4 P principles: predictive, preventive, personalised and participatory—all referring to the grouping of patients based on their risk of disease or response to therapy, using diagnostic tests or techniques [1]. This medical model offers patients and healthcare providers the opportunity to benefit from more targeted and effective treatments, which can lead to improved health outcomes and greater efficiency for the healthcare system. This approach also supports the expansion of the market for specialised and more effective treatments [1]. Systemmedicine and its interdisciplinary approach is both the basis and an essential component of precision medicine. Leroy Hood was one of the pioneers of systems medicine—the application of systems biology (the umbrella term) to tackle human disease. Twenty years ago, however, he and other advocates of systems medicine were struggling to gain acceptance for this approach [2].

More specifically, systems medicine is an interdisciplinary field of study that considers the systems of the human body as part of an integrated whole, including biochemical, physiological, and environmental interactions. Drawing on systems science and systems biology, systems medicine considers the complex interactions within the human body in the light of a patient's genomics, behaviour, and environment [3]. The term began to be used in the early 1990s in publications explaining the link between systems biomedicine and pharmacology [4].

Systems biology is the study of biological systems as collections of networks at multiple levels, ranging from the molecular level, through cells, tissues and organisms, to the population level [5]. In 2009, the US National Research Council

T. Akhrymenka (✉)
GETEC Group/IIF Fund/Capital Investment and M&A, Frankfurt, Germany
e-mail: tatsiana.akhrymenka.emba-s18@said.oxford.edu

P. Plugmann, D. Portius (eds.), *Innovations in Healthcare and Outcome Measurement*, https://doi.org/10.1007/978-3-031-77302-0_2

recognised the importance of systems biology, reporting that years of research have produced detailed information about the components of the complex systems that characterise life—genes, cells, organisms and ecosystems—and this knowledge has begun to coalesce into a better understanding of how all these components work together as systems [6]. The US National Research Council had pointed out that "looking at biological networks as a whole is much more powerful and fruitful than the traditional or "limited" way of studying disease based on a single gene or protein at a point in time", mentioning that "integration within biology and increasingly fruitful collaborations with physical, earth and computational scientists, mathematicians and engineers are making it possible to predict and control the activities of biological systems in ever greater detail" [5].

Systems biology and systems medicine use computational approaches to address biological complexity. Systems medicine utilises large datasets to track complex biological networks, building a network of networks to better understand human biology. For example, DNA (static picture of what a cell or organism might become) and RNA (measures what cells or organisms are doing at a specific moment) techniques are used [5]. With large amounts of data and analysis of biological networks, more precise conclusions and predictions can be made about individual health or disease conditions based on individual genetic structure and environment.

Conditions dealt with systems medicine can be addressed by either molecular or organismal systems medicine. Molecular systems medicine uses biological "omics" disciplines such as genomics, proteomics, metabolomics, metagenomics, phenomics, and transcriptomics, and is a "bottom-up" approach to the study of conditions, diseases and physiological processes, in which the description of molecular processes is analysed, simulated, synthesised and integrated to provide an explanation of an organ system or organism as a whole. Organismal systems medicine is a top-down approach that analyses complex processes from the top level (e.g. neural networks) and attempts to match the corresponding conditions at the molecular level [7].

2.2 The Link Between Precision and Systems Medicine

The US Institute of Medicine (IOM) and the US National Academy of Scientists published several reports in 2009–2012 that integrated the P4 approach to medicine and built on the identification of the core elements of systems medicine and the associated strengths, opportunities and risks [8].

In its reports, the IOM refers to precision medicine as one of the key benefits of systems medicine—stratifying or creating a risk profile of diseases and individuals based on genetic, molecular and cellular indicators and markers related to the causes rather than symptoms of disease [8]. The Institute for Systems Biology (ISB) criticised the term "precision" as being generic and not representing modern new medicine. The ISB argued that the goal of medicine or biology, in general, is to achieve precision in its various approaches, whereas systems medicine focuses on the integration of various large datasets (genomic, metabolic, transcriptomic, lifestyle and behaviour, etc.) for individuals, groups of individuals or populations to classify or stratify health and disease conditions into different groups [8, 9]. Thus, the IOM has suggested that systems medicine should be utilised as a systematic and more holistic approach to basically reclassify all diseases based on their causes [8, 9].

However, the view of P4 or precision medicine has evolved over the years. P4 medicine has emerged as an intersection of the megatrends (Fig. 2.1, 2013):

- Improved capability of systems medicine and systems biology to decode the complexity of medical conditions and diseases.
- Digitalisation enables the collection, storage, analysis, conclusion-drawing, and sharing of information and large amounts of data.
- Patient-driven interest and involvement in improving their own health. Access to better quality information allows patients to have more influence on their own health and lifestyle.

The term "big data" has been used since the late 1990s. In 2005 the first open-source framework for storing and analysing large amounts of data was created (Hadoop). It was another 5 years before Data Lakes, which allowed data to be stored in its raw or natural format in a large repository, appeared. From then on, big data and data analytics began to become a discipline in their own right [10].

P4 medicine has continued to evolve, and big data and analytics have become an integral part of its representation (Fig. 2.1).

The integration of consumer and patient participation in healthcare is one of the most important levers for the sustainable transformation of healthcare. Consumers' willingness to manage their own health using the internet and social media channels

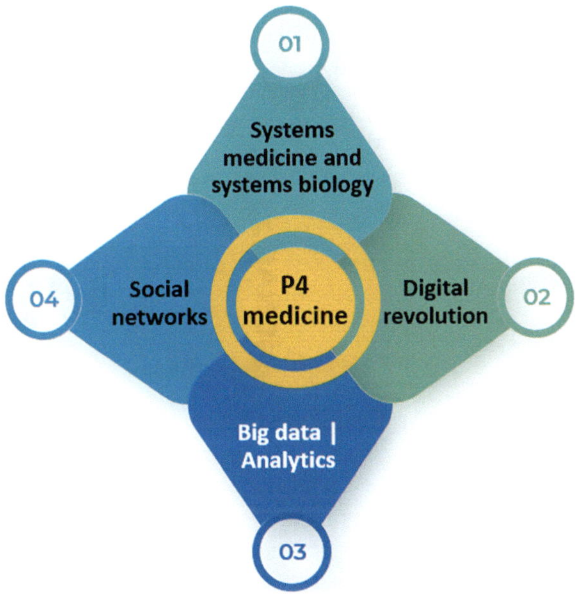

Fig. 2.1 Evolution of P4 medicine: 2018 social networks were integrated [8, 9] (www.researchgate.net; www.ncbi.nlm.nih.gov)

is rapidly accelerating, and as technology improves, so is the pace of this transformation process. The ever-increasing number of digital health applications and the number of consumers using these application tools support the enhancement of big data and data analytics with expanded and higher-quality data and information feeds.

Big data and analytics speed up the innovation cycle of systems medicine—the fundamental pillar of P4 medicine—and support consumers and patients in their health through better lifestyle choices, and more importantly, with those choices, contribute to scaling up the combat process of widespread medical conditions and diseases such as diabetes. Ultimately, this cycle of efficiency relieves the healthcare costs for patients and eases the financial burden on the entire healthcare system [5].

As mentioned above, the terms personalised and precision are often used interchangeably. Personalised medicine is the use of diagnostic tests to identify the most appropriate and optimal prevention, diagnosis and treatment of a disease based on the patient's genetics and molecular/cellular characteristics. In the past, personalised medicine was mainly associated with genetics, but it now encompasses various personalisation measures, e.g. imaging analysis and nanoparticle-based theragnostics [9, 11, 12].

Thus, P4 medicine (Fig. 2.2) is fundamentally based on the pillars shown above: systems medicine and systems biology, increasing digitalisation, social networks that impact and influence patients' health-related decisions and promote proactive patient participation, and big data analytics with ever-improving data quality and analysis tools/outcomes.

The combination of scientific and technological strength of systems medicine with the active participation of the consumers will not only have a positive effect on

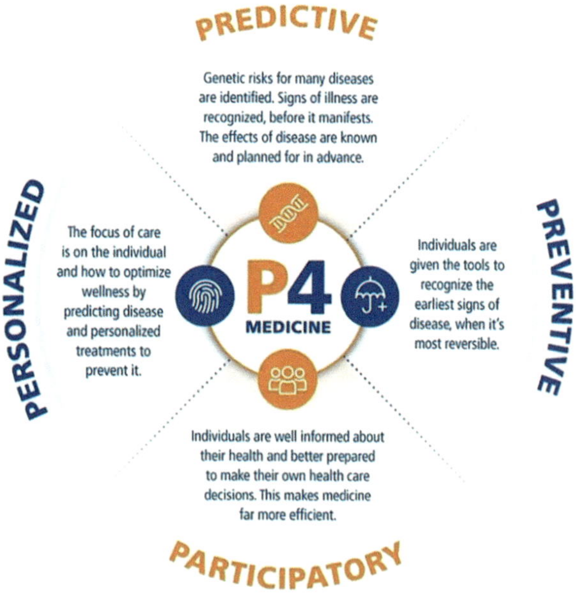

Fig. 2.2 4P medicine [13]. (Federoff HJ, Gostin LO (September 2009), Evolving from reductionism to holism: is there a future for systems medicine?)

reduced disease prevalence and reduced healthcare cost but also create a "learning healthcare system" and "learning society" [5].

For systems medicine to work as part of P4, it will require new infrastructure, including

- Cutting-edge technologies that collect and generate data based on multiple dimensions of an individual's experience of disease and health conditions.
- Digital infrastructure that can directly connect participating discovery science, data, and data analytics from clinical institutions and patients.
- Personalised clouds that can store and analyse information and data from the personal journey of disease and health experience, such as genetic and phenotypic information, medical history, demographics and other relevant data.
- Analytical techniques, tools and technologies to support prevention, including AI.

The effectiveness of systems medicine, and ultimately P4 medicine, requires data from as many people as possible, covering biological complexity and allowing inferences about healthy behaviours, and sophisticated computational tools, intelligence and thinking to analyse that data.

While "personalised" and "predictive" in P4 (Fig. 2.2) stand for predictive identification and personalised treatment of disease, "participatory" and "preventive" consider the crucial role of patient and consumer participation in the transformation of healthcare.

An important topic in systems medicine and biomedicine is the development of computational models that describe disease progression and the effects of therapeutic interventions.

More recent approaches include redefining disease phenotypes based on common mechanisms rather than symptoms. These then provide therapeutic targets, including network pharmacology and drug repurposing.

2.3 Status Quo Applications of Precision Medicine and Use Cases

2.3.1 Interview with Entrepreneur, Global Healthcare and AI Expert: Dr. Usman Lashari (MD, MBA, FACHE FAAD)

As precision medicine applications grow, the approach promises to revolutionise healthcare by offering more effective and personalised treatment options than traditional one-size-fits-all approaches.

Dr. Usman Lashari, MD, MBA, FACHE, FAAD, a healthcare and AI expert and long-time practitioner and entrepreneur, discusses the current state of AI in precision medicine: "Precision medicine is most advanced in oncology. Techniques such as genetic profiling of tumours allow for the identification of specific mutations, enabling the use of targeted therapies. For example, drugs such as trastuzumab for HER2-positive breast cancer have shown remarkable success. In addition, initiatives such as the National Institutes of Health's All of Us Research Program, which aims to collect diverse health data from one million participants, are further advancing research in this area.

Despite these advances, the transition from traditional to precision medicine in all areas of healthcare will take time. Several challenges need to be addressed, including the need for large-scale genetic data, the integration of new technologies into clinical practice, and the establishment of robust regulatory and ethical frameworks. In addition, healthcare providers will need to be trained in genomics and personalised treatment strategies.

Over the next decade, I expect to see a significant shift towards precision medicine in more medical disciplines. As genomic technologies become more affordable and data integration improves, personalised treatments will become standard practice. However, full integration into routine healthcare is likely to take 15–20 years, given the pace of technology adoption, regulatory processes and the need for extensive clinical validation."

AI will be a cornerstone of precision medicine, improving diagnostic accuracy, personalising treatments and accelerating drug discovery.

Some examples of AI applications/use cases:

1. Genomic Data Interpretation—Foundation Medicine
   (a) Foundation Medicine uses AI-driven genomic profiling to identify mutations in cancer patients. Its comprehensive genomic profiling (CGP) tests, such as FoundationOne CDx, analyse the DNA of cancer cells to identify genetic alterations and match them to targeted therapies. This approach enables personalised treatment plans tailored to the genetic profile of each patient's cancer [14].
2. Predictive Analytics and Disease Risk Assessment—Cardiogram
   (a) Cardiogram uses AI algorithms to analyse data from wearable devices, such as Apple Watch and Fitbit, to predict cardiovascular risks like atrial fibrillation, sleep apnea, and hypertension. The app provides users with real-time health insights and alerts, enabling proactive management of heart health [15].
3. Drug Discovery and Development—BenevolentAI and Insilico Medicine
   (a) BenevolentAI leverages AI to accelerate the drug discovery process. Their platform integrates vast amounts of biomedical information to identify potential drug candidates and predict their efficacy. Notably, BenevolentAI identified a potential treatment for COVID-19, baricitinib, which was later tested in clinical trials [16].
   (b) Insilico Medicine uses AI for drug discovery and development, focusing on aging and age-related diseases. Their AI-driven platform has identified novel compounds for various diseases, including fibrosis and cancer, significantly reducing the time and cost of preclinical drug development [17].

   It is worth noting that AI in drug discovery can bring significant efficiencies through literature mining, genomic databases, and case history analysis, shortening drug discovery to clinic timelines; through drug repurposing: combining 2–3 existing drugs helping to identify and to formulate the most effective treatment quickly [18].

4. Medical Imaging and Diagnostics—Zebra Medical Vision and Aidoc
   (a) Zebra Medical Vision utilises AI to analyse medical imaging data and detect conditions such as cancers, cardiovascular issues and liver diseases. Their AI algorithms assist radiologists by providing automated, accurate readings of medical images, enhancing diagnostic efficiency and accuracy [19].
   (b) Aidoc offers AI solutions that support radiologists detect critical conditions in medical images. Their AI platform analyses imaging data in real-time, flagging urgent cases such as intracranial haemorrhages and pulmonary embolisms, allowing for quicker diagnosis and treatment [20].

   In addition, the use of AI is transforming the disciplines of pathology, dermatology and radiology in particular. In pathology, for example, AI is improving the efficiency and accuracy of diagnostic processes. Some examples are digital platforms such as PathAI and Google Health's AI or automated analysis tool PageAI [21]:

   (c) PathAI: This platform uses machine learning algorithms to assist pathologists in diagnosing diseases from tissue samples. It can identify cancerous cells with high accuracy, reducing diagnostic errors and improving patient outcomes.
   (d) Google Health's AI: Google Health has developed an AI system that can detect breast cancer in mammograms with greater accuracy than human radiologists. The system analyses histopathological images to identify malignancies, significantly aiding pathologists in their diagnostic processes [22].
   (e) Paige.AI: This AI tool automates the analysis of pathology slides, particularly for cancer diagnosis. It assists pathologists by highlighting areas of interest and providing quantitative analysis, which speeds up the diagnostic process and increases accuracy.

   In dermatology, AI is being used to improve the diagnosis and treatment of skin conditions, with examples including AI-powered diagnostic apps and teledermatology platforms:

   (f) SkinVision: This app uses AI to analyse photos of skin lesions and moles, assessing the risk of skin cancer. It provides users with a risk indication, urging them to seek professional advice if necessary.
   (g) Dermatology AI by Google Health: Google Health has developed an AI model capable of identifying skin conditions from images. The model can recognise a wide range of dermatological issues, assisting clinicians in making accurate diagnoses.
   (h) VisualDx: This tool uses AI to provide clinical decision support for dermatologists. It helps diagnose skin conditions by analysing clinical images and patient data and offering differential diagnoses and treatment recommendations.

   AI has also made significant strides in radiology by enhancing image analysis, diagnostic accuracy, and workflow optimisation.

(i) Aidoc's AI platform analyses medical images in real time, assisting radiologists in detecting critical conditions such as intracranial haemorrhages and pulmonary embolisms. The system flags urgent cases, ensuring timely diagnosis and treatment.
(j) Zebra Medical Vision—AI tool scans radiology images to detect various conditions, including liver disease, cardiovascular issues and cancers. It provides automated, accurate readings, enhancing radiologist efficiency and diagnostic accuracy.
(k) Arterys provides AI-powered solutions for radiology that streamline workflow by automating tasks such as image segmentation and quantification. This allows radiologists to focus on interpretation and decision-making, improving overall productivity and accuracy.

The above-mentioned AI applications demonstrate the potential of integrating advanced technologies into medical practice, paving the way for more precise and efficient healthcare.

2.4 Potential and Advantages of Systems Medicine and P4 Medicine

Precision medicine offers many advantages over traditional medicine, particularly its ability to provide more personalised and effective treatments. In oncology, genetic profiling of tumours enables targeted therapies that can be more effective and have fewer side effects than conventional treatments. Similarly, AI-driven predictive analytics can predict disease risk and treatment response, allowing for earlier intervention and personalised care plans [23]. In cardiology, predictive models such as those developed by IBM Watson Health can predict cardiovascular events and guide preventive measures [24].

Systems medicine as part of P4 medicine can lead to cost-effective healthcare by arranging people and diseases into distinct subgroups. Genomic analysis stratifies people into subgroups with different reactions to medication, treatments, and drugs, various disease risk groups, and other clinical factors. Diseases such as breast cancer, once classified as a single disease, are being stratified into clinically relevant subgroups based on genetic, molecular, and cellular network interactions [5]. Reclassification into subgroups allows for more accurate diagnoses and more cost- and outcome-effective treatments based on the underlying causes of disease [5]. The most notable successes of targeted therapies based on genetic profiling, such as trastuzumab for HER2-positive breast cancer, have been in oncology.

Surgery and other aspects of traditional medicine will be influenced by the stratification of disease and, where appropriate, people. Focusing on the causes rather than the symptoms of disease will allow intervention much earlier in the disease process, and in many cases prevent disease from occurring in the first place [5].

Artificial intelligence will also have a significant impact on genetics and genomics [25]. Deep genomics aims to identify patterns in huge datasets of genetic information and medical records, looking for mutations and links to disease. They are

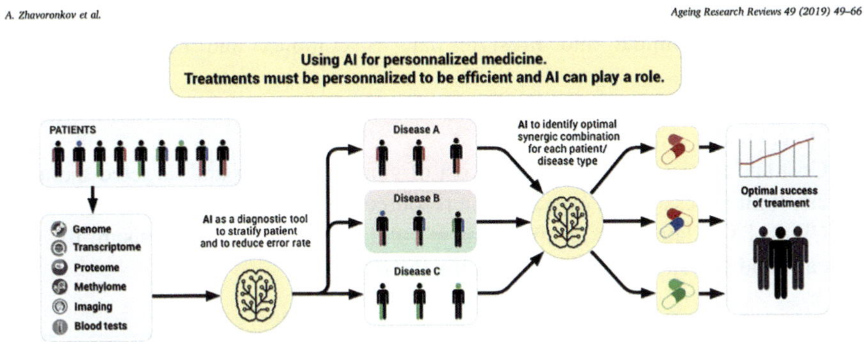

Fig. 2.3 Using AI for personalised medicine. (From [26] Aging research reviews 49, Zhavorankov et al., 2019, 49–66, licensed under CC-BY 4.0)

inventing a new generation of computational technologies that can tell doctors what happens inside a cell when DNA is altered by genetic variation, whether natural or therapeutic. AI has the greatest potential to analyse vast amounts of data and provide insights to create personalised solutions and targeted treatments. AI also plays a huge role in drug discovery (see companies BenevolentAI and Insilico Medicine above), reducing the time and cost of bringing new treatments to market.

Some noteworthy trends in precision medicine [23, 24]:

- Increased use of AI and machine learning: AI will continue to improve precision medicine by enhancing data analytics and predictive capabilities.
- Expansion beyond oncology: Precision medicine is expected to make significant inroads into other areas such as cardiology, neurology and infectious diseases.
- Integration with conventional medicine: Rather than completely replacing traditional medicine, precision medicine will likely integrate with it, enhancing traditional approaches with personalised strategies.
- Regulatory and ethical frameworks: The development of robust regulatory and ethical frameworks will be essential to guide the use of precision medicine.

In addition, the trend in preventive medicine, in which AI will play a crucial role, is to classify "ageing" as a disease and to work on increasing healthy longevity while looking at patience in different age groups. Figure 2.3 shows how stratification into groups according to specific conditions or age can lead to more accurate diagnoses, reducing error rates and providing effective treatments [26].

2.5 Potential Risk Areas Within Precision Medicine

Despite its promising positive impact, precision medicine also faces several challenges that may hinder its ability to fully replace traditional medicine in the near future [25]:

- Data integration and standardisation: Integrating and standardising vast amounts of genetic, clinical and lifestyle data is complex and requires a robust infrastructure.
- Ethical and privacy concerns: Managing patient data while ensuring privacy and ethical use is critical.
- Cost and accessibility: The high cost of genomic testing and targeted therapies can limit accessibility, especially in resource-poor settings.
- Clinical validation: Extensive clinical validation is required to ensure the efficacy and safety of precision medicine interventions.

2.6 Future Outlook and Conclusion

Precision medicine has immense potential to transform healthcare. The transformation process will take time and is interdependent on the advancement of systems medicine, digital transformation in medicine and infrastructure requirements, increasing solutions using data analytics and AI tools while improving the quality of outcomes, and social networks actively contributing to the transformation process.

While the transition from traditional to precision medicine is underway, a complete shift will require continued innovation, investment and collaboration across the healthcare community.

Though precision medicine is poised to transform healthcare by offering more personalised and effective treatments, it is unlikely to completely replace traditional medicine in the foreseeable future. Instead, we can expect a synergistic integration where precision medicine complements traditional approaches, leading to a more comprehensive and personalised healthcare system. The future of medicine lies in this integration, leveraging the strengths of traditional and precision methods to improve patient outcomes and healthcare efficiency. (Selected inputs out of: [23].)

References

1. Stratified medicines report final docx.pdf, 2015.
2. Hood L, Balling R, Auffray C. Revolutionizing medicine in the twenty-first century through systems approaches. Biotechnol J. 2012;7(8):992–1001.
3. Federoff HJ, Gostin LO. Evolving from reductionism to holism: is there a future for systems medicine? JAMA. 2009;302(9):994–6.
4. Kamada T. System biomedicine: a new paradigm in biomedical engineering. Front Med Biol Eng. 1992;4(1):1–2.
5. P4 medicine: how systems medicine will transform the healthcare sector and society—PMC (nih.gov). www.ncbi.nlm.nih.gov/pmc/articles/PMC4204402/y.
6. A new biology for the 21st century: ensuring the United States leads the coming biology revolution. Washington, DC: National Academies Press; 2009.
7. www.ncbi.nlm.nih.gov/pmc/articles/PMC6523452/.
8. https://www.researchgate.net/.

9. Personalized medicine 101. Personalized medicine coalition. Archived from the original on 10 May 2019. PMC_The_Personalized_Medicine_Report_Opportunity_Challenges_and_the_Future.pdf (personalizedmedicinecoalition.org).
10. The origin of big data analytics—analytics Vidhya. https://www.analyticsvidhya.com/blog/2022/09/the-origin-of-big-data-analytics/.
11. Priyadharshini VS, Teran LM. Personalized medicine in respiratory disease: role of proteomics. Adv Protein Chem Struct Biol. 2016;102:115–46.
12. Xie J, Lee S, Chen X. Nanoparticle-based theranostic agents. Adv Drug Deliv Rev. 2010;62(11):1064–79.
13. Rodríguez G. How P4 medicine will transform the healthcare sector and society. Medium; 2023. www.medium.com.
14. Foundation Medicine, FoundationOne CDx.
15. Cardiogram, Cardiogram AI.
16. BenevolentAI, BenevolentAI Drug Discovery.
17. (14) Insilico Medicine, Insilico Medicine.
18. Trotsyuk A. AI in healthcare and drug development, 2024.
19. Zebra Medical Vision, Zebra Medical Vision AI.
20. Aidoc, Aidoc AI.
21. PathAI.
22. https://health.google/health-research/imaging-and-diagnostics/.
23. The Lancet, www.thelancet.com/ebiom-digital-health-collection.
24. https://publichealth.jmir.org/2016/2/e157/.
25. Interview Usman Lashari, a healthcare and AI expert.
26. Zhavorankov A, et al. Artificial intelligence for aging and longevity research: recent advances and perspectives. Aging Res Rev. 2019;49:49–66.

Tatsiana Akhrymenka (Executive MBA Oxford University, Said Business School; Group M&A Leader in Infrastructure and Energy sector: GETEC Group Capital Deployment/M&A Lead) has many years of experience in strategic development and investments, cross-border transactions and post-merger integrations in various sectors across geographical boundaries. Her expertise includes the introduction, definition and implementation of inorganic corporate strategies in medium and large companies as well as establishment and development of family office investment activities in various asset classes from venture capital to growth capital. In addition, Tatsiana is the founder and is involved in various entrepreneurship activities as an investor and value contributor in early-stage companies; she is also highly engaged in innovation, digitalisation and sustainability aspects of various disciplines, including personalised and longevity medicine, exploring the untapped potential with data-driven technologies and innovations of these disciplines. Tatsiana is also the editor and author of various books and publications.

Unlocking the Potential: Cloud Computing's Impact on Healthcare

3

Rakesh Margam

3.1 Methodology of the Study

Literature Review—A key element of this research project will be a thorough and methodical examination of academic and commercial literature on the application of cloud computing in the healthcare sector. This literature study seeks to act as the conceptual framework for the ensuing analysis and conclusions.

Keyword Search—With the goal of facilitating the systematic evaluation of the literature, a thorough search will be done using pertinent keywords that include the main ideas of the investigation. To thoroughly search academic databases, research repositories, and industry publications, keywords like "cloud computing in healthcare," "Software as a Service (SaaS) in healthcare," and "Platform as a Service (PaaS) applications in healthcare" will be used. The use of these precise keywords will guarantee the discovery of important publications, studies, and resources that have a direct bearing on the area of research

Selection Criteria—A strict set of selection criteria will be used to ensure the accuracy and relevance of the literature used in this review. We will carefully choose literature that offers in-depth analysis of the various cloud service models (SaaS PaaS and IaaS) and their observable effects on the healthcare ecosystem. The criteria will take into account things like how recently the paper was published how reliable the source is how comprehensive the study was and how in-depth the analysis was. This careful selection procedure will make it possible to include academic papers and industry reports that considerably advance knowledge of the complex interaction between cloud computing and healthcare.

Data Extraction—To ensure the acquisition of significant insights, the necessary material will be painstakingly extracted from the chosen literature. The most important facts, such as the benefits, difficulties, and effects of using cloud computing in healthcare settings, will be painstakingly extracted. In addition, pertinent case

R. Margam (✉)
SecureKloud Technologies Inc., Pleasanton, CA, USA

P. Plugmann, D. Portius (eds.), *Innovations in Healthcare and Outcome Measurement*, https://doi.org/10.1007/978-3-031-77302-0_3

studies showcasing actual applications and results will be examined and included in the study. This literature analysis will provide a thorough perspective on the changing state of cloud computing in healthcare by methodically removing these crucial elements, promoting a better grasp of its transformational potential and related implications.

Data Analysis—The study project's analysis phase is anticipated to be a thorough and extensive process that will produce insightful findings and shed light on the complex interactions between cloud computing and the healthcare industry. The examination will include numerous crucial dimensions, including:

1. Thematic Analysis—The retrieved data will be subjected to a thorough thematic analysis, during which it will be methodically divided into overarching topics that are specifically connected to the effect of cloud computing on the healthcare industry. Finding repeating themes, motifs, and patterns in the literature will be a part of this approach. The study will offer a detailed picture of how cloud computing is affecting many elements of healthcare delivery, management, and patient outcomes by grouping the data into six thematic groups. These topics will act as the framework for the analysis that follows.
2. Comparison—The comparison of the three main cloud computing service models—Software as a Service (SaaS), Platform as a Service (PaaS), and Infrastructure as a Service (IaaS)—in the context of healthcare will be a key component of the data analysis. This side-by-side comparison will examine the unique qualities, benefits, and drawbacks of each service type. The report attempts to provide useful insights into the strategic issues that healthcare organisations must navigate when choosing a particular cloud service model by highlighting the differences and synergies between these models.
3. A thorough investigation of certain case studies, particularly those included in the study's opening, would enhance the data analysis. To find real-world applications, results, and lessons gained, these real-world cases will go through a thorough study. The analysis will shed light on the concrete effects of cloud computing on healthcare organisations and clarify its transformational potential through a thorough examination of these case studies. The analysis will include both successful implementations and possible difficulties encountered in these scenarios, giving a balanced view of the real-world effects of cloud adoption in healthcare.

3.2 Introduction

The concept of cloud computing, which allows remote access to pooled computer resources over the internet, has arisen as a disruptive force that is transforming businesses all over the world [1]. Particularly significant is how it affects the healthcare services industry, a field that faces many complicated problems and offers several opportunities. In-depth analysis of the complex link between cloud computing and healthcare is undertaken in this study, along with an explanation of the fundamental principles of cloud computing and how it may completely transform the healthcare industry. The healthcare industry has faced several challenges in recent years, from the need to increase accessibility to medical services to the effective administration of enormous patient data banks. A potential solution to these problems is cloud computing, which offers a flexible, scalable, and economically feasible infrastructure [2]. Cloud computing has the potential to spark new methods to patient care, medical research, and administrative tasks by enabling safe data storage, smooth data processing, and quick information exchange. This rigorously organised article examines all of the various ways that cloud computing is being used in the healthcare industry. To highlight the transformational potential of cloud-based solutions, it specifically explores the administration of Electronic Health Records (EHR), telemedicine, remote patient monitoring, and medical imaging [3]. The particular benefits and accompanying difficulties of integrating cloud computing are visible in each of these fields, necessitating a thorough understanding of its implications. The dual-edged aspect of cloud computing—which offers benefits while creating challenges—commands attention in the context of healthcare's continual growth. The following sections of this chapter, a painstaking synthesis of research and exposition, explore the benefits of cloud computing, embracing scalability, collaborative healthcare, and strong disaster recovery mechanisms, while assiduously examining the complex environment of data security, privacy preservation, and regulatory adherence [4]. In conclusion, this chapter aims to give a comprehensive picture of cloud computing's disruptive potential within the realm of healthcare. The goal is to provide discerning insights into the nuanced interaction of cloud computing and healthcare services, thereby enhancing understanding of this dynamic symbiosis, by navigating through its fundamental principles, practical applications, inherent merits, and associated challenges [5].

3.3 Cloud Computing in Healthcare: An Overview

Cloud computing is a significant technical development that presents several prospects for change in the modern healthcare scene. Cloud computing, which is the delivery of computer services through the internet, has developed into a crucial instrument for improving healthcare services in a variety of ways. Three main service models have arisen under this paradigm: software as a service (SaaS), platform as a service (PaaS), and infrastructure as a service (IaaS). Each of these models has been developed to meet the specific needs of healthcare organisations and patients [6].

The underlying technology of cloud computing, Infrastructure as a Service (IaaS), provides virtualised computer resources through the internet. IaaS in healthcare provides access to scalable and adaptable infrastructure that can meet the needs of processing and storing healthcare data [7]. This architecture is the basis for data backup, storage, and computing, relieving healthcare organisations of the burden of physical hardware upkeep.

A cornerstone of cloud computing, software as a service (SaaS), offers pre-built programmes that are available through web browsers. SaaS models cover a wide range of healthcare-related products, including telemedicine platforms, practise management software, and electronic health record (EHR) systems. These apps' cloud hosting lessens the load of local installs and frees up healthcare practitioners to concentrate on giving patients the best treatment possible.

Another aspect of cloud computing is Platform as a Service (PaaS), which offers developers a dynamic environment in which to build, distribute, and manage programmes. PaaS gives developers the ability to create unique medical apps, analytical tools, and creative solutions in the field of healthcare [2]. PaaS speeds up the development cycle and encourages the creation of customised apps to match the constantly changing demands of the healthcare industry by abstracting infrastructural complexity.

The underlying technology of cloud computing, Infrastructure as a Service (IaaS), provides virtualised computer resources through the internet. IaaS in healthcare provides access to scalable and adaptable infrastructure that can meet the needs of processing and storing healthcare data [8]. This architecture is the basis for data backup, storage, and computing, relieving healthcare organisations of the burden of physical hardware upkeep.

The centralisation of data, resources, and services on distant computers is the basis of cloud computing's operational mechanism. When compared to previous methods, this paradigm shift away from on-premises infrastructure has several benefits [9]. The scalability that cloud computing offers is the most significant of these benefits, allowing healthcare organisations to dynamically alter resources in response to changing demand. This flexibility prevents the inefficiencies of overprovisioning and guarantees peak performance. Beyond resource optimisation, cloud computing offers other advantages [10]. Because cloud service providers are now in charge of maintaining physical infrastructure, healthcare institutions that use it will see simplified operations and lower operating costs [3]. The simplicity of exchanging patient data between institutions and departments enhances collaborative treatment and encourages a holistic approach to healthcare delivery.

Cloud-enabled solutions bring in a new era of patient involvement from the standpoint of the patient. Individuals are given access to their own health records that are safely maintained in the cloud, promoting a sense of ownership and active engagement in their treatment plans. Additionally, telemedicine powered by the cloud and remote patient monitoring overcome geographic limitations to provide healthcare in off-the-grid and underprivileged places. The many service models meet a range of demands, completely changing how healthcare services are provided and accessed. The cloud's immense influence on healthcare organisations and patients alike is highlighted by its scalability, adaptability, collaborative potential, and better patient involvement.

3.4 Applications of Cloud Computing in Healthcare

The fusion of cloud computing with healthcare creates a diverse ecosystem of applications that go beyond limitations and improve the effectiveness and calibre of medical care. The contributions of cloud computing are outlined in a larger context in this part, which also covers telemedicine, remote patient monitoring, medical imaging and examinations, investigation and data analytics, and health information exchange [11]. Electronic health records (EHR) and health information management are also included.

3.4.1 Medical Records Management and Electronic Health Records (EHR)

The dynamics of patient record management are transformed by the integration of cloud computing into EHR systems. A new era of safe data storage, unrestricted access, and centralised record-keeping is ushered in by cloud-based technologies [10]. Medical professionals have quick access to thorough patient histories, fostering coordinated care delivery and well-informed clinical judgement. Additionally, cloud solutions ease the problems brought on by data silos, promoting interoperability and data sharing among healthcare organisations [12]. However, strict steps are required to protect data privacy and security as a result of the digitalisation of sensitive medical data into cloud platforms. In order to protect patient confidentiality and maximise the effectiveness of cloud-integrated EHR systems, encryption procedures, authentication mechanisms, and regulatory conformance emerge as essential elements [13].

3.4.2 Remote Monitoring and Telemedicine

Remote patient monitoring and other innovative healthcare techniques are made possible by cloud computing. Telemedicine solutions enabled by the cloud enable virtual consultations, giving patients access to medical advice and treatment from a distance [14]. Patients in remote or rural areas benefit most from this, as it removes barriers to accessing treatment. In line with this, cloud-based remote patient monitoring uses IoT sensors and wearable technology to continuously collect and transmit patient data, giving healthcare practitioners the ability to proactively monitor patient health indicators [15].

3.4.3 Diagnostics and Imaging in Medicine

The processing power of cloud computing has significant advantages for the field of medical imaging. The restrictions of physical storage mediums are eliminated by cloud-based storage, resulting in a centralised repository for medical photographs [1]. The communication between radiologists and specialists is sped up and treatment strategies are improved because to this easy accessibility. Furthermore, the processing capacity of the cloud enables complex image analysis algorithms, enhancing diagnostic accuracy and reducing the time needed for important evaluations [16].

3.4.4 Data Analytics and Research

The elastic architecture of cloud computing proves to be extremely helpful for research and data analytics. In order to examine large datasets and carry out complex studies, researchers may take advantage of the cloud's enormous processing power [17]. This speeds up the hunt for new drugs, genomics research, and epidemiological investigations. Creating safe, collaborative spaces for academics from many geographical areas to collaborate on complex topics is made possible by cloud platforms.

3.4.5 Exchange of Health Information

The role of a conduit for efficient health information transmission is taken on by the cloud. By allowing various healthcare systems to safely communicate patient data, it promotes interoperability. This is of utmost importance in emergency situations where quick access to patient records is crucial to saving lives. Additionally, cloud-anchored health information exchange platforms improve the continuity of treatment by giving healthcare professionals access to up-to-date patient data [18].

In conclusion, there are several uses of cloud computing in the healthcare industry. The cloud's transformational potential is almost limitless, from enhancing diagnostics and research to allowing telemedicine and health data interchange. To fully capitalise on the array of advantages that cloud computing bestows upon the healthcare industry, however, constant attention must be paid to data security, privacy laws, and ethical issues.

3.5 Advantages and Challenges

3.5.1 Health Care Benefits of Cloud Computing

The use of cloud computing in the healthcare industry brings about a slew of benefits that penetrate many aspects of medical services [19]. The main advantages of cloud computing in healthcare are explained in this section, including scalability, cost-effectiveness, flexibility, shared treatment, immediate information sharing, recovery from disasters, and continuity of operations.

3.5.2 Flexibility, Affordability, and Scalability

The scalability that distinguishes cloud computing enables healthcare organisations to dynamically modify their resource distribution in response to changing demands. This flexibility prevents overprovisioning's inefficiencies while avoiding bottlenecks during moments of high demand. The pay-as-you-go concept also correlates to cost-effectiveness since cloud services allow organisations to optimise spending based on real consumption [12]. The inherent flexibility of the cloud further improves operational agility by enabling healthcare organisations to quickly react to changing requirements without requiring time-consuming transfers.

3.5.3 Sharing Real-Time Data and Collaborative Care

Collaboration in healthcare undergoes a fundamental leap thanks to cloud computing. The centralised database of patient data speeds up interdepartmental dialogue and well-informed clinical judgement [19]. Real-time access to patient records by professionals in various places promotes the provision of comprehensive treatment. In addition to bridging temporal gaps, this real-time data exchange leads to more coordinated treatment plans, quicker diagnoses, and improved patient satisfaction [20].

3.5.4 Recovery from Disasters and Business Continuity

Healthcare organisations are protected against unanticipated disruptions via the cloud. In the case of system failures or natural disasters, vital patient data is protected through reliable disaster recovery procedures and automatic backups [21]. Thus, business continuity is protected, preventing data loss and interruption for operations. Continuity planning driven by the cloud reduces interruptions and strengthens the dependability of healthcare services, inspiring trust in both patients and providers.

3.6 Challenges and Concerns

3.6.1 Privacy and Data Security Issues

Despite the abundance of advantages, cloud computing in healthcare raises fundamental questions about data security and privacy. Concerns regarding unauthorised access, data breaches, and cyberattacks arise as a result of moving sensitive patient data to distant computers. To protect patient confidentiality and combat possible intrusions, strict encryption, multifactor authentication, and persistent monitoring are essential.

3.6.2 Compliance with Regulations, Such As HIPAA in the US

A maze of regulatory frameworks that preserve patient rights and data integrity govern how the healthcare industry functions. Due to its accessibility throughout the globe, cloud computing presents difficulties in complying with many laws, such as the Health Insurance Portability and Accountability Act (HIPAA) in the United

States [22]. To guarantee that patient data is protected from legal risks, healthcare organisations must carefully evaluate the compliance of cloud providers with local laws.

3.6.3 Reliance on Uninterrupted Internet Connectivity

The operational dependency introduced by cloud computing's reliance on internet access deserves consideration. Internet connectivity issues or downtime might interfere with medical treatment by making it difficult to obtain vital patient data. To lessen the effects of erratic connectivity, redundancy measures, backup connectivity options, and local caching systems are crucial.

Numerous benefits that improve operational effectiveness and patient care are delivered when cloud computing is implemented in the healthcare industry. However, difficulties with data security, legal compliance, and infrastructure resilience highlight the significance of carefully navigating the cloud environment. Harnessing the revolutionary potential of cloud computing in healthcare depends critically on finding equitable solutions to these problems [18] (Table 3.1).

Table 3.1 Advantages and challenges

Serial no.	Aspect	Advantages of cloud computing in healthcare	Challenges and concerns in healthcare cloud computing
1	Scalability, flexibility, affordability	Dynamic resource allocation enables healthcare organisations to adjust resources based on demand, reducing inefficiencies. The pay-as-you-go cost model ensures cost-effectiveness	Privacy concerns may arise due to storing sensitive patient data off-site. Data security measures, such as encryption and authentication, are essential. Compliance with regulations like HIPAA is critical
2	Real-time data sharing and collaboration	Centralised patient data accelerates interdepartmental communication, resulting in more informed clinical judgements. Real-time access to patient records improves treatment coordination and speeds up diagnoses	Uninterrupted internet connectivity is crucial for real-time data access. Downtime or connectivity issues can lead to data breaches and operational disruptions
3	Recovery from disasters and business continuity	Reliable disaster recovery procedures and automatic backups safeguard critical patient data. This ensures business continuity even during system failures or natural disasters. Cloud-driven continuity planning minimises interruptions and enhances dependability	Dependence on uninterrupted internet connectivity is a potential vulnerability. Lack of connectivity can disrupt medical treatment and operations
4	Enhanced patient satisfaction	Quick access to medical records and well-informed clinical judgement lead to faster diagnoses and improved patient satisfaction	Privacy and data security concerns must be addressed to maintain patient trust

(continued)

Table 3.1 (continued)

Serial no.	Aspect	Advantages of cloud computing in healthcare	Challenges and concerns in healthcare cloud computing
5	Cost-effectiveness	The pay-as-you-go cost model allows healthcare organisations to optimise spending based on actual resource consumption, reducing unnecessary costs	Adequate cost management and monitoring are required to maximise cost-effectiveness
6	Accessibility and remote monitoring	Remote access to patient records and telemedicine improve healthcare accessibility. However, ensuring data privacy during remote access is essential	Remote access introduces potential privacy risks that need to be mitigated through proper safeguards
7	Data analytics and informed decision-making	Centralised patient data facilitates health data analytics, leading to more data-driven and effective healthcare decisions	Analysing data effectively and ensuring data accuracy are essential for informed decision-making

3.7 Case Studies

The deployment of cloud computing inside healthcare organisations has culminated in observable success stories that highlight this technology paradigm's capacity for transformation. This section goes into example case studies, illuminating the results, accomplishments, and difficulties these institutions faced while also emphasising key best practises and learnings from their experiences.

1. Cleveland Clinic—When the famous Cleveland Clinic switched its EHR system to a cloud-based platform, it started a transformational journey. This change not only sped up data accessibility and sharing but also encouraged teamwork in the provision of healthcare. The results were striking: increased care coordination, simpler procedures, and a decrease in medical mistakes thanks to more accurate data [23]. Despite these successes, the clinic still had data security issues, which were overcome by implementing strong encryption techniques and carefully choosing vendors. The need of coordinating cloud integration with strict security guidelines is shown by this scenario.
2. Mercy Health—A major healthcare organisation, Mercy Health, used cloud computing to improve telemedicine services. They increased their geographic reach by integrating cloud-powered telemedicine tools, providing medical services in off-the-grid and underserved regions. The result was not just increased access to healthcare but also significant cost savings due to the reduction in the demand for physical infrastructure. Mercy Health [24] has to come up with creative solutions, such offline means for consultations, in response to the problem of connection gaps in rural areas. This instance demonstrates the strategic significance of modifying cloud technology to get beyond regional constraints.
3. Beth Israel Deaconess Hospital—By utilising cloud-based medical imaging and diagnostics, Beth Israel Deaconess Medical Centre has significantly improved the storage, retrieval, and analysis of medical images. This change sped up

diagnostics and enabled prompt treatment choices. The centre also had to deal with the issue of data sovereignty since it was necessary for the data of patients from other countries to adhere to a variety of data protection laws [25]. They were able to preserve efficiency while customising data storage based on regulatory requirements by implementing hybrid cloud solutions. This instance illustrates how important it is to match cloud strategy with local regulatory regimes.

4. Massachusetts General Hospital—To improve its research efforts, Massachusetts General Hospital utilised cloud-based tools. The hospital accelerated intricate genetic analysis and simulations using the computational power of the cloud, spurring advances in personalised treatment. This resulted in quicker medication development and more customised treatment plans, which had a big influence on patient outcomes [18]. The university had difficulties with data transfer speeds for large genomic datasets while enjoying these advantages. This demonstrated the necessity for flexible solutions and led the hospital to improve its data transmission methods.
5. Philadelphia Children's Hospital—To support its attempts to exchange health information, The Children's Hospital of Philadelphia used cloud computing. Care coordination was expedited and decision-making was made more quickly thanks to cloud-powered data exchange between multiple departments and associated healthcare organisations. The facility proved successful in streamlining patient care and minimising unnecessary medical examinations [26]. However, it became difficult to guarantee data correctness and integrity across several platforms. The need of data standardisation and strong integration protocols in maximising the potential of cloud-enabled information interchange is shown by this scenario.
6. Mayo Clinic—Mayo Clinic used the cloud to improve its capacity for disaster recovery. The institution made sure that patient care would continue even in the event of a natural disaster or technology failure by moving its crucial patient data to the cloud. The results were significant: fewer service interruptions, less downtime, and continuous patient care [22]. The Health Insurance Portability and Accountability Act (HIPAA) compliance was one of the problems that this project faced. The Mayo Clinic overcame issue by working with cloud providers that provided comprehensive HIPAA-compliant services, highlighting the importance of careful provider evaluation.
7. The Royal Free London NHS Foundation—the Royal Free London NHS Foundation Trust used cloud computing to improve patient access to medical imaging. The institution sped up picture sharing and diagnosis by centralising medical images on the cloud. This resulted in more rapid treatment choices and better patient care results. However, issues with data privacy and patient permission surfaced, particularly in light of the delicate nature of medical pictures [27]. In response, the institution put in place strict access restrictions and improved permission management, highlighting the meeting point of moral concerns and cloud solutions (Fig. 3.1 and Table 3.2).

Optimal Techniques and Lessons Learned—These case studies highlight some essential guidelines for effective cloud adoption in the healthcare industry. To

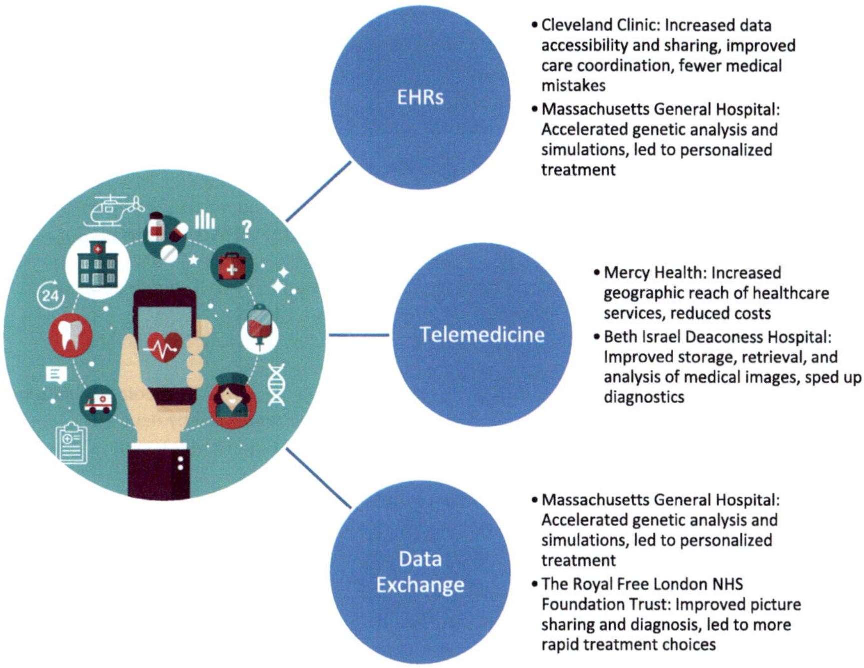

Fig. 3.1 Learnings from case studies

Table 3.2 Summary of case studies

Serial number	Healthcare organisation	Use of cloud computing	Outcomes and challenges
1	Cleveland Clinic	EHR system migration to the cloud	– Improved data accessibility and sharing – Enhanced teamwork in healthcare delivery – Increased care coordination – Reduced medical errors – Data security challenges overcome with strong encryption and vendor selection
2	Mercy Health	Cloud-powered telemedicine tools	– Expanded geographic reach for healthcare services – Cost savings due to reduced infrastructure demands – Creative solutions for connectivity gaps in rural areas
3	Beth Israel Deaconess Hospital	Cloud-based medical imaging and diagnostics	– Accelerated storage, retrieval, and analysis of medical images – Prompt treatment decisions – Data sovereignty challenges addressed through hybrid cloud solutions

(continued)

Table 3.2 (continued)

Serial number	Healthcare organisation	Use of cloud computing	Outcomes and challenges
4	Massachusetts General Hospital	Cloud-based tools for research	– Accelerated genetic analysis and simulations – Advances in personalised treatment – Challenges with data transfer speeds for large genomic datasets, leading to improvements in data transmission methods
5	Philadelphia Children's Hospital	Cloud-powered data exchange	– Streamlined care coordination and decision-making – Reduced unnecessary medical examinations – Challenges with data correctness and integrity addressed by data standardisation and integration protocols
6	Mayo Clinic	Disaster recovery in the cloud	– Ensured patient care continuity during disasters or tech failures – Reduced service interruptions and downtime – HIPAA compliance challenges addressed through careful cloud provider selection
7	The Royal Free London NHS Foundation	Centralised medical imaging on the cloud	– Accelerated picture sharing and diagnosis – Improved patient care outcomes – Data privacy and patient permission challenges mitigated with strict access restrictions and permission management

protect patient privacy, stringent data security procedures are essential. These include encryption, multi-layer authentication, and thorough vendor inspections. Additionally, tailoring cloud solutions to meet certain institutional requirements, such offline functionality and data residency concerns, is essential for maximising cloud advantages. The cases also teach us important lessons. First, successful integration of cloud technology necessitates institutional cultural changes in addition to technological ones. Second, the dynamic nature of the healthcare industry demands an adaptable cloud strategy that can change with the requirements of patients and the regulatory environment [28]. Finally, to guarantee continuous healthcare delivery, strong contingency planning is essential. This includes redundancy measures for connectivity shortages. These many case studies provide light on the cloud computing's wide-ranging effects on healthcare. Although the advantages are clear, difficulties with data transfer rates, interoperability, regulatory compliance, and ethical issues highlight how complicated cloud integration is. The most effective techniques and insights gained from these experiences emphasise the significance of careful planning, adaption, and alignment of cloud initiatives with institutional goals.

3.8 Future Directions and Trends

The trajectory of cloud computing's use in healthcare heralds a future rife with opportunity, changing patient interaction, healthcare delivery, and research. This section makes an effort to forecast the changing role of cloud computing in healthcare, to foresee new technical improvements, and to critically examine the ethical and societal repercussions that may result from more cloud integration.

3.8.1 Cloud Computing's Changing Role in Healthcare

The use of cloud computing in healthcare will likely go beyond its current uses. Diagnostics are about to undergo a revolution thanks to the rising convergence of cloud computing, artificial intelligence, and the Internet of Things (IoT). AI algorithms that are driven by the cloud can quickly analyse medical pictures, find abnormalities, and help physicians diagnose illnesses with previously unheard-of precision. This combination improves both diagnostic accuracy and the speed of therapy selection. Predictive analytics will also play a bigger part in proactive healthcare management, powered by patient data stored on the cloud [5]. Cloud-based prediction algorithms can recognise individuals who are at high risk for developing chronic diseases, enabling early therapies that slow the spread of the disease and reduce the need for hospitalisation.

3.8.2 Innovations and Advances in Technology

New developments in personalised medicine are promised by advances in cloud-based genomic sequencing. The scale and processing power of cloud computing may enable quick genome analysis, accelerating the discovery of genetic variables impacting illness and therapeutic responses. Genome databases driven by the cloud can hasten the development of new drugs and improve treatment strategies. A revolution in telemedicine is anticipated, helped along by augmented reality (AR) and virtual reality (VR). Cloud-hosted AR/VR systems will make it possible to conduct immersive virtual consultations that cross geographic boundaries and simplify complex procedures with remote expert supervision. Integrating blockchain technology with cloud computing will strengthen data privacy and integrity [29]. Blockchain's decentralised ledger improves the security of patient data and makes it possible for institutions to share it easily while yet preserving patient control.

3.8.3 Societal and Ethical Ramifications

Ethics discussions are sparked by the rising use of cloud computing in healthcare. To protect patient confidentiality and autonomy, issues around data ownership, patient permission, and sharing must be resolved. Institutions must strike a delicate balance between protecting patient rights and maximising the possibilities of cloud-enabled collaborative care. Additionally, when massive volumes of patient data are gathered by cloud-based healthcare systems, concerns about data monetisation and potential biases in AI algorithms surface. To sustain public confidence and justice, ethical issues around data monetisation and algorithmic transparency are crucial [30]. The digital gap becomes more prominent in society as people with less dependable internet connectivity have less access to healthcare. Particularly in impoverished areas, efforts must be made to provide fair access to cloud-based medical services [31].

3.9 Conclusion

Through its numerous uses, cloud computing has evolved from an ethereal idea to a fundamental force. Electronic health records (EHR) and medical records management have undergone a revolution that makes it possible for patients to get collaborative treatment and have easy access to their records. Geographical limitations have been removed via telemedicine and remote patient monitoring, democratising access to healthcare. Medical imaging and diagnostic analysis have reached previously unheard-of levels of precision and efficiency in their storage, sharing, and analysis. The cloud's processing power has been welcomed by research and data analytics, accelerating technological advances in medicine. Transcending conventional limitations, health information exchange has made it possible for data sharing to be seamless. Scalability, cost-effectiveness, and collaborative care are benefits, but they have been accompanied by difficulties with data security, privacy, and regulatory compliance. Case studies from actual organisations, such the Cleveland Clinic, Mercy Health, and Beth Israel Deaconess Medical Centre, have shed light on the transformational effects of cloud computing. These incidents have brought to light the benefits, difficulties, and priceless lessons that come with cloud adoption. Future developments in cloud computing for healthcare will undoubtedly change how we think about medicine. Diagnostic and therapeutic possibilities will be expanded with the convergence of cloud computing, AI, and the Internet of Things. Healthcare delivery is set to change as a result of technological developments in genetic analysis, telemedicine using augmented reality, and data security supported by blockchain. However, as the use of cloud computing in healthcare grows, ethical and societal issues must get constant attention. Ownership of patient data, permission, openness, and equal access become fundamental principles in this digital change. The ethical ramifications of algorithmic biases and data monetisation highlight the need for prudent controls. In conclusion, cloud computing continues to have unmatched promise in the healthcare industry. A patient-centric, cooperative, and technologically advanced healthcare environment is ushered in by the real advantages illustrated by case studies. In addition to technological brilliance, the path to this future requires a strong dedication to preserving patient rights, privacy, and equal access. The use of cloud computing in healthcare paves the way for a more connected and healthy society as we proceed along this route.

References

1. Banimfreg BH. A comprehensive review and conceptual framework for cloud computing adoption in bioinformatics. Healthc Anal. 2023;3:100190.
2. Wang X, Gui Q, Liu B, Jin Z, Chen Y. Enabling smart personalized healthcare: a hybrid mobile-cloud approach for ECG telemonitoring. IEEE J Biomed Heal Inf. 2014;18(3):739–45.
3. Sultan N. Making use of cloud computing for healthcare provision: opportunities and challenges. Int J Inf Manag. 2014;34(2):177–84.
4. Piette JD, Mendoza-Avelares MO, Ganser M, Mohamed M, Marinec N, Krishnan S. A preliminary study of a cloud-computing model for chronic illness self-care support in an underdeveloped country. Am J Prev Med. 2011;40(6):629–32.
5. Griebel L, Prokosch HU, Köpcke F, Toddenroth D, Christoph J, Leb I, et al. A scoping review of cloud computing in healthcare. BMC Med Inform Decis Mak. 2015;15(1):1–16.
6. Margam R. Importance of cybersecurity in electronic health records. Int J Innov Sci Res Technol. 2023;8(7).
7. Margam R. Connecting healthcare ecosystems: the journey of interoperability. Int J Bioinforma Blockchain Technol. 2023;1(1):1–9.
8. Ali O, Shrestha A, Soar J, Wamba SF. Cloud computing-enabled healthcare opportunities, issues, and applications: a systematic review. Int J Inf Manag. 2018;43:146–58.
9. Margam R. The importance of EHR in revolutionizing healthcare delivery and financial success. Artic Int J Comput Trends Technol. 2023;71:52–5.
10. Javaid M, Haleem A, Singh RP, Rab S, Suman R, Khan IH. Evolutionary trends in progressive cloud computing based healthcare: ideas, enablers, and barriers. Int J Cogn Comput Eng. 2022;3:124–35.
11. Shashi DP. Role of cloud computing for improvement in healthcare services. Int J Recent Technol Eng. 2022;11(2):88–95.
12. Kabachinski J. What's the forecast for cloud computing in healthcare? Biomed Instrum Technol. 2011;45(2):146–50.
13. Tortorella GL, Saurin TA, Fogliatto FS, Rosa VM, Tonetto LM, Magrabi F. Impacts of Healthcare 4.0 digital technologies on the resilience of hospitals. Technol Forecast Soc Change. 2021;166:120666.
14. Rejeb A, Rejeb K, Treiblmaier H, Appolloni A, Alghamdi S, Alhasawi Y, et al. The Internet of Things (IoT) in healthcare: taking stock and moving forward. Internet of Things. 2023;22:100721.
15. Elhoseny M, Abdelaziz A, Salama AS, Riad AM, Muhammad K, Sangaiah AK. A hybrid model of Internet of Things and cloud computing to manage big data in health services applications. Futur Gener Comput Syst. 2018;86:1383–94.
16. Lv Z, Qiao L. Analysis of healthcare big data. Futur Gener Comput Syst. 2020;109:103–10.
17. Zhu Z, Su P, Zhong S, Huang J, Ottikkutti S. Using a VAE-SOM architecture for anomaly detection of flexible sensors in limb prosthesis. J Ind Inf Integr. 2022;35:100490.
18. Aceto G, Persico V, Pescapé A. A survey on information and communication technologies for industry 4.0: state-of-the-art, taxonomies, perspectives, and challenges. IEEE Commun Surv Tutorials. 2019;21(4):3467–501.
19. Aceto G, Persico V, Pescapé A. Industry 4.0 and health: Internet of Things, Big Data, and cloud computing for healthcare 4.0. J Ind Inf Integr. 2020;18:100129.
20. Kaur PD, Chana I. Cloud based intelligent system for delivering health care as a service. Comput Methods Prog Biomed. 2014;113(1):346–59.
21. Cao H, Leung V, Chow C, Chan H. Enabling technologies for wireless body area networks: a survey and outlook. IEEE Commun Mag. 2009;47(12):84–93.
22. Narkhede BE, Raut RD, Narwane VS, Gardas BB. Cloud computing in healthcare—a vision, challenges and future directions. Int J Bus Inf Syst. 2020;34(1):1.
23. Hartman K, Phillips SC, Sornberger L. Computer-assisted coding at the cleveland clinic: a strategic solution: addressing clinical documentation improvement, ICD-10-CM/PCS implementation, and more. J AHIMA. 2012;83(7):24–8.

24. Wu P, Jackson C, Hunt M. Information technology electronic health record physician adoption strategies.
25. Mertz L, Hospital CIO. Explains blockchain potential: an interview with Beth Israel Deaconess Medical Center's John Halamka. IEEE Pulse. 2018;9(3):8–9.
26. Nigam VK, Bhatia S. Impact of cloud computing on health care. Int Res J Eng Technol. 2016;3(5):2804–10.
27. Gao F, Sunyacv A. Context matters: a review of the determinant factors in the decision to adopt cloud computing in healthcare. Int J Inf Manag. 2019;48:120–38.
28. Minh Dang L, Piran MJ, Han D, Min K, Moon H. A survey on Internet of Things and Cloud computing for healthcare. Electron. 2019;8(7):768.
29. Kagadis GC, Kloukinas C, Moore K, Philbin J, Papadimitroulas P, Alexakos C, et al. Cloud computing in medical imaging. Med Phys. 2013;40(7):070901.
30. Kuo AMH. Opportunities and challenges of cloud computing to improve health care services. J Med Internet Res. 2011;13(3):e67.
31. Fong EM, Chung WY. Mobile cloud-computing-based healthcare service by noncontact ECG monitoring. Sensors (Basel). 2013;13(12):16451–73.

AI in Healthcare

4

Jan Beger

Artificial Intelligence will be the most significant platform shift of the decade, revolutionizing industries by streamlining processes and enriching decision-making through the smart analysis of large amounts of information. Its rapid advancements are opening new opportunities that were previously unimaginable, especially in healthcare. AI is expected to drastically improve patient care and treatment outcomes by enabling personalized medicine and more accurate diagnostics. Additionally, by automating routine tasks, AI enhances human abilities, allowing healthcare professionals to focus more on patient care and less on administrative duties. This transformative role of AI underscores its potential to revolutionize healthcare.

4.1 Drowning in Data

The exponential increase in medical information places a significant cognitive load on doctors. In 1950, a newly trained physician could practice for their entire career without witnessing a doubling in medical knowledge [1]. However, today, medical knowledge doubles approximately every 72 days [2]. New medical articles are being published at a rate of at least one every 26 s. If a physician were to attempt to read every medical journal published, they would need to go through 5000 articles per day. Specifically for dermatologists, there are 3900 publications to read per year [3]. Furthermore, to stay current with Primary Care literature, a General Practitioner would need to dedicate 21 h every day to reading [4]. As a result, even the most skilled and intelligent physicians across various specialties struggle to keep up with this overwhelming amount of information, making it increasingly challenging to make well-informed decisions.

J. Beger (✉)
GE HealthCare, Chicago, IL, USA

P. Plugmann, D. Portius (eds.), *Innovations in Healthcare and Outcome Measurement*, https://doi.org/10.1007/978-3-031-77302-0_4

Today, the healthcare industry generates approximately 30% of the world's total data volume [5]. The expected growth rate is notably higher than that of other major industries, indicating the rapid expansion of health-related data and its increasingly significant role in the global data ecosystem. The amount of information in a single mammogram—an X-ray of the breast used to detect breast cancer and abnormalities—is greater than what you would find in the entire New York phone book, assuming such a physical book still exists. A digital mammography study can be as large as 1 GB [6]. But this is almost nothing compared to the dimensions of images in digital pathology. Here, a high-resolution digitized microscope slide can boast dimensions of 100,000 × 100,000 pixels, translating to about 50 GB of uncompressed data [7]. Annually, hospitals carry out 3.6 billion imaging procedures, producing an immense volume of data [8]. The workload of today's radiologists reflects this exponential growth in data. During a 12-h shift, a radiologist may analyze up to 50,000 images—a tenfold increase from about 500 images reviewed 15 years ago [9, 10].

While the "data explosion" has affected all aspects of life, the healthcare sector is no exception, and there's no sign that this trend will slow down. It is fueled by advances in technology and data collection methods. Astonishingly, only 3% of healthcare data is actively used to generate meaningful insights [8]. The remaining 97% remains largely untapped, unused, and underexplored. This underutilization represents not just missed opportunities but a substantial financial drain. Maintaining, securing, and managing this data requires investment, yet without the corresponding return on investment one might expect in terms of improved patient outcomes or operational efficiencies.

4.2 Medical Errors and Their Consequence

Every year, a staggering 42 million medical errors occur worldwide, a figure that remains stubbornly high despite advancements in modern medicine [11]. Diagnostic errors alone affect more than 12 million Americans each year. For every 100 hospital admissions, approximately 14 adverse events occur. A striking half of Europeans fear receiving improper treatment in their hospitals [12].

EU statistics unveil that nearly a quarter of Europeans have faced a medical error directly or through a relative [13]. Among these, 18% encountered serious errors in hospitals, and 11% received incorrect medication prescriptions. Europe witnesses up to 163,000 deaths annually from medication errors alone, comparable to the populations of cities like Basel, Oxford, and Ghent [14].

Statistics indicate that strategies aimed at mitigating the risks of medical errors in the European Union alone could prevent more than 750,000 patients from experiencing harmful and health-altering medical errors each year. This would result in 3.2 million fewer days of hospitalization, 260,000 fewer incidents of permanent disability, and 95,000 fewer deaths per year [15].

The impact of these errors varies widely, from minor to fatal. Misdiagnosis is common, and there's a high chance you or someone close has been affected.

Furthermore, delays in cancer testing have become a global issue, with about 7% of abnormal results not promptly shared with patients, causing critical diagnostic delays [16].

4.3 The Healthcare Workforce Crisis

The global healthcare sector is grappling with a critical shortage of seven million healthcare professionals, a number that the World Health Organization (WHO) predicts will escalate to ten million by 2030 [17]. This looming crisis is largely attributed to an aging workforce, a lack of young professionals entering the field, and low job satisfaction. The problem is particularly severe in low- and lower-middle-income countries.

Further exacerbating the issue is the rising demand for healthcare services, fueled by an aging global population and a surge in chronic diseases. The complexity of healthcare delivery has also increased, making care pathways more intricate than ever before.

In Europe, the healthcare workforce crisis is reaching a tipping point, necessitating immediate intervention. This urgency is underscored by frequent strikes and industrial actions among healthcare workers, spotlighting the challenging work conditions and inadequate resources available. A regional report from WHO/Europe sounds the alarm on a "ticking timebomb" that threatens the stability of health systems. This is due to a combination of factors: an aging population, a rise in chronic illnesses, and the ongoing impact of the COVID-19 pandemic. Alarmingly, the report reveals that in 13 of the 44 countries surveyed, 40% of medical doctors are already 55 years of age or older, posing a significant risk to the long-term sustainability of the healthcare workforce [18].

4.4 Aging Populations and Growing Cost

Population aging is one of the most significant trends of the twenty-first century, having profound implications across all aspects of society, especially healthcare. Every second, two people celebrate their sixtieth birthday, summing up to an eye-watering total of nearly 58 million sixtieth birthdays annually [19]. One in nine people globally is 60 years or older, expected to rise to one in five by 2050 [20]. This demographic shift is exerting considerable strain on healthcare systems already under pressure.

The rise in healthcare expenses can be largely attributed to this shift, as the number of people aged 65 and older is anticipated to double by 2050 [21], in contrast to those under the age of 5. Data from OECD countries reveal that in 2022, the ratio of healthcare spending to GDP was highest in the United States (16.6%), followed by Germany (12.7%) and France (12.1%). Moreover, an additional 14 high-income nations, including Canada and Japan, allocated over 10% of their GDP to healthcare in the same year [22].

Despite this increase in spending, there is no corresponding improvement in the quality or efficiency of healthcare services. Simply put, the increase in healthcare costs is not translating into better health outcomes.

4.5 Interconnected Challenges

As described above, the healthcare industry is currently confronting numerous interconnected challenges that significantly impact care globally. The "data explosion" is overwhelming medical professionals, who now face the daunting task of navigating an ever-growing ocean of medical information and patient data. Despite the vast amount of data generated, only a small fraction is effectively used, leaving valuable insights untapped.

High rates of medical errors, including diagnostic inaccuracies and medication errors, have severe consequences, impacting millions of people. These errors lead to unnecessary hospitalizations, permanent disabilities, and fatalities [23].

The global healthcare workforce crisis is severely limiting access to quality healthcare. This crisis, characterized by workforce shortages, an aging workforce, and declining job satisfaction, hamper the sector's ability to meet growing care demands [24]. Complicating matters, the intertwined challenges of an aging population, and a surge in chronic diseases—both fueled by demographic shifts and lifestyle changes—add significant strain and complexity to healthcare provision.

Healthcare costs are skyrocketing without corresponding improvements in outcomes. Globally, countries are witnessing a substantial increase in healthcare expenditures as a percentage of GDP, but this heightened investment doesn't always translate to enhanced healthcare services or healthier populations [25].

These issues demand novel solutions and systemic innovation to ensure the sustainability and effectiveness of healthcare systems globally. Utilizing data for enhanced outcomes and innovative healthcare solutions is pivotal for the future of healthcare. Artificial Intelligence stands at the forefront of this transformation, offering a multifaceted role. Beyond specific applications, AI's most significant contribution is its ability to augment the capabilities of healthcare professionals, empowering them to deliver superior care and make more informed decisions. Additionally, AI can free up valuable time for healthcare providers, allowing for more meaningful patient interactions and facilitating the delivery of real-time insights directly to the point of care.

4.6 The Current State of AI

In the field of healthcare, AI has seen significant advancements, highlighted by the increase in approvals of AI/ML-enabled medical devices since 2018, with radiology standing out [26].

Radiology's adoption of AI is a pioneering example of its transformative impact across healthcare specialties. With radiologists being a scarce yet highly sought-after resource, the growing accessibility and advancement of medical imaging technology have led to an increased demand for top-tier radiology diagnostics [27]. This surge in demand places considerable strain on the available radiology workforce, driving the search for innovative solutions to bridge this gap. Technology, especially AI, emerges as a key player in addressing this challenge.

AI algorithms are crafted to augment radiologists' ability to interpret medical images swiftly and with greater precision. Beyond enhancing interpretation accuracy, AI also plays a pivotal role in improving the quality of images themselves, reducing scan times, and enhancing the overall patient experience. Additionally, one of the critical benefits of AI in medical imaging is its ability to help reduce radiation exposure without compromising image quality [28]. This advancement ensures a safer diagnostic process, further prioritizing patient safety alongside comfort, and represents a significant leap forward in patient-centric care.

These AI tools are not only speeding up the diagnostic process but are also increasing the accuracy with which conditions such as breast cancer, lung nodules, and numerous other medical conditions are identified [29, 30]. This capability to detect anomalies in X-rays, MRIs, and CT scans more effectively allows for the early diagnosis of diseases, extending the benefits of early detection to a broader population than ever before. Consequently, AI plays a pivotal role in improving patient care by identifying health issues at a stage when they are more treatable, thereby improving the likelihood of successful outcomes and demonstrating the far-reaching impact of AI across the healthcare landscape [31].

Beyond radiology, AI transforms healthcare through innovative applications that enhance patient care, streamline workflows, and improve [32]. For instance, in predictive analytics, AI is instrumental in analyzing vast amounts of patient data to forecast health events, such as predicting which patients are at higher risk of developing conditions like sepsis or heart failure [33]. This foresight enables early interventions, potentially saving lives and reducing hospital stays.

AI also plays a crucial role in personalized medicine, which includes analyzing genetic information to tailor treatments to individual patients. This approach is particularly impactful in oncology, where AI-driven analyses of tumor genetics can guide the selection of the most effective therapies, improving survival rates and reducing side effects [34].

Furthermore, AI assists in drug discovery and development by predicting the efficacy of new compounds, significantly cutting down the time and cost of bringing new medicines to market. It automates and refines drug screening, identifies potential treatment pathways, and uncovers new uses of existing drugs [35].

Within patient care and management, AI-powered chatbots and virtual health assistants provide round-the-clock support and monitoring, offering advice, answering patient queries, and reminding patients to take their medication, thereby enhancing patient engagement and adherence to treatment plans [36].

The deployment of AI has predominantly centered on highly specialized tasks, utilizing unimodal data sources. This has led to the development of AI systems that excel in performing distinct functions, such as analyzing radiological images, genetic sequences, or electronic health records. This focused approach yields exceptional accuracy and efficiency in specific applications, including diagnosing particular conditions through radiology imaging or predicting patient risks based on historical health data [37].

However, this specialization also brings a significant limitation: it narrows the scope of AI's applicability in healthcare. By relying on point solutions that focus on a single data type, AI's ability to engage with the complex and multimodal nature of patient information is underutilized. As a result, these specialized AI models often struggle to generalize beyond their training data, which restricts their broader use in healthcare [37].

AI in healthcare—despite its significant potential—has not been broadly adopted across health systems for several reasons. Less than 5% of healthcare organizations used AI tools as of 2022 [38]. One of the main hurdles is the perception of AI, which is often considered a futuristic concept rather than a present reality, despite the FDA's approval of more than 880 medical AI systems by mid-2024 [26]. This slow uptake can be attributed to a variety of factors, including misaligned incentives, reimbursement policies, regulatory and data challenges, lack of trust and understanding, and economic pressures.

Despite these challenges, there's an increasingly acknowledged potential for AI not just to support the work of medical professionals but also to fully automate specific tasks or processes. This doesn't mean AI is set to replace human roles entirely. Rather, it highlights AI's capability to handle routine, repetitive tasks or those that benefit from the consistency and scalability AI offers. This shift allows healthcare professionals to concentrate on more complex and nuanced aspects of patient care. Viewing AI's role as an augmentation and enhancement rather than a replacement reflects a cautious yet optimistic stance on its integration into healthcare. The concept of a human-in-the-loop approach champions a symbiotic partnership between AI and human expertise, aiming to optimize outcomes. Such collaboration fosters an environment of continuous learning and improvement, with AI systems and healthcare providers benefiting from mutual insights [39].

4.7 The Future

Electronic health records (EHRs) are inherently multimodal and include provider notes, billing codes, lab data, images, vitals, and increasingly, genomic data and information from wearable devices. The complexity and multimodality of EHRs have significantly increased, underscoring that no single data type can offer a complete view of a patient's health [40]. For example, accurately interpreting medical images requires consultation with structured records for context.

AI is often described as the "new electricity" because it serves as a general-purpose technology [41]. Much like electricity, its applications are incredibly versatile and not limited to a single domain. Despite the wealth of data available, AI's potential remains partially untapped, focusing predominantly on single modalities such as CT scans. The current focus of AI in healthcare so far is on specific tasks using single data modalities, like CT scans. However, true clinical practice involves a complex interplay of diverse data, necessitating dynamic, multimodal AI systems [42].

Incorporating multiple data types could lead to more accurate representations of patient health and expand the ways AI can assist healthcare providers [43]. For instance, clinicians might use natural language queries to search medical imaging databases or generate synthetic medical images based on textual descriptions of abnormalities.

The transition towards harnessing and interpreting multimodal data marks a significant leap forward in AI development. By tapping into the complex and diverse nature of healthcare data, AI can provide a more comprehensive understanding of patient health, significantly expanding its influence across the healthcare industry. This evolution from unimodal to multimodal AI systems is set to improve the precision and efficiency of healthcare services while paving the way for novel approaches to patient care and treatment [44].

These advancements offer concrete benefits for both healthcare providers and patients, initiating a new era of personalized and streamlined care. Imagine the convenience of Google search applied within the healthcare domain; multimodal search capabilities enable medical professionals to inquire using natural language, such as identifying female patients aged 40–60 with a specific diagnosis in the last 6 months. This technology swiftly sifts through patient data, eliminating the time-consuming manual search processes of the past.

Equipping clinicians with accurate information precisely when and where they need it significantly expedites various processes [45]. Such progress could lead to faster, more accurate diagnoses and improved predictions about how individual patients might respond to different treatments. As a result, healthcare professionals can tailor treatments more specifically to individual patient needs, increasing the likelihood of successful outcomes.

Foundation models are advanced AI systems trained on diverse data like text, images, and audio, which can understand and generate content like human intelligence. In healthcare, these models are invaluable for analyzing complex, multimodal medical data such as patient records, radiology images, and lab results [46]. For instance, AI foundation models can accurately predict patient outcomes following heart surgery by integrating and analyzing information from clinical notes, visual patterns in radiology images, and data from lab results [47]. This capability allows healthcare professionals to provide more personalized and effective treatment plans, transforming patient care by efficiently interpreting and leveraging vast amounts of diverse data. Foundation models introduce innovative ways to interact with AI, offering natural language interfaces and the possibility for dialogue, making them more user-friendly and adaptable [48].

The future of healthcare is deeply intertwined with the advancement and integration of AI. The development and adoption of foundational AI technologies are central to this transformation. By focusing on flexible, general-purpose AI models, we enable quick adaptation to a wide variety of tasks and data types, significantly reducing the dependence on extensively labeled data. This change is vital in healthcare, where data acquisition is notably costly and time-consuming.

At this critical moment of significant progress, today's innovations set the stage for tomorrow's breakthroughs. These advancements address pressing issues such as clinician burnout, fragmented healthcare delivery, and patients' challenges in accessing care quickly and efficiently. AI's contribution goes beyond the mechanics of data collection and prediction generation. It addresses the organizational challenge of enabling informed decision-making at crucial moments and the strategic imperative of using enhanced information to transform decision-making processes. Essentially, AI amplifies human capabilities, reshaping what is possible in healthcare and beyond.

The healthcare sector faces pressing challenges: the overwhelming growth of data, widespread medical errors, a critical shortage of professionals, and the pressures of an aging population, all compounded by escalating costs. These issues, significant on their own, collectively threaten the quality of care and the sustainability of healthcare systems worldwide. Amidst these challenges, AI stands out as a source of hope, offering a practical pathway to overhaul and improve the system. Leveraging AI allows us to navigate through complex data for actionable insights, reduce medical errors with advanced diagnostics and decision support, and address workforce shortages by automating routine tasks. AI also offers a way to mitigate the effects of an aging population through personalized and preventive care, potentially lowering the costs associated with chronic and age-related diseases.

Healthcare stands as one of the most stringently regulated sectors, and rightfully so. Implementing technological solutions in healthcare, including AI, demands thorough validation [49]. Our primary mandate is to ensure patient safety, adhering to the foundational principle of "do no harm." This is especially pertinent for AI applications, where the stakes of accuracy and reliability are exceptionally high. In this context, the concept of "responsible AI" is of critical importance [50]. It emphasizes the need for AI systems to be ethical, transparent, and accountable, ensuring they enhance healthcare delivery without compromising patient well-being. Responsible AI champions the creation of technology that is not only advanced but also aligned with the highest standards of care and ethics [51].

Integrating AI into healthcare represents a profound shift, reimagining our approach to meet the sector's most pressing challenges. This path towards an AI-enhanced future is driven by the combination of technological innovation and human creativity, striving to create a more efficient, accessible, and sustainable healthcare ecosystem. Embracing AI is crucial for overcoming today's obstacles and preparing for future challenges, ensuring a healthier future for generations to come.

At the heart of this shift lies a crucial call to action for everyone, especially healthcare professionals, to cultivate AI literacy. Grasping the basics of AI and acknowledging its crucial role in healthcare goes beyond simple professional development; it's a fundamental step in gearing up for the future.

Healthcare professionals, in particular, have a unique responsibility to embrace AI literacy. By familiarizing themselves with AI's capabilities and potential, they enhance their own practices and pave the way for improved patient outcomes. This knowledge allows them to leverage AI technologies effectively, guiding the future of medical practice toward more efficient and impactful patient care.

Moreover, understanding AI equips healthcare professionals to lead by example in adopting these technologies. They become advocates for AI, showcasing how it can enhance health outcomes and streamline healthcare processes. This leadership is crucial in demystifying AI for the broader public and highlighting its potential benefits, especially when individuals interact with the healthcare system as patients or consumers.

Embracing AI with an open and inquisitive mindset ensures its benefits extend across all aspects of our global community. This approach not only transforms personal health experiences but also broadens our understanding of possible advancements in healthcare. By championing AI literacy and adoption, healthcare professionals play a pivotal role in steering this technological revolution, making health experiences richer and more accessible for everyone.

References

1. Densen P. Challenges and opportunities facing medical education. Trans Am Clin Climatol Assoc. 2011;122:48–58. PMID: 21686208; PMCID: PMC3116346. https://www.ncbi.nlm.nih.gov/pmc/articles/PMC3116346/.
2. American Medical Association. The future of AI in medicine and what it means for physicians and practices with Tom Lawry. Philadelphia: American Medical Association; 2023. https://www.ama-assn.org/practice-management/digital/future-ai-medicine-and-what-it-means-physicians-and-practices-tom-lawry.
3. PubMed query. https://pubmed.ncbi.nlm.nih.gov/?term=%27skin%27+AND+%27disease%27+OR+%27dermatology%27&filter=dates.2022%2F1%2F1-2022%2F12%2F31&sort=datee.
4. Elsevier. What are the 4 biggest challenges facing the healthcare sector? 2018. https://www.elsevier.com/en-au/connect/what-are-the-4-biggest-challenges-facing-the-healthcare-sector.
5. Thomason J. Big tech, big data and the new world of digital health. Global Health J. 2021;5(4):165–8. ISSN 2414-6447. https://doi.org/10.1016/j.glohj.2021.11.003.
6. Maidment ADA. Digital mammography. Semin Roentgenol. 2003;38(3):216–30. https://www.imagephysics.com/201.pdf.
7. Linder E, Lundin M, Thors C, Lebbad M, Winiecka-Krusnell J, et al. Web-based virtual microscopy for parasitology: a novel tool for education and quality assurance. PLoS Negl Trop Dis. 2008;2(10):e315. https://doi.org/10.1371/journal.pntd.0000315.
8. World Economic Forum. 4 ways data is improving healthcare. 2019. https://www.weforum.org/agenda/2019/12/four-ways-data-is-improving-healthcare/.
9. Bruls RJM, Kwee RM. Workload for radiologists during on-call hours: dramatic increase in the past 15 years. Insights Imaging. 2020;11:121. https://doi.org/10.1186/s13244-020-00925-z.
10. Applied Radiology News Briefs. The radiologist's gerbil wheel: interpreting images every 3-4 seconds eight hours a day at Mayo Clinic. 2024. https://appliedradiology.com/articles/the-radiologist-s-gerbil-wheel-interpreting-images-every-3-4-seconds-eight-hours-a-day-at-mayo-clinic#.
11. World Health Organization. Patient safety. 2019. https://www.who.int/news-room/facts-in-pictures/detail/patient-safety.
12. Harvard School of Public Health. Millions harmed each year from unsafe medical care. 2023. https://www.hsph.harvard.edu/news/press-releases/millions-harmed-each-year-from-unsafe-medical-care/.
13. European Commission. Special eurobarometer report on medical errors. 2005. https://ec.europa.eu/health/ph_information/documents/eb_64_en.pdf.

14. European alliance for access to safe medicines. PRESS RELEASE: medication errors—the most common adverse event in hospitals threatens patient safety and causes 160,000 deaths per year. 2022. https://eaasm.eu/en-gb/2022/09/13/press-release-medication-errors-the-most-common-adverse-event-in-hospitals-threatens-patient-safety-and-causes-160000-deaths-per-year/.
15. World Health Organization Europe. Patient safety, data and statistics. https://who-sandbox.squiz.cloud/en/health-topics/Health-systems/patient-safety/data-and-statistics.
16. The Joint Commission. Quick safety issue 52: advancing safety with closed-loop communication of test results. 2019. https://www.jointcommission.org/resources/news-and-multimedia/newsletters/newsletters/quick-safety/quick-safety-issue-52-advancing-safety-with-closed-loop-communication-of-test-results/.
17. World Health Organization. Health workforce: the health workforce crisis. 2009. https://www.who.int/news-room/questions-and-answers/item/q-a-on-the-health-workforce-crisis.
18. World Health Organization. Ticking timebomb: without immediate action, health and care workforce gaps in the European Region could spell disaster. 2022. https://www.who.int/azerbaijan/news/item/14-09-2022-ticking-timebomb%2D%2Dwithout-immediate-action%2D%2Dhealth-and-care-workforce-gaps-in-the-european-region-could-spell-disaster.
19. HelpAge International, UNFPA. Ageing in the twenty-first century: a celebration and a challenge. 2012. https://socialprotection-humanrights.org/resource/ageing-in-the-twenty-first-century-a-celebration-and-a-challenge/.
20. World Health Organization. Decade of healthy ageing 2020-2030. 2019. https://www.who.int/docs/default-source/documents/decade-of-health-ageing/decade-ageing-proposal-en.pdf.
21. United Nations. UN report calls for re-thinking social protection as the world ages. 2023. https://news.un.org/en/story/2023/01/1132392.
22. OECD Health Statistics. Health expenditure. 2023. https://www.oecd.org/els/health-systems/health-expenditure.htm.
23. Domer G, Gallagher TM. Patient safety: preventing patient harm and building capacity for patient safety. London: IntechOpen; 2021. https://www.intechopen.com/chapters/79011.
24. McKinsey & Company. Care for the caretakers: building the global public health workforce. 2022. https://www.mckinsey.com/industries/social-sector/our-insights/care-for-the-caretakers-building-the-global-public-health-workforce.
25. World Health Organization. Global spending on health: rising to the pandemic's challenges. 2022. https://www.who.int/publications/i/item/9789240064911.
26. FDA. Artificial intelligence and machine learning (AI/ML)-enabled medical devices. 2024. https://www.fda.gov/medical-devices/software-medical-device-samd/artificial-intelligence-and-machine-learning-aiml-enabled-medical-devices.
27. Najjar R. Redefining radiology: a review of artificial intelligence integration in medical imaging. Diagnostics. 2023;13(17):2760. https://www.mdpi.com/2075-4418/13/17/2760.
28. Jo GD, Ahn C, et al. 75% radiation dose reduction using deep learning reconstruction on low-dose chest CT. BMC Med Imaging. 2023;23(1):121. https://bmcmedimaging.biomedcentral.com/articles/10.1186/s12880-023-01081-8.
29. CancerNetwork. MammoScreen AI tool improves diagnostic performance of radiologists in detecting breast cancer. 2020. https://www.cancernetwork.com/view/mammoscreen-ai-tool-improves-diagnostic-performance-of-radiologists-in-detecting-breast-cancer.
30. Kanan M, Alharbi H, et al. AI-driven models for diagnosing and predicting outcomes in lung cancer: a systematic review and meta-analysis. Cancers (Basel). 2024;16(3):674. https://www.mdpi.com/2072-6694/16/3/674.
31. Mayo Clinic Press. AI in healthcare: the future of patient care and health management. 2024. https://mcpress.mayoclinic.org/healthy-aging/ai-in-healthcare-the-future-of-patient-care-and-health-management.
32. World Economic Forum. How AI can transform patient care and treatment. 2024. https://www.weforum.org/agenda/2024/01/how-ai-can-transform-patient-care-and-treatment.
33. CAP Today. Using predictive analytics to gauge sepsis risk. 2019. https://www.captodayonline.com/using-predictive-analytics-to-gauge-sepsis-risk/.

34. Demetriou D, Hull R, Kgoebane-Maseko M, Lockhat Z, Dlamini Z. AI-enhanced digital pathology and radiogenomics in precision oncology. In: Dlamini Z, editor. Artificial intelligence and precision oncology. Cham: Springer; 2023. https://link.springer.com/chapter/10.1007/978-3-031-21506-3_5.
35. Mak KK, Wong YH, Pichika MR. Artificial intelligence in drug discovery and development. In: Hock FJ, Pugsley MK, editors. Drug discovery and evaluation: safety and pharmacokinetic assays. Cham: Springer; 2023. https://link.springer.com/referenceworkentry/10.1007/978-3-030-73317-9_92-1.
36. Software Streets. Virtual health assistants: how chatbots are improving patient support. 2023. https://softwarestreets.com/blog/virtual-health-assistants/.
37. Techopedia. Elevating healthcare: the promise of generalist medical AI (GMAI). 2023. https://www.techopedia.com/elevating-healthcare-the-promise-of-generalist-medical-ai-gmai.
38. Johns Hopkins University, Hopkins Business of Health Initiative. AI in healthcare is here, but uptake is slow. 2022. https://hbhi.jhu.edu/news/ai-healthcare-here-uptake-slow.
39. Jarrahi MH, Askay D, Eshraghi A, Smith P. Artificial intelligence and knowledge management: a partnership between human and AI. Bus Horizons. 2023;66(1):87–99. https://www.sciencedirect.com/science/article/pii/S0007681322000222.
40. Liu Z, Zhang J, et al. Machine learning for multimodal electronic health records-based research: challenges and perspectives. 2023. https://link.springer.com/chapter/10.1007/978-981-19-9865-2_10.
41. Stanford Graduate School of Business. Andrew Ng: why AI is the new electricity. 2017. https://www.gsb.stanford.edu/insights/andrew-ng-why-ai-new-electricity.
42. Google Research. Multimodal medical AI. 2023. https://research.google/blog/multimodal-medical-ai/.
43. Sachin DN, Annappa B, et al. A multimodal contrastive federated learning for digital healthcare. SN Comput Sci. 2023;4:674. https://link.springer.com/article/10.1007/s42979-023-02124-1.
44. Chen X, Xie H, et al. Artificial intelligence and multimodal data fusion for smart healthcare: topic modeling and bibliometrics. Artif Intell Rev. 2024;57:91. https://link.springer.com/article/10.1007/s10462-024-10712-7.
45. Gong Y, Kang H. Usability and clinical decision support. In: Berner E, editor. Clinical decision support systems. Health informatics. Cham: Springer; 2016. https://link.springer.com/chapter/10.1007/978-3-319-31913-1_4.
46. Stanford University, Human-Centered Artificial Intelligence. How foundation models can advance AI in Healthcare. 2022. https://hai.stanford.edu/news/how-foundation-models-can-advance-ai-healthcare.
47. Christensen M, Vukadinovic M, et al. Vision–language foundation model for echocardiogram interpretation. Nat Med. 2024;30:2959. https://www.nature.com/articles/s41591-024-02959-y.
48. Ada Lovelace Institute. Foundation models in the public sector. 2023. https://www.adalovelaceinstitute.org/evidence-review/foundation-models-public-sector/.
49. Sujan M, Smith-Frazer C, et al. Validation framework for the use of AI in healthcare: overview of the new British standard BS30440. BMJ Health Care Inform. 2024;30(1):e100749. https://informatics.bmj.com/content/30/1/e100749.
50. OECD. Collective action for responsible AI in health. 2024. https://www.oecd.org/health/collective-action-for-responsible-ai-in-health-f2050177-en.htm.
51. World Health Organization. WHO calls for safe and ethical AI for health. 2023. https://www.who.int/news/item/16-05-2023-who-calls-for-safe-and-ethical-ai-for-health.

The Importance of Production Innovation for the Success of Medical Supplies and Devices

5

Karl H. Ohlberg

5.1 Introduction

The rise of global supply chains in manufacturing industries since the early 1980s and the sharp increase in production in Asia, particularly in recent decades, have reshaped the global economy. This has been compounded by rapidly evolving technologies such as the Internet of Things, 3D printing, advanced robotics and artificial intelligence, whose significant impact on the traditional role of manufacturing is increasingly leading to structural change in many economies.

Immediately after the unexpected COVID-19 pandemic subsided, there were other less expected influences such as geopolitical crises, the war in Ukraine and the Israel-Hamas war, as well as raw material shortages and sustainability regulations.

In addition to these unexpected upheavals, the following changes have been observed for a long time:

- The middle class is growing in some parts of the world. This also means more consumption of medical products and therefore business opportunities for manufacturers. However, these must be developed with resources, which can pose risks.
- More and more emerging countries, including smaller ones, have the opportunity to compete through production and are doing so. Established manufacturers are facing more competition as a result.
- On the Internet, options, prices and services are becoming increasingly transparent, which also increases competition.
- Customers' needs are becoming increasingly individualized.
- Country regulations are becoming more diverse. In the past, a U.S. FDA approval in the healthcare sector was sufficient for distribution in large parts of the world, but today there is a wide variety of regional/national regulation.

K. H. Ohlberg (✉)
EmpraGlob GmbH, Düsseldorf, Germany
e-mail: karl@empraglob.com

P. Plugmann, D. Portius (eds.), *Innovations in Healthcare and Outcome Measurement*, https://doi.org/10.1007/978-3-031-77302-0_5

Last but not least, there is the global sustainability challenge, in which manufacturers have a major responsibility and are increasingly being challenged by competitors, investors, customers, governments and NGOs.

In this situation, manufacturing companies, whose business models are predominantly traditional, must master not only all the challenges described above but also the digital transformation.

The environment described has a profound impact on the practice of all board areas, especially in the context of innovation.

On the one hand, manufacturing industries will require much more new approaches for radical innovation, i.e. they will have to invest and accept risks in order to remain competitive. On the other hand, they will need to achieve increased efficiency in existing business through appropriate innovative approaches to ensure short-term profitability. These two very different capabilities need to be reconciled in business strategy, which is referred to as organizational ambidexterity, or ambidexterity for short [1].

From the perspective of a practitioner in innovation consulting for medium-sized and large manufacturers, the chapter has the following objectives:

- Classifying the topic of production innovation in the wider context of innovation management.
- Demonstrating the importance of production innovation.
- Raising awareness of the topic in the business world and in academia.
- Supporting strategic management in companies, especially with regard to explorative production innovation.
- Using the example of medical supplies and devices to assess how production innovation can contribute to the success of products.

5.2 Types of Innovation from a Technical Perspective

Before we go into more detail about production innovation, here is an overview of some different types of innovation that are important for manufacturers from a technical perspective. Specific details of production innovation will be discussed in the next section.

Innovation is the successful exploitation of new ideas or ones that are adopted from other sectors or organizations [2]. Despite this simple and generally valid definition, the term innovation is an umbrella term involving a myriad of innovation types [3] with a large number of scientific publications and practical applications.

Terms relating to innovation, especially with regard to types of innovation, are not used uniformly, making it difficult to maintain an overview. Various taxonomies and frameworks exist for categorizing types of innovation [4–7], each of which focuses on different aspects and is designed to be industry-unspecific. However, even these are not complete, as new concepts of innovation are constantly emerging in the academic, consultancy, corporate and administrative spheres.

For the practical implementation of successful innovation projects, it is therefore essential that all participants first develop a common understanding of the approach and a common conceptual model, including the terms used. This section is intended to contribute to this.

With a focus on manufacturing industries, an attempt will therefore be made below to classify production innovation in the context of other types of innovation. The priority is to provide an abstract overview of innovation types and associated resources in as simple and practically applicable a form as possible, ignoring some details and accepting inconsistencies (Fig. 5.1).

The significance of the technical innovation types quickly becomes clear from the innovation terms and the consideration of resources. In the case of resources, the terms are broadly defined. For example, the term *production equipment* in Fig. 5.1 refers not only to the manufacturer's equipment but also to current and potential suppliers of such equipment as well as service providers of all kinds, including knowledge suppliers. Modern production is characterized by the fact that all these resources, including supply chain resources, work together in a network that must be orchestrated by the manufacturer for its benefit and with the aim of innovation.

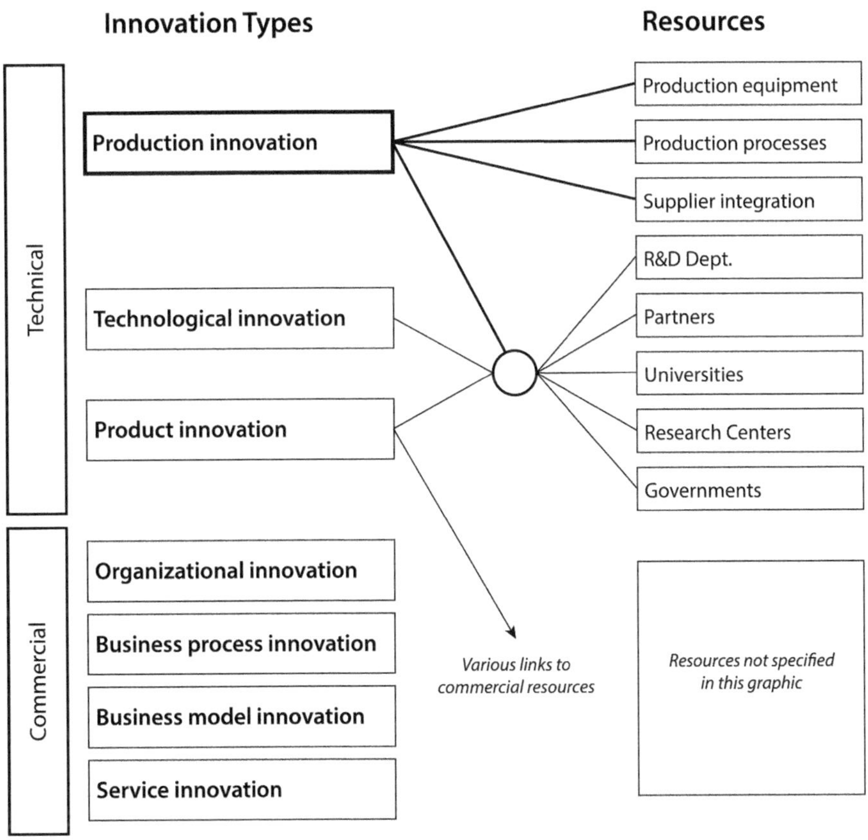

Fig. 5.1 Innovation types and allocated resources. (Source: authors)

The allocation of resources to the innovation types in the abstracted diagram (Fig. 5.1) already gives an indication of the prominent position of production innovation, namely in that not only the resources directly required for production (equipment, processes and suppliers) are allocated but also all other technical resources. In practice, fewer resources may be allocated, but the R&D department, for example, is still dependent on coordination with production during product development in order to be able to manufacture new products economically. Product innovation and production innovation must work hand in hand in these cases. It should be noted that the terms *production innovation* and *product innovation* are sometimes used interchangeably in the scientific literature, whether due to a typing error or carelessness. This is fatal because they are completely different concepts.

All other technical resources can become important depending on the innovation activity. Even the government resource can play a role in production innovation if new regulations need to be complied with and their coordination or change needs to be worked towards, or if the manufacturer wishes to participate in government innovation projects.

Among the commercial innovation types, organizational innovation in particular can have an impact on all areas of a company, including the technical areas [8, 9]. Organizational innovation is often overlooked or not systematically addressed in companies. The fact is, however, that suitable, innovation-promoting organizational structures are the prerequisite for all other forms of innovation.

Organizational innovation can also be understood as a mindset to support innovation processes in an agile manner. It is closely linked to innovation management, a structured process that ensures that developed concepts are implemented and contribute to the economic success of the company. Innovation management is standardized in ISO 56000 and is ideally evaluated and optimized through KPIs. It is used with all the types of innovation described above.

In innovation management, a distinction is made between various strategies that define the form in which internal or external ideas, knowledge and concepts are integrated into the innovation process or used for risk assessment:

- **Closed innovation** [10] is the traditional and still predominant innovation strategy in manufacturing industries, in which ideas, knowledge and concepts are developed and exploited within the company's own closed environment, with particular attention paid to IP protection.
- **Regional innovation clusters** [11] are strategic cooperations between companies and institutions that work together along a value chain or within a sector in close proximity but are legally independent of each other. This helps opening up the innovation process.
- **Open innovation** [12] is a renowned concept by Henry Chesbrough for integrating external sources into the innovation process, which today represents the standard in practically all nonmanufacturing industries and enables high value creation in innovation processes. In the "reluctant manufacturing industries"—as Chesbrough calls them—Open Innovation is largely rejected. The main reasons for this are concerns about IP protection and incompatibility with the processes in the traditional Closed Innovation strategy.

- **Proposal-based innovation** [13] is a new data-driven concept that will use AI to generate concrete proposals for external innovation resources and identify risks of innovation activities without changing the existing innovation process—which is usually very complex for manufacturers—while maintaining IP protection. Proposal-based Innovation has already received attention in the scientific community and among companies and is now seeking further support for practical implementation. Proposal-based Innovation can be a long-term path to Open Innovation for manufacturers by helping overcome concerns and making the benefits of openness visible in practice.

5.3 Production Innovation and Ambidexterity

In the following, fundamental aspects of production innovation are explained, followed by a focus on ambidexterity.

In manufacturing industries, product innovation (not to be confused with production innovation) is traditionally given the greatest attention and priority. Ideally, product innovation is based on technological innovation, which can mean higher added value or competitive advantages. There is usually innovation management based on the work of the departments involved (e.g. R&D, pre-development, development, start-up cooperation). Other types of innovation such as business model innovation or service innovation have become increasingly important in recent years and are often integrated into manufacturers' business processes.

Production innovation, on the other hand, occupies a special position in innovation management. This is reflected in the following points:

- In contrast to product innovation, production innovation does not have to be successful on the market, but must support success within the company.
- Production innovation takes place exclusively in the environment of manufacturing industries, which differ from service industries in terms of innovation in many areas [13].

This special position means that the area of production innovation is often not included at all in systematic considerations of innovation activities, or is simply overlooked.

In terms of innovation management, production innovation can be seen as part of process innovation, which has received little attention to date and has been the subject of little research [14]. It is worth noting, however, that its importance has increased significantly in recent years (more on this below).

In the traditional view, production and production innovation are seen as a cost factor that has negative consequences (material consumption, energy, machine costs, personnel costs, buildings) that must be minimized. The focus is therefore on efficiency, i.e. using fewer resources. In today's business environment, however, production innovation can make a significantly higher, decisive contribution to a company's success, as described below.

5.3.1 Fundamental Considerations on Production Innovation

The concept of production innovation is basically easy to explain. The goal is to introduce new methods in production for the benefit of the company.

The traditional benefits of production innovation are:

- To make production more cost-effective.
- To improve product characteristics and quality.

Today, manufacturers find themselves in an increasingly fast-paced and unforgiving competitive environment in which they must constantly review their strategies. In this respect, production innovation is a great opportunity to support business objectives.

The extended benefits of production innovation are therefore:

- Meet emerging regulatory obligations.
- Achieve sustainability goals.
- Enable a wide range of product variants.
- Realize small batch sizes, up to batch size 1.
- Utilizing global markets in terms of production technologies (not the traditional concept of suppliers, but bringing in technologies from remote locations).

Another point may be that extended, more innovative production solutions make improved or even new products possible in the first place and thus contribute to the success of a company [14].

However, successful production innovation depends on successful implementation. This is the hardest part of a complex topic. The most important prerequisite is that the internal structures of a company's production environment are able to recognize production innovation as an issue and provide it with resources and a priority. In most cases, manufacturers lack these organizational structures. Experience has shown that there is usually a significant gap between intention and implementation.

As complex systems, production environments are characterized by the internal and external networking of resources and equipment as well as the long service life of large parts of the equipment combined with more rapidly changing individual equipment components. Manufacturers usually have little experience with production innovation processes. That's the challenge.

5.3.2 The Ambidexterity Challenge

From a bird's eye view, the following picture emerges in companies:

- Strategic management is responsible for the target-oriented design of sustainable corporate success.
- Operational management is responsible for immediate success and securing liquidity.

- The task of the entire management is to convert the strategically defined potential for success into business.

From this perspective, it becomes clear that the sustainable goals of strategic management often conflict with quarterly operational goals, especially when it comes to innovation. Or to put it another way, a company is maximally successful in the short term if it does not innovate or only innovates a little (incrementally) and concentrates entirely on proven strengths. This is exactly what happens time and again and in many cases leads to a company's downfall in the long term.

The implementation of innovations requires an organization geared towards innovation management with appropriate control and monitoring. With regard to production innovation, the special feature of innovation management lies in the high complexity of the subject area combined with the high demands on the predictability of the production process. This necessary predictability is often incompatible with an experimental character of new solutions and the associated risk.

In order to illustrate the challenges of production innovation in this area of tension in more detail and to identify solutions, the topic of ambidexterity [1] is explained below in a simplified and practical form.

Ambidexterity (a special field of organization science) refers to a company's ability to balance and harness the power of both exploration and exploitation—exploring new opportunities (e.g. technologies, partners, markets) while exploiting existing resources, capabilities and knowledge. This balance is crucial for sustaining competitiveness and achieving long-term success in dynamic environments. Ambidexterity is manifested in organizations through three primary forms, temporal, contextual and structural [15], which are explained in the following:

- **Temporal ambidexterity** suggests that an organization shifts its focus back and forth between exploitation and exploration over time, depending on strategic priorities, market conditions, or availability of resources. This form of ambidexterity is often used in production innovation by exploiting ongoing production processes over a long period of time and integrating exploration for a short period of time when needed.
- **Contextual ambidexterity** involves the duality of exploitation and exploration, i.e. their simultaneous application in business execution. This requires the creation of a flexible organizational context in which employees can switch between exploration and exploitation modes depending on the requirements of their work. This approach relies on a strong organizational culture and leadership that encourages employees to divide their time as autonomously as possible between these competing demands in order to foster innovation while maintaining operational excellence.
- **Structural ambidexterity** refers to the organization's structural separation of units or teams dedicated to exploration and those focused on exploitation. An example is large companies exploring new approaches with startups. This separation (e.g. between company and startup) allows for specialized processes and cultures to develop within each unit, suited to the unique challenges of

exploration or exploitation. Synergies can be utilized and separated units can be integrated at a later stage.

Most successful manufacturers today realize—at least to some extent—one or more forms of ambidexterity. In terms of production innovation, the picture from practical experience is as follows:

- Structural ambidexterity plays virtually no role in production innovation. It would mean outsourcing a production process. This is basically a make-or-buy decision that will not be pursued further here.
- Contextual ambidexterity is still rarely used in production innovation, but has great potential in dynamic production environments when production requirements are changing ever more rapidly. More details follow below.
- Temporal ambidexterity is the most frequently implemented ambidexterity in production innovation.

5.3.2.1 The Strategy of Temporal Ambidexterity

We begin with the concept of temporal ambidexterity because it facilitates understanding of contextual ambidexterity.

With a strategy of temporal ambidexterity (Fig. 5.2) there is a long phase of exploitation in which a well-functioning production is not or only slightly changed. After setup and testing, the production runs at a certain output, which is gradually increased incrementally over time through tuning and small changes. After a certain period of production (often several years), a further increase in performance using existing methods or technologies is hardly possible. This results in a typical s-curve [16] with regard to performance (Production environment 1 in Fig. 5.2).

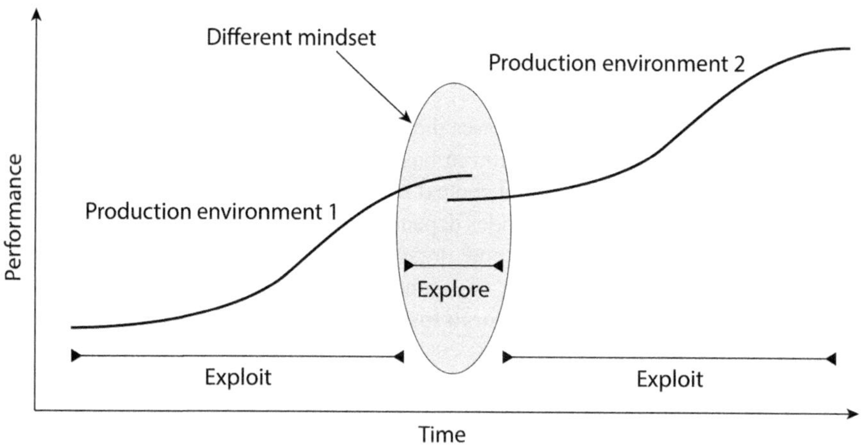

Fig. 5.2 Temporal ambidexterity in production innovation. Principle of s-curves from Foster [16]. (Source: authors)

When additional performance is needed, a phase of exploratory production innovation follows, where new methods and techniques (radical innovation) are researched and implemented. This is followed by another phase of exploitation (Production environment 2 in Fig. 5.2).

However, a completely different mindset is required in the exploration phase than in the exploitation phase. While the focus in this first phase is on efficiency and security, the priority in the exploration phase is experimentation, innovation and growth, which requires a fundamentally different mindset and is associated with risk [17].

This change of mindset (Table 5.1) is a huge challenge for everyone involved. It cannot be emphasized enough how great these challenges are in practice. The organizational basis for an explorative mindset is not in place and strategic management requires leaders who bring together various groups within an organization to develop actions. Employees and stakeholders need to be led in an unfamiliar explorative environment, which requires a completely different approach to management and leadership (Table 5.2). For this reason, many projects in this transition phase do not have the desired success. Experience has shown that delays occur, budgets are not adhered to or projects even fail.

5.3.2.2 The Strategy of Contextual Ambidexterity

The concept of temporal ambidexterity described above was mostly acceptable in the past, despite the major challenges, because many manufacturers worked in an environment of slow product innovation cycles with little change in production conditions, meaning that changeover was rare. The associated difficulties had to be accepted.

Table 5.1 Mindset for exploration and exploitation in comparison. Adapted from Weibler and Keller [17]

	Exploitation mindset	Exploration mindset
Main focus	Benefit, optimize, preserve	Searching, experimenting, rethinking
Strategic focus	Efficiency and profit	Innovation and growth
Results	Predictable, immediately visible	Uncertain, visible in the long term
Structural features	Formalization, centrality, control	Autonomy, decentralization, agility
Cultural characteristics	Security mindset	Risk tolerance

Table 5.2 Management and leadership roles in ambidextrous organizations

	Exploitative management role	Explorative leadership role
Process	Exploitation (execution)	Exploration
Action	Doing things right	Doing the right things
Innovation type	Incremental	Radical
Time horizon	Short-term	Long-term
Managerial style	Authoritative	Visionary

Today, one of the most important questions from a company's perspective is the question of the future competitive landscape. Depending on the analysis, the need for explorative production innovation can arise quickly.

The reason is that due to increasing process complexity, shorter product and innovation cycles and smaller production volumes, more flexibility and faster changes in production environments are required. Another trend is towards more customization in manufacturing and individualized products, which means that the need for production innovation has increased in principle and is likely to increase further. Issues such as corporate sustainability goals and a switch to alternative energy sources may also necessitate significant changes in production and therefore require innovation.

It is therefore an obvious choice to realize explorative production innovation in a strategy of contextual ambidexterity, i.e. to allow exploitation and exploration to run simultaneously. However, due to the requirement for stable production processes in a complex production environment, experiments and changes are not possible in regular production.

To give an example of contextual ambidexterity in action, let's take a brief look at a non-manufacturing sector, namely retail. In the supermarket, one can experience an ideal field for the application of simultaneous exploitation and exploration every day. For example, in addition to the traditional checkouts (exploit), individual checkouts are installed for customers to scan and pay themselves (explore). Product locations are changed daily to analyze how consumers behave (explore) while sales are in progress (exploit).

It is immediately clear that such an explorative playing field is not available in production innovation. Production environments are unique and must be geared towards exploitation.

Since the successful implementation of this type of innovation must be a key competence of many manufacturers in the future, the task is therefore to find an approach to combine explorative production innovation with exploitative production. In this respect, the author has developed a concept in his practical work in the m_bridge project (www.m-bridge.io), which is described below.

It is proposed that, in addition to their existing exploitative production environments, manufacturers set up additional explorative environments in parallel, in which corresponding future production topics are developed in series. The results of this work are stored until they are needed at a suitable time (explore–store–implement). A transition from production environment 1 to production environment 2 then takes place at this desired point in time (Fig. 5.3). This may be, for example, the introduction of a product successor, variants or special market requirements.

In his practical work, the author has learned that there is no other way than to address the concept of explorative production innovation at the strategic level of a company, whereby the understanding of the topic varies greatly depending on the company.

Explorative production innovation is always associated with experimentation and risk [14]. The usual goal of increasing performance in the short term cannot be pursued. Resistance in internal processes must be taken into account [14], precisely because the ideas and concepts are not yet tangible. Focusing on opportunities and pursuing future potential must be the driver.

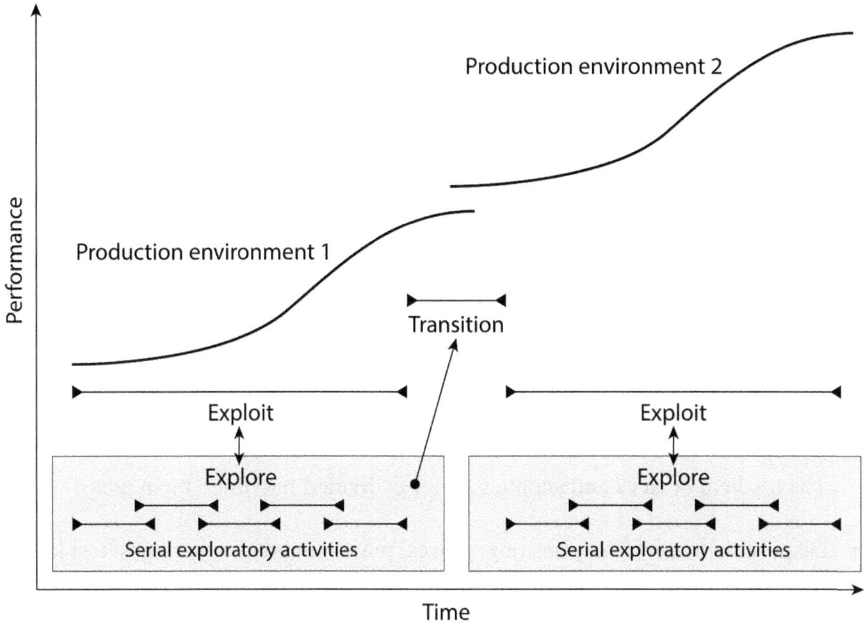

Fig. 5.3 Proposal for contextual ambidexterity in production innovation. Principle of s-curves from Foster [16]. (Source: authors)

Furthermore, financial and human resources must be allocated, especially for operational staff and decision-makers. Some employees in the production department must be given a time budget to work on new solutions, ideally supported by KPIs linked to personal business goals. External resources may need to be involved if internal resources are not available to the extent required.

Overall, the implementation of the concept depends on multidisciplinary and cross-departmental collaboration and an adaptable and innovative culture. Even more than in other areas of the company, contextual ambidexterity in the production department requires skillful leadership that conveys a clear strategic vision.

Everyone involved must be aware that explorative production innovation is usually not immediately measurable, especially not with established measurement methods, and long-term thinking is required. All in all, the balance between Exploit and Explore is crucial.

To summarize:

- By effectively integrating exploration and exploitation, manufacturers can navigate complex production environments and ensure both short-term efficiency and long-term innovation.
- It must be clear that the acquisition of new innovation skills in production does not represent an immediate advantage, as newly acquired skills need to mature and be mastered in order to turn them into a real competitive edge [18].

Finally, an appeal: "There is a need for focused research on production innovation generally, and exploration of explorative production innovation particularly" [14].

5.4 The Impact of Production Innovation on the Success of Medical Devices and Supplies

As described in the previous sections, production innovation is a complex topic and can have an impact on the success of products in many manufacturing industries. This section uses the example of the medical devices and supplies industry to describe the impact that production innovation can have.

Qualitative assessments are made, as there are no concrete scientific studies and there has been insufficient focused research on the topic of production innovation to date [14].

The medical devices and supplies sector is divided into three main areas:

- Disposable medical supplies (e.g. gloves, masks, bandages, syringes, test kits).
- Durable medical equipment (e.g. wheelchairs, hospital beds, oxygen concentrators).
- Medical devices (e.g. pacemakers, defibrillators, ultrasound machines, ventilators).

The following two questions are essential for assessing the impact of production innovation:

- What does the future competitive landscape look like?
- What is the rate of change in the respective industry?

The question of the competitive landscape depends on each individual company and its specific products, as well as the markets in which it is sold. The answer to this question is therefore very individual. It is therefore advisable for every company to carry out and continuously update analyses in all target geographies, e.g. according to Porter's Five Forces framework [19]. However, this chapter will not go into this in detail.

The question of the rate of change in industries can be answered more generally because it is not specific to a particular company. In addition, changes, even if they initially only take place locally, can quickly have an impact on the global market. Of course, every company is advised to carry out appropriate analyses here too, with a particular focus on technological innovations.

As a comment on the priority of this question, there is hardly a more apt statement than the following quote from Jack Welch, the former Chairman and CEO of General Electric: "If the rate of change on the outside exceeds the rate of change on the inside, the end is near". Especially in the current times of upheaval, business strategists should keep the meaning of this statement in mind and, above all, bear in mind that changes are not just about products, services and business models, but also about production.

Changes in products or product details, even inconspicuous ones such as their packaging, bring about a change in the production process that is often so far-reaching that innovations are required. An example is plastic packaging for a sterile product that has to be switched to paper due to regulations.

The qualitative assessments of production innovation are described in the following sections.

5.4.1 Disposable Medical Supplies

These disposable products (e.g. gloves, masks, bandages, syringes, test kits) are either simple mass-produced products or advanced mass-produced products (e.g. with hypoallergenic materials or embedded technologies).

For **simple mass products**, quality (specification) and price matter. The rate of change is quite low.

The following is an assessment of production innovation. This is similar for all products in this area, which is why specific products are not discussed.

As product innovation is practically impossible due to fixed standards and regulations, production innovation (apart from logistics optimization) is the only option for improving the competitive situation. There is no other field of application to reduce costs and increase profitability.

Examples of the potential of production innovation:

- Reduce production line downtime.
- Optimize all forms of automation in the production process.
- Identify high-maintenance production components and replace them with new technologies where possible.
- Identify unstable processes and replace them with new technologies where possible.
- Reduce material and energy consumption through changes to the manufacturing process.
- Implement new environmental and sustainability standards.

These simple products already show the potential of production innovation, which is technically the only way to increase business success.

With **advanced mass products**, all of the above points apply and there are further opportunities for production innovation. The rate of change is higher.

To realize the following innovations, the product development and production departments must work together. This concept is called product-driven production innovation [14]. Only with intensive cooperation and effective input from production the full innovation potential can be utilized. The following are examples in which production innovation can play a major role:

- Material innovations, e.g.:
  - Biodegradable and sustainable materials.
  - Antimicrobial and hypoallergenic materials.
- Intelligent disposables, e.g.:
  - Embedded technologies such as biosensors in wound dressings that can monitor the healing process.
  - Temperature-sensitive labels that indicate the sterility of packaged instruments.
  - QR codes or RFID tags to enable better tracking and inventory management.
- Color-coded safety features, e.g.:
  - Color-coding of disposables so that healthcare workers can quickly identify sizes or types.

Some of the innovations mentioned seem simple to implement. However, experience has shown that with medical supplies, every detail is a challenge to implement due to regulations and quality requirements, which can make the production innovation particularly valuable.

5.4.2 Durable Medical Equipment

These durable products (e.g. wheelchairs, hospital beds, oxygen concentrators) are also either simple mass products or advanced mass products with a medium rate of change.

With regard to the potential of production innovation, the scaling of production has a high priority. Efforts must be made to scale production and reduce costs without compromising quality, making products more affordable. This is particularly important if products are to be distributed in developing countries, where cost is a significant barrier to access. But price is also an important criterion in developed countries. Economic success is difficult to achieve without production innovation.

As in the previous section, product-driven production innovation [14] is also the key to success in this area of advanced mass products. The following are examples of areas in which the production department can contribute to the increased success of products in combination with product development:

- Technological progress
  - Connectivity and IoT: The integration of Internet-of-Things (IoT) functions into products (e.g. wheelchairs and respiratory therapy devices) is a strong trend.
  - Wearable technology: Advances in wearable technology for devices (e.g. prostheses) or wearable devices for rehabilitation represent a potential for innovation.
- Material innovations
  - New materials that are both lighter and more durable.
  - Antimicrobial coatings to reduce the risk of infection.

- Customization
  - Advances in technology to adapt to the individual needs of patients.
- Changes in regulations
  - Regulatory bodies around the world are setting stricter safety and efficacy standards that can only be achieved through innovation.
- Sustainability efforts
  - Reducing environmental impact (longer lifespan, improving energy efficiency, recycling old devices) is a strong trend.

5.4.3 Medical Devices

These devices form the highest technological class in this section. The rate of change tends to be at a high level. The units require the highest level of product innovation as well as production innovation.

As before, the potential of production innovation can be used to scale production and optimize prices. A particularly important key to success here is the aforementioned product-driven production innovation [14].

The following are examples of products in connection with topics that can be particularly relevant to the production process.

- Pacemakers
  - Leadless and miniaturized designs
  - Longer battery life and energy efficiency.
- Defibrillators
  - Integration with wearable technology for at-risk patients.
- Ultrasound machines
  - Portable and handheld devices, enhanced image quality and functionality.
- Ventilators
  - Home use designs, more user-friendly, portable ventilators.
- Dialysis machines
  - Wearable kidney devices to allow greater mobility for patients.
  - Enhancements in dialysate cleansing and recycling to reduce water and energy usage.
- Endoscopes
  - High-definition and 3D imaging.
  - Disposable options: Development of single-use endoscopic accessories.
- Infusion pumps
  - Wireless communication, integration with hospital systems.
  - Enhanced mechanisms to prevent free flow and ensure accurate dosing.

5.5 Conclusion

When it comes to technical innovation of products, the sole focus is often on product innovation, as production must be efficient and stable. The resulting mindset is characterized by risk aversion, control and efficiency.

However, in times of changing markets, increasing product diversity and growing competition, it is precisely production innovation (not to be confused with product innovation) that offers potential for improvement. Unfortunately, this potential has often been insufficiently exploited because the opportunities are not recognized or the structures are too rigid.

Analyses are necessary to recognize the competitive situation and the rate of change and, based on this, to set targets for innovation. If a need for major innovations in production is recognized, an explorative production innovation approach can be a way of tapping into this potential.

However, for this to be possible, the company's structures and processes must be adapted to a mindset of flexibility and openness without sacrificing efficiency (ambidexterity).

Strong leadership is required to create the necessary acceptance and achieve the goals, supported by the top strategic decision-making level, or more precisely the decision-makers. The greatest challenge lies in the implementation of such a change.

The examples from the medical supplies and devices sector provide insight into the areas where implementation can be beneficial. It is reasonable to assume that this approach can be applied to other industries with mass production.

References

1. O'Reilly CA, Tushman ML. Organizational ambidexterity in action: how managers explore and exploit. Calif Manag Rev. 2011;53(4):5–22. https://doi.org/10.1525/cmr.2011.53.4.5.
2. Taylor SP. What is innovation? Insight. 2017. https://insight.cumbria.ac.uk/id/eprint/3475/.
3. Edwards-Schachter M. The nature and variety of innovation. Int J Innov Stud. 2018;2(2):65–79. https://doi.org/10.1016/j.ijis.2018.08.004.
4. Keeley L, Pikkel R, Quinn B, Walters H. Ten types of innovation: the discipline of building breakthroughs. New York: Wiley; 2013.
5. Moore GA. Dealing with Darwin: how great companies innovate at every phase of their evolution. New York: Portfolio; 2008.
6. Satell G. The 4 types of innovation and the problems they solve. Harv Bus Rev. 2017. https://hbr.org/2017/06/the-4-types-of-innovation-and-the-problems-they-solve.
7. Ziemnowicz C. Joseph A. Schumpeter and innovation. In: Carayannis EG, editor. Encyclopedia of creativity, invention, innovation and entrepreneurship. New York, NY: Springer; 2013. https://doi.org/10.1007/978-1-4614-3858-8_476.
8. Alharbi I, Jamil R, Mahmood N, Shaharoun A. Organizational innovation: a review paper. Open J Bus Manag. 2019;7:1196–206. https://doi.org/10.4236/ojbm.2019.73084.
9. Jacob C. Innovative, agile Führungsansätze – Resilienz von Menschen und Systemen fördern. In: Kastner C, Jacob C, Hesmer D, Plugmann P, editors. Innovative Unternehmensführung. Wiesbaden: Springer Gabler; 2023. https://doi.org/10.1007/978-3-658-40943-2_2.
10. Vrontis D. Innovative business practices prevailing a turbulent era. Newcastle upon Tyne: Cambridge Scholars Publishing; 2013.

11. Bröcker J, Dohse D, Soltwedel R, editors. Innovation clusters and interregional competition. Berlin: Springer; 2003. https://doi.org/10.1007/978-3-540-24760-9.
12. Chesbrough HW. Open innovation: the new imperative for creating and profiting from technology. Boston, MA: Harvard Business School Press; 2003.
13. Ohlberg KH, Salmeron JL. Proposal-based innovation: a new approach to opening up the innovation process. In: Future of business and finance. Berlin: Springer International Publishing; 2020. p. 201–31. https://doi.org/10.1007/978-3-030-41309-5_14.
14. Larsson L. A conceptual framework for production innovation. PhD dissertation, Luleå University of Technology; 2020. https://urn.kb.se/resolve?urn=urn:nbn:se:ltu:diva-77589.
15. Gibson CB, Birkinshaw J. The antecedents, consequences, and mediating role of organizational ambidexterity. Acad Manag J. 2004;47(2):209–26. https://doi.org/10.2307/20159573.
16. Foster R. Innovation: the attacker's advantage. New York: Summit Books; 1986.
17. Weibler J, Keller T. Führungsverhalten im Kontext von Ambidextrie. In: Trends der Psychologischen Führungsforschung. Göttingen: Hogrefe Verlag; 2015.
18. Romero D, Larsson L, Rönnbäck AÖ, Stahre J. Strategizing for production innovation. In: Advances in production management systems. The path to intelligent, collaborative and sustainable manufacturing. Berlin: Springer International Publishing; 2017. p. 3–12. https://doi.org/10.1007/978-3-319-66923-6_1.
19. Porter ME. Competitive strategy: techniques for analyzing industries and competitors. New York: Free Press; 1980.

Part II

Multidisciplinary Perspectives on Health and Well-Being

Beyond Limits: The Fusion of Nature and Technology in Achieving Optimal Health—The Truth of Biohacking

6

Dorothea Portius

6.1 Introduction

Throughout human history, the quest for health optimization and prolonged lifespans has been a fundamental endeavor. This pursuit has primarily seen advancements through significant improvements in medical and pharmaceutical interventions [1]. Despite these advancements extending the human lifespan, they have paradoxically led to a reduction in healthspan due to the increased prevalence of chronic diseases. Specifically, the rise of age-related chronic conditions, such as cardiovascular diseases (CVD), nonalcoholic fatty liver disease (NAFLD), cancers, type-2 diabetes mellitus (T2DM), hypertension, as well as neurodegenerative diseases such as Alzheimer's disease and Parkinson's disease, has become a notable concern.

In recent years, there has been expanding interest in exploring longevity, focusing on biochemical research aimed at mitigating the functional decline of cellular metabolism and overall physical fitness, preserving reproductive capabilities, and significantly decelerating the mortality rate associated with advancing age [1, 2]. These explorations encompass strategies such as exercise, diet and nutrition, cold therapy, and other alternative modalities collectively referred to as biohacking [2]. These efforts represent a holistic approach to extending human longevity while concurrently enhancing the overall quality and well-being of individual life experiences, reflecting a nuanced approach to health optimization.

D. Portius (✉)
Institute for Agriculture and Nutritional Sciences, Martin-Luther-University Halle-Wittenberg, Halle (Saale), Germany
e-mail: dorothea.portius@landw.uni-halle.de

P. Plugmann, D. Portius (eds.), *Innovations in Healthcare and Outcome Measurement*, https://doi.org/10.1007/978-3-031-77302-0_6

6.2 Defining Biohacking

The concept of biohacking encapsulates a broad spectrum of practices, yet its exact definition still needs to be discovered within academic discourse. This ambiguity is noteworthy given the term's infrequent appearance in scholarly literature. An investigation in PubMed shows that between 2009 and February 2024, there were only 31 articles in which "biohacking" was mentioned, indicating that it plays only a minor role in the scientific discussion. Conversely, a simple query of "biohacking" on Google yields an overwhelming array of websites predominantly offering services aimed at health optimization. Such disparity presents a significant challenge for nonexperts attempting to discern methods and approaches that are both scientifically substantiated and evidence-based.

Examining the etymology of the term "biohacking" reveals its roots: "bio-" deriving from biology, indicative of life and living systems, and "hack" implying gaining access or modifying systems in unconventional ways. Biohacking is identified as a global movement premised on the conviction that one can achieve unparalleled control over one's biology through the deliberate modification of one's external environment and internal physiological processes [3]. For many adherents, the concept of "control" goes beyond basic sufficiency, evolving into a pursuit for enhanced well-being and superior performance. Thus, biohacking emerges as an interdisciplinary domain combining elements of art and science to optimize one's physiology and neurological functions for peak efficiency, intellectual capacity, and operational effectiveness. Typically, the term is applied to describe the practice of "do-it-yourself" biology, wherein individuals proactively engage in manipulating their biological systems [4, 5].

6.3 Integrative Biohacking: A Holistic Perspective on Self-Optimization

A "holistic" approach in health optimization and biohacking encompasses a broad integrative perspective emphasizing the interconnected nature of physical, mental, and emotional health. This approach promotes a synergistic consideration of various facets of well-being rather than isolating them as independent elements.

Within the context of biohacking, adopting a holistic strategy means employing a variety of "natural" methods to enhance health across several dimensions. These methods can be grounded by three pillars of health and well-being:

- **NUTRITION**: Prioritizing a balanced diet rich in nutrients that fuel the body, support metabolic processes, and mitigate disease risk. Emphasis is placed on whole foods with a tailored approach to meet individual dietary needs and goals.
- **EXERCISE**: Incorporating regular physical activity tailored to one's fitness level and preferences. This includes strength training, cardiovascular workouts, flexibility exercises, and movement practices that foster physical resilience, enhance performance, and improve mental health.

- **MINDSET**: Cultivating a positive mental attitude, stress management techniques, and mindfulness practices. This pillar recognizes the critical role of psychological well-being in achieving overall health. It involves developing resilience, fostering a growth mindset, and incorporating practices such as meditation, journaling, walking in nature, and cognitive-behavioral strategies to enhance emotional regulation and mental clarity.

The integration of these holistic pillars forms a foundational framework for understanding and enhancing health and well-being. However, significant advancements in health-tracking technologies and the widespread availability of digital tools have markedly increased the practicality of incorporating and overseeing these pillars at the individual level.

This ease of integration and monitoring in daily life is pivotal as it allows individuals to take a more active and informed role in managing their health. Consequently, the act of **MONITORING** itself emerges as a critical fourth component enveloping the core pillars (Fig. 6.1).

Monitoring not only facilitates the continuous assessment of one's health status but also enables the adjustment of personalized strategies in real time. It also refers to data collection using IoT digital apps and wearables for continuous control of health data like vital parameters from interstitial fluid, blood pulse detection, diet, movement, or sleep [6, 7]. In essence, the concept of "monitoring" serves as a comprehensive health dashboard, displaying individual key performance indicators (KPIs) and offering actionable insights to maintain and enhance health management.

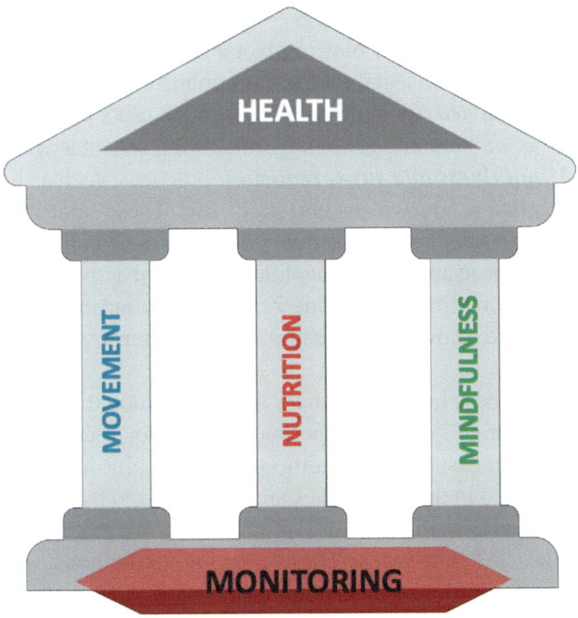

Fig. 6.1 The house of health. Holistic four pillars, nutrition, exercise, and mindfulness, carry the roof HEALTH, stabilized by the integration of Monitoring. Own representation

A holistic approach to biohacking transcends mere symptom management and the targeting of specific health outcomes. It involves a complete lifestyle overhaul, addressing the root causes of health issues, encouraging preventive care, and boosting the body's natural healing abilities. Additionally, biohacking extends to improving mental health and fostering an ethical mindset. It emphasizes the importance of a balanced and mindful strategy in self-improvement, promoting a comprehensive uplift in both physical and mental health for a better quality of life [8].

6.4 The Gold Standard of Holistic Biohacking: The Blue Zones

The Blue Zones are compelling examples of holistic biohacking, regions globally renowned for high concentrations of centenarians and lower rates of chronic diseases [9–11]. One Blue Zone region is Icaria in Greece, with 80% of the people between ages 65 and 100 without pharmaceutical requirements. The Blue Zones represent quintessential examples of holistic biohacking, embodying a lifestyle-centric approach to fostering longevity and overall well-being. These regions encompass next to Icaria, Sardinia (Italy), Okinawa (Japan), Nicoya (Costa Rica), and Loma Linda (California, USA). Individuals adopt a range of practices that contribute to their extended health spans and overall vitality [9]. Based on the biohacking pillars, it combines dietary, social, exercise, and mental aspects.

Dietary patterns in Blue Zones revolve around plant-centric choices (whole foods), emphasizing vegetables, legumes, and whole grains. Lean proteins (meat, fish, and dairy products) are consumed in moderation, locally sourced, and minimally processed.

Social connectivity plays a pivotal role in Blue Zones, where strong community ties and regular social interactions contribute to emotional well-being and resilience.

Physical activity integrated into routine tasks involves low-intensity exercises such as walking and gardening, mitigating sedentary lifestyles.

Mindfulness and stress reduction practices, such as meditation, prayer, or contemplation, are woven into daily life. These contribute to mental well-being and stress resilience, essential components of holistic health. In addition, a sense of purpose and engagement in meaningful activities, even in later stages of life, is a common thread in Blue Zones. This contributes to mental and emotional resilience, showcasing the importance of purpose-driven living.

As these holistic practices are deeply rooted in ancient traditions, the monitoring component becomes superfluous or is not used here. Instead, people in the Blue Zones measure their health via intuitive physical well-being. The health practices observed in the Blue Zones are characterized by intentional behaviors, distinct from the reactive engagements prompted by digital applications on mobile phones or other IoT interfaces. These populations demonstrate a lifestyle penetrated with health-promoting behaviors from an early age, a phenomenon attributed to cultural norms and environmental factors rather than technological interventions. Notably, despite their geographical separation from the highly stressed, achievement-oriented ethos prevalent in Western societies, these "longevity regions" are situated within countries integral to the global industrial complex, such as Italy, Japan, and the United States. This controversy prompts a critical examination of biohacking methodologies.

Moreover, the significance of individual genetic and metabolic profiles must also be taken into account. Not only is this longevity lifestyle transmitted from generation to generation, but the epigenetic effects of this lifestyle must also be considered [12].

6.5 Western Perspectives on Biohacking Today: Digital Integration and Its Impact

In our Westernized and fast-paced world, we are increasingly distancing ourselves from the Blue Zone lifestyle. Contemporary diets often consist of highly processed foods, readily available to satisfy hunger or provide convenient snacks. Our reliance on automobiles, trams, and trains supersedes walking or biking due to their perceived efficiency. Although technological advancements have significantly improved various aspects of life, they have simultaneously altered our social behaviors. Face-to-face interactions have diminished, resulting in fewer genuine personal connections. Recent studies indicate that residents of large cities frequently experience loneliness [13]. Despite technological and medical innovations, there is a paradoxical increase in societal health issues.

Given these modern challenges, it is imperative to explore alternative approaches to health and well-being. Biohacking, as previously detailed, encompasses a diverse array of practices, each targeting specific facets of human biology. The subsequent figure (Fig. 6.2) delineates various biohacking domains, including digital components, and notes that certain areas may overlap or convey similar concepts. This observation underscores the necessity for a consistent definition and highlights the predominantly nonscientific approach to biohacking.

Lifestyle Biohacking: This domain focuses on adopting behaviors and lifestyles that promote peak biological performance and longevity. Accessible avenues for initiating biohacking, such as dietary modifications, breathwork, meditation, and physical exercise, fall under this category. These practices activate biological pathways conducive to enhanced performance and extended lifespan.

Molecular Biohacking: This branch involves leveraging both natural and synthetic molecules to modulate one's biology. It includes the intake of supplements, such as vitamins, minerals, and peptides, aimed at eliciting specific biological responses to optimize bodily functions.

Biologics in Biohacking: Biologics refer to cellular or biological entities intended to augment biological processes. This category includes various forms of cellular materials or informational entities like exosomes, which are complexes

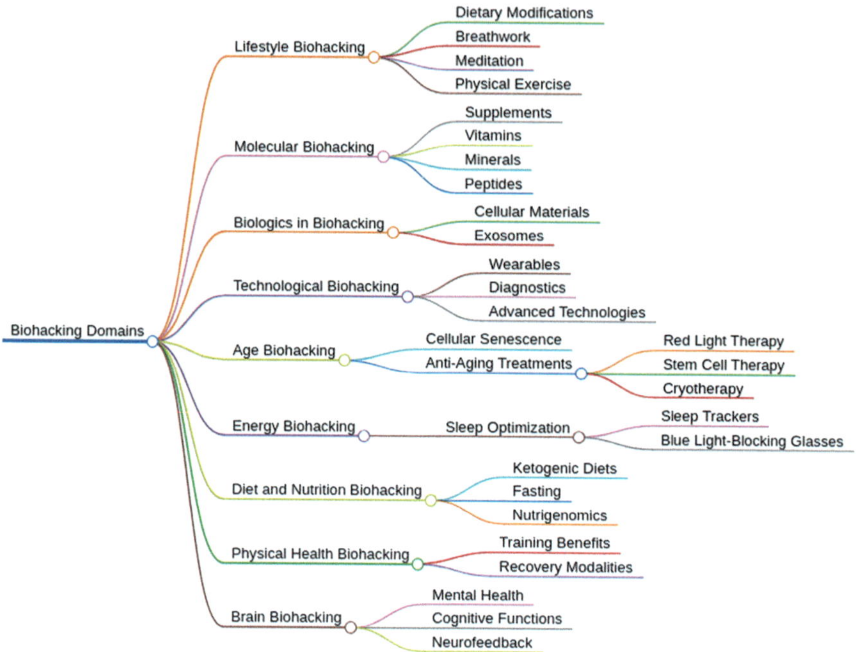

Fig. 6.2 Biohacking domains. This figure provides an overview of major biohacking domains, highlighting key examples of current interest in longevity and biohacking. (Own figure adapted from [14])

comprising DNA, mRNA, proteins, and growth factors. These biologics can be administered through ingestion, injection, or intravenous methods, and they may range from FDA-approved medications to nonmedical therapies available in specialized facilities.

Technological Biohacking: This segment utilizes devices such as wearables and diagnostics to gather physiological data, enabling individuals to fine-tune their health strategies for optimal performance. Advanced technologies like hyperbaric chambers or electromagnetic stimulators are employed to expedite physiological alterations or healing processes.

Age Biohacking: As individuals age, they often turn to biohacking to mitigate the signs of aging. This involves understanding and influencing cellular senescence and the body's efficiency in removing damaged cells. Strategies like red light therapy, stem cell therapy, cryotherapy, and the consumption of anti-aging supplements are employed to promote cellular health and regeneration.

Energy Biohacking: Aims to enhance vitality, often integrating sleep optimization as rest is crucial for energy levels. Techniques include the use of sleep trackers, blue light-blocking glasses, and light therapy for circadian rhythm regulation, alongside meditation apps and specific supplements to boost energy.

Diet and Nutrition Biohacking: This aspect focuses on tailoring one's diet to enhance cellular nutrition and metabolic function. Approaches like ketogenic diets or fasting regimens are explored to influence cellular metabolism, with an emphasis on understanding the interaction between nutrients and genetics (nutrigenomics).

Physical Health Biohacking: Athletes and fitness enthusiasts often employ biohacking to enhance training, performance, and recovery. This includes leveraging exercise-induced cellular benefits, high-intensity interval training, and various modalities like cold plunging, heat therapy, and vibration therapy to optimize physical health.

Brain Biohacking: Focuses on managing and training the brain to improve mental health and cognitive functions. Strategies include using nootropics, psychotropics, brainwave entrainment, neurofeedback therapy, and regular physical activity to stimulate the production of brain-derived neurotrophic factor, enhancing brain function and neuroplasticity.

These categories illustrate the diverse methodologies, each contributing to the overarching aim of biological enhancement and optimization through a combination of lifestyle adjustments, molecular interventions, technological advancements, and a deeper understanding of the body's intrinsic mechanisms [8, 15–19].

6.6 Biohacking: Synergy with Advanced Technology

In the face of modern health innovation, biohacking is converging with digital elements and biotech, ushering in a new era of individualized strategies to transform health. It's crucial to navigate this frontier with caution, given the nascent stage of many biohacking methodologies. The scientific accuracy and safety of these methods demand rigorous control. Moreover, ethical issues, the safeguarding of personal health data, and the prospect of unforeseen effects require a balance between enthusiasm for innovation and adherence to evidence-based practices [20].

The current renaissance in health technology, marked by the advent of wearable health devices, the integration of the Internet of Things (IoT), and the application of artificial intelligence (AI), has become the cornerstone of personalized health and wellness enhancement. Wearable technology, encompassing devices from smartwatches and fitness bands to rings, plays an instrumental role in biohacking by providing continuous health metrics that empower customized health and fitness regimens [21].

The penetration of wearables into the health and fitness sector is unprecedented. Instruments such as smartwatches, equipped with a myriad of sensors for cardiac rhythm, sleep tracking, and kinetic activity, provide a snapshot of an individual's metabolic and physiological status. There is evidence that wearables could enhance cardiac health and overall fitness. However, the long-term benefits of these devices require further study to establish a sustained impact on health and activity levels [22].

The integration of IoT into clinical research has fundamentally transformed data collection methods, marking a significant shift towards personalized health monitoring and interventions. This evolution is particularly evident in the increasing popularity of the bring-your-own-device (BYOD) model in recent years [23, 24]. Unlike traditional research designs that provide participants with specific devices or resources for data collection, BYOD studies utilize data from individuals' personal smart devices. The COVID-19 pandemic has further propelled the use of the BYOD model in digital health research, as efforts to expedite illness detection, facilitate remote medical care, and prevent further spread have benefited from leveraging personal device data [25]. Additionally, the digital health tools sector has seen a significant surge in interest from healthcare providers eager to learn about and employ these tools in patient care [23].

In this context, there's a growing interest in leveraging IoT applications not only for point-of-care diagnostics but also as a preventive measure to enhance lifestyle and thereby improve an individual's health. This approach heralds the era of precision medicine, where tracking individual parameters allows for tailored recommendations and outcomes. By closely monitoring and analyzing these parameters, there is potential to gain a deeper understanding of an individual's metabolism and overall well-being, customizing health interventions to their unique physiological makeup. This personalized approach promises to revolutionize our current approach to health care, making it more responsive to the individual needs of each patient.

For instance, wearable technology has demonstrated the potential to improve sleep quality. They can provide real-time and real-life (avoiding being in a sleep laboratory) data on sleep patterns, informing lifestyle adjustments such as diet, exercise, and mindfulness techniques to improve sleep quality. AI algorithms may analyze sleep data to recommend personalized dietary changes that enhance sleep [26], such as increasing magnesium-rich foods for better relaxation. In a study focusing on breast cancer survivors, a wearable-based physical activity intervention led to improvements in sleep disturbances as measured by wrist-worn actigraphy. These improvements were sustained over a longer period, suggesting that wearables may have a lasting positive impact on sleep quality. Furthermore, the study found that the intervention seemed to provide greater benefits to those initially poor sleepers [27].

Similarly, data on physical activity and heart rate can guide personalized exercise regimens aligned with holistic health principles, ensuring that physical exertion matches the body's natural rhythms. Innovative biofeedback techniques can further enhance this integration. For instance, heart rate variability (HRV) monitoring, a key indicator of autonomic nervous system balance, can guide personalized stress management practices [28]. By integrating HRV data with mindfulness practices, individuals can adopt their meditation routines to optimize stress reduction and enhance overall well-being.

Wearable devices are playing an increasingly pivotal role in metabolic health management by providing continuous real-time monitoring of health and metabolic status. As ongoing and longitudinal tracking, it proves especially advantageous in managing conditions such as altered glucose metabolism, including insulin resistance, which serves as the silent harbinger of fully developed and medication-dependent T2DM. The importance of monitoring blood glucose levels lies in understanding individual responses to dietary intake, physical activity, and stress, enabling early comprehensive interventions aimed at reducing the risk for more severe health complications.

Emerging evidence from mobile health (mHealth) interventions underscores the significance of glucose monitoring in the effective management of obesity and diabetes. These interventions offer crucial insights into everyday health management beyond the confines of clinical settings [29, 30]. By incorporating wearable technology, healthcare becomes more tailored to individual needs, significantly enhancing the management and prevention of comorbidities.

Advanced microbiome analysis represents another frontier in biohacking integration. By analyzing gut flora through noninvasive stool tests, individuals can receive personalized dietary recommendations that support gut health, immunity, and mental well-being. This integration of microbiome science with holistic nutrition practices can lead to more effective personalized dietary interventions [31].

There are several other techniques and practices that have gained interest in both the scientific and commercial fields. Services such as genetic and epigenetic testing, as well as sweat analysis, are becoming increasingly popular among biohackers and consumers. However, it is crucial to approach these offerings with caution, as many products and services lack robust scientific evidence. It is important to understand that no single factor—be it genes, blood, or microbiome—can provide a comprehensive solution for personalized treatment. Instead, a holistic health approach necessitates the integration of multiple biological and anthropometric measures to effectively guide personalized health strategies.

Despite their widespread use and integration into daily routines, a critical question remains: do wearable devices genuinely foster improved lifestyle choices and health outcomes? While successful and practical use of wearables for health monitoring should ideally lead to a decrease in chronic health conditions, the opposite seems true as chronic diseases continue to rise.

The core issue lies in the interpretation and analysis of the data collected by these devices. Without proper contextualization, this data is meaningless. Often, the pursuit of perfection colors the data's interpretation. Does failing to meet daily step goals motivate individuals to adopt personalized strategies, or does it lead to diminished self-esteem and feelings of failure? The constant barrage of notifications may also disconnect individuals from their intrinsic bodily cues. Should one follow the "technical" recommendation of high-intensity interval training (HIIT) or a long-distance run, or should one instead listen to their body's own needs?

Understanding and addressing these questions is essential to realizing the true potential of wearable devices in promoting health and well-being.

6.7 Supporting Preventive Measures Against Chronic Diseases

The integration of holistic and technological biohacking holds significant potential for preventing chronic diseases. Continuous monitoring through wearables allows for early detection of health issues such as irregular heartbeats, sleep disturbances, or abnormal glucose levels. Early intervention strategies can then combine technological insights with holistic practices to address these issues before they develop into chronic conditions [32].

For instance, as mentioned above, regular monitoring of blood glucose levels using continuous glucose monitors (CGMs) can identify prediabetic states. This data, combined with personalized dietary advice based on genetic and microbiome analysis, can guide interventions that prevent the onset of diabetes. Studies have shown that personalized nutrition advice based on genetic markers and gut microbiome composition can significantly improve glycemic control and metabolic health [31, 33].

Similarly, integrating stress monitoring technologies with holistic stress management techniques can enhance cardiovascular health. Wearables that track HRV and cortisol levels can alert individuals to rising stress levels, prompting timely interventions such as mindfulness practices, yoga, or breathwork [34]. Research indicates that regular mindfulness meditation can reduce blood pressure and improve HRV, thereby lowering the risk of cardiovascular diseases [35].

Furthermore, combining technological tools with traditional exercise regimens can optimize physical health. For example, wearables that monitor muscle oxygenation and fatigue can help tailor strength training programs to an individual's unique physiology, maximizing efficiency and reducing injury risk. Personalized exercise programs that consider genetic predispositions can improve fitness outcomes and reduce the likelihood of exercise-related injuries [36, 37].

6.8 Conclusion and Outlook

The future of biohacking lies in the seamless integration of holistic and technological approaches, creating a comprehensive and multifaceted framework for health optimization. Throughout human history, the pursuit of extended health spans and improved quality of life has driven advancements in both natural and technological innovations. Holistic biohacking, drawing inspiration from practices observed in Blue Zones, emphasizes the importance of diet, exercise, social interaction, and mindfulness. These practices foster a deep connection to natural rhythms and promote a balanced, nutrient-rich lifestyle that enhances physical, mental, and emotional well-being.

In contrast, technological biohacking leverages advanced tools such as wearables, IoT devices, and AI to provide real-time insights into physiological functions. This data-driven approach allows for precise adjustments to health strategies, enabling individuals to monitor and optimize various health metrics from heart rate and sleep patterns to blood glucose levels and genetic markers. By combining the strengths of both methodologies, a synergistic approach emerges, offering a more comprehensive understanding and optimization of health.

Despite the promise and potential of digital biohacking and precision medicine, they still need to be at the forefront of research or effectively integrated into our healthcare system. Several barriers contribute to this status quo. First, the rapid pace of technological advancement often outstrips the slower processes of scientific validation and regulatory approval. This lag creates a gap between innovation and clinical application. Second, the integration of vast amounts of health data requires robust infrastructure and stringent data privacy measures, which are still developing. Third, there is a need for interdisciplinary collaboration to bridge the gap between technology developers, healthcare providers, and researchers to ensure practical and effective implementation.

Incorporating digital biohacking and precision medicine into mainstream healthcare holds the potential to decrease the risk of several chronic diseases, increase healthspan, and, in turn, reduce healthcare costs. Continuous monitoring and personalized interventions can detect and address health issues early, preventing them from progressing into more serious conditions. By fostering a proactive rather than reactive approach to health management, we can shift the focus from treating diseases to maintaining wellness.

As we continue to advance in both holistic practices and technological innovations, the potential for achieving optimal health becomes increasingly attainable. The convergence of these two paradigms not only enriches our understanding of human biology but also empowers individuals to take an active role in their health journey. This integrated approach fosters a balanced and precise method of health optimization, enhancing quality of life and preventing chronic diseases. With concerted efforts in research, infrastructure, and interdisciplinary collaboration, the vision of a healthcare system that seamlessly integrates digital biohacking and precision medicine can become a reality, ushering in a new era of personalized and preventive healthcare.

References

1. Liu J-K. Antiaging agents: safe interventions to slow aging and healthy life span extension. Nat Prod Bioprospect. 2022;12:18. https://doi.org/10.1007/s13659-022-00339-y.
2. Devito LM, Barzilai N, Cuervo AM, et al. Extending human healthspan and longevity: a symposium report. Ann N Y Acad Sci. 2022;1507:70–83. https://doi.org/10.1111/nyas.14681.
3. Asprey D. Smarter not harder—the biohackers's guide to getting the body and mind you want. New York, NY: HarperCollins; 2023.
4. Landrain T, Meyer M, Perez AM, et al. Do-it-yourself biology: challenges and promises for an open science and technology movement. Syst Synth Biol. 2013;7:115–26. https://doi.org/10.1007/s11693-013-9116-4.
5. Gaspar R, Rohde P, Giger JC. Unconventional settings and uses of human enhancement technologies: a non-systematic review of public and experts' views on self-enhancement and DIY biology/biohacking risks. Hum Behav Emerg Technol. 2019;1:295–305. https://doi.org/10.1002/hbe2.175.
6. Bai J, Shen L, Sun H, et al. Physiological informatics: collection and analyses of data from wearable sensors and smartphone for healthcare. Singapore: Springer Singapore; 2017. p. 17–37. https://doi.org/10.1007/978-981-10-6041-0_2.
7. Gambhir SS, Ge TJ, Vermesh O, et al. Toward achieving precision health. Sci Transl Med. 2018;10:eaao3612. https://doi.org/10.1126/scitranslmed.aao3612.
8. Sandua D. BIOHACKING: the science of optimizing the human body. Seattle: Kindle Direct Publishing; 2024.
9. Buettner D, Skemp S. Blue Zones. Am J Lifestyle Med. 2016;10:318–21. https://doi.org/10.1177/1559827616637066.

10. Pes GM, Dore MP, Tsofliou F, et al. Diet and longevity in the blue zones: a set-and-forget issue? Maturitas. 2022;164:31–7. https://doi.org/10.1016/j.maturitas.2022.06.004.
11. Ungvari Z, Fazekas-Pongor V, Csiszar A, et al. The multifaceted benefits of walking for healthy aging: from Blue Zones to molecular mechanisms. GeroScience. 2023;45:3211–39. https://doi.org/10.1007/s11357-023-00873-8.
12. McEwen LM, Morin AM, Edgar RD, et al. Differential DNA methylation and lymphocyte proportions in a Costa Rican high longevity region. Epigenetics Chromatin. 2017;10:21. https://doi.org/10.1186/s13072-017-0128-2.
13. Hammoud R, Tognin S, Bakolis I, et al. Lonely in a crowd: investigating the association between overcrowding and loneliness using smartphone technologies. Sci Rep. 2021;11(1):24134. https://doi.org/10.1038/s41598-021-03398-2.
14. Health F. Biohacking: what is it and how does it work? Forbes; 2024.
15. Almeida M, Diogo R. Human enhancement. Evol Med Public Health. 2019;2019:183–9. https://doi.org/10.1093/emph/eoz026.
16. Asprey D. The bulletproof diet: lose up to a pound a day, reclaim energy and focus, upgrade your life. Emmaus: Rodale Books; 2014.
17. Cooper ID, Kyriakidou Y, Petagine L, et al. Bio-hacking better health—leveraging metabolic biochemistry to maximise healthspan. Antioxidants. 2023;12:1749. https://doi.org/10.3390/antiox12091749.
18. Gangadharbatla H. Biohacking: an exploratory study to understand the factors influencing the adoption of embedded technologies within the human body. Heliyon. 2020;6:e03931. https://doi.org/10.1016/j.heliyon.2020.e03931.
19. Zettler PJ, Guerrini CJ, Sherkow JS. Regulating genetic biohacking. Science. 2019;365:34–6. https://doi.org/10.1126/science.aax3248.
20. Yeung AWK, Torkamani A, Butte AJ, et al. The promise of digital healthcare technologies. Front Public Health. 2023;11:1196596. https://doi.org/10.3389/fpubh.2023.1196596.
21. Huhn S, Axt M, Gunga H-C, et al. The impact of wearable technologies in health research: scoping review. JMIR Mhealth Uhealth. 2022;10:e34384. https://doi.org/10.2196/34384.
22. Tang MSS, Moore K, McGavigan A, et al. Effectiveness of wearable trackers on physical activity in healthy adults: systematic review and meta-analysis of randomized controlled trials. JMIR Mhealth Uhealth. 2020;8:e15576. https://doi.org/10.2196/15576.
23. Shandhi MMH, Singh K, Janson N, et al. Assessment of ownership of smart devices and the acceptability of digital health data sharing. NPJ Digit Med. 2024;7(1):44. https://doi.org/10.1038/s41746-024-01030-x.
24. Demanuele C, Lokker C, Jhaveri K, et al. Considerations for conducting bring your own "device" (BYOD) clinical studies. Digital Biomarkers. 2022;6:47–60. https://doi.org/10.1159/000525080.
25. Baumgart DC. Digital advantage in the COVID-19 response: perspective from Canada's largest integrated digitalized healthcare system. NPJ Digit Med. 2020;3:114. https://doi.org/10.1038/s41746-020-00326-y.
26. Gallucci D, Ho ECY, Geraci J, et al. Respondents of health survey powered by the innovative NURO app exhibit correlations between exercise frequencies and diet habits, and between stress levels and sleep wellness. Front Psychiatry. 2022;13:945780. https://doi.org/10.3389/fpsyt.2022.945780.
27. Nguyen NH, Vallance JK, Buman MP, et al. Effects of a wearable technology-based physical activity intervention on sleep quality in breast cancer survivors: the ACTIVATE Trial. J Cancer Surviv. 2021;15:273–80. https://doi.org/10.1007/s11764-020-00930-7.
28. Gullett N, Zajkowska Z, Walsh A, et al. Heart rate variability (HRV) as a way to understand associations between the autonomic nervous system (ANS) and affective states: a critical review of the literature. Int J Psychophysiol. 2023;192:35–42. https://doi.org/10.1016/j.ijpsycho.2023.08.001.
29. Keshet A, Reicher L, Bar N, et al. Wearable and digital devices to monitor and treat metabolic diseases. Nat Metab. 2023;5:563–71. https://doi.org/10.1038/s42255-023-00778-y.

30. Rodriguez-León C, Villalonga C, Munoz-Torres M, et al. Mobile and wearable technology for the monitoring of diabetes-related parameters: systematic review. JMIR Mhealth Uhealth. 2021;9:e25138. https://doi.org/10.2196/25138.
31. Song E-J, Shin J-H. Personalized diets based on the gut microbiome as a target for health maintenance: from current evidence to future possibilities. J Microbiol Biotechnol. 2022;32:1497–505. https://doi.org/10.4014/jmb.2209.09050.
32. Shajari S, Kuruvinashetti K, Komeili A, et al. The emergence of AI-based wearable sensors for digital health technology: a review. Sensors. 2023;23:9498. https://doi.org/10.3390/s23239498.
33. Bermingham KM, Linenberg I, Polidori L, et al. Effects of a personalized nutrition program on cardiometabolic health: a randomized controlled trial. Nat Med. 2024;30:1888–97. https://doi.org/10.1038/s41591-024-02951-6.
34. Jerath R, Syam M, Ahmed S. The future of stress management: integration of smartwatches and HRV technology. Sensors. 2023;23:7314. https://doi.org/10.3390/s23177314.
35. Chen Q, Liu H, Du S. Effect of mindfulness-based interventions on people with prehypertension or hypertension: a systematic review and meta-analysis of randomized controlled trials. BMC Cardiovasc Disord. 2024;24(1):104. https://doi.org/10.1186/s12872-024-03746-w.
36. Nasb M, Wei M, Lin B, et al. Unraveling precision exercise: a journey from efficacy to molecular insights. Adv Exercise Health Sci. 2024;1:3–15. https://doi.org/10.1016/j.aehs.2024.01.004.
37. Seçkin AÇ, Ateş B, Seçkin M. Review on wearable technology in sports: concepts, challenges and opportunities. Appl Sci. 2023;13:10399. https://doi.org/10.3390/app131810399.

The Biohacking-Code: An Eternal Pursuit of Perfection—The Myth About Living Forever?! From the Fine Line of Self-Optimization to Self-Destruction

7

Stefan Odenbach-Wanner

7.1 Relevance of Biohacking

Biohacking is not only en vogue, but meanwhile a fast-growing industry, because due to the fuzzy definition of the term many miracle cures or methods are labeled, e.g. 20 min. Strength training with power vests or sitting in freeze-rooms or breathe pure Oxygen. In addition to numerous blogs, podcasts, and social media channels, there are more and more providers in major cities who sell paid programs, aids, or tools for self-optimization—sometimes at horrendous prices and especially for anti-aging. As with many other concepts, it is worth taking a closer look at the details of biohacking, because there is still no "magic pill" with an overnight effect and some measures even require an extremely high degree of self-discipline and patience during implementation until a certain state is achieved.

The most prominent example worldwide is the tech millionaire Bryon Johnsons from the USA [1]. He invests 1–2 million every year in his "Blueprint" project in order not only to stop his own aging process, but even to reverse it completely and sell these experimental insights to other people. According to the motto "Forever Young" he tries to get back the body of an 18-year-old at the age of over 40. His daily routine consists of a very strict program, consisting of training, nutrition, regeneration, and all kinds of aids from inside and outside, as well as countless doctors and (blood) tests every day (24/7). He goes far beyond natural limits and accepts pain and asceticism for his personal goal achievement.

The direct comparison with a healthy lifestyle according to the "80/20 method" is also interesting and many people could already achieve much positive for their own health, if certain routines are integrated into everyday life without turning the complete (bio) system upside down. With biohacking, one should also delimit the

S. Odenbach-Wanner (✉)
Faculty of Management, Comenius University, Bratislava, Slovakia
e-mail: odenbach1@uniba.sk

P. Plugmann, D. Portius (eds.), *Innovations in Healthcare and Outcome Measurement*, https://doi.org/10.1007/978-3-031-77302-0_7

target group, because basically people from competitive sports react differently to certain stimuli than the hobby athlete.

This chapter is intended to show the different facets of biohacking and to highlight the opportunities and risks using real examples, as well as to show alternatives.

7.2 Definition of Biohacking

The human body consists of hardware (genes) and software (nerves), which can be controlled by certain stimuli. Under certain conditions, this stimulation can actually cause the body to be reprogrammed and learn a different behavior. For example, a marathon runner can still run faster on fewer calories because he or she has learned to tap into other (energy) sources in the body rather than through pure carbohydrates. In a study with cancer patients, it was investigated how to activate "killer cells" to animate self-healing by destroying the malignant cancer cells.

On the one hand, the whole concept sounds like proven training methods from competitive sports, and on the other hand, some strategies lack the necessary evidence. This is often the case with certain herbal supplements (so-called nootropics), which are supposed to improve mental performance in particular, and this is usually not proven by clinical studies or only over a very small cohort in a short period of time.

Although "biohacking" sounds positive for many individuals (especially on social media) and something worth testing out, the term "hack" also contains some risks to healthy living. If a virus hacks your PC or body, it can be harmful and dangerous [2]. It is the same issue when someone "jailbreak" his or her smartphone, then you lose the warranty in the best case, and in the worst case, the device could be useless [3]. A machine can easily be replaced for some extra money, but the loss of health due to a failed biohack could become a big problem and influence the quality of the rest of a human's life [4].

Therefore, it is mandatory that every biohacking approach informs about the pros and cons of special treatment because often, the actual gain is lower compared to the efforts in time and money [5].

A quote from a US-Health expert Mark Moschel describes biohacking like this:

> ***What sets biohackers apart from the rest of the self-optimization world is their systemic approach to our own biology*** [6].

The following figure shows the bride field of Biohacking at a glance (Fig. 7.1):

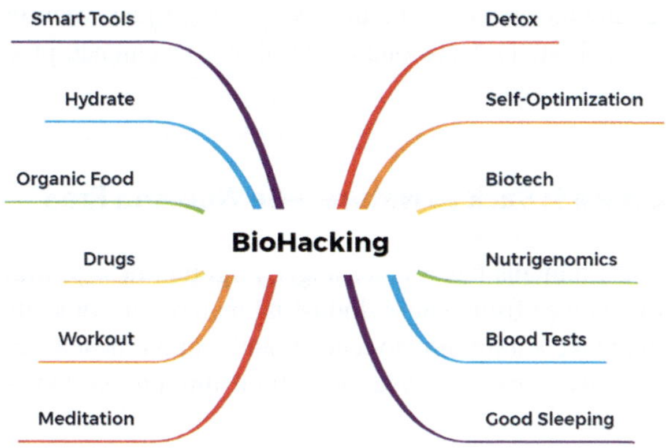

Fig. 7.1 Overview of biohacking (own presentation)

7.3 Seven Principles of Biohacking

As with any method, biohacking also follows a certain pattern, which can be more or less successful if used correctly. Each sub-area can be used in whole or in part, as not every human reacts in the same way to external and internal stimuli. Monitoring, therefore, plays a special role in biohacking, as "gains" can only be detected and visualized if input and output are measured correctly over a certain period of time.

7.3.1 Principle #1: Move Your Body More Often

As the saying goes, "Stagnation is death" and "He who rests, rusts"—the principle of movement is the epitome of progress. If you train your body, muscles, and brain harder and more often, they generally become stronger, provided they don't break under the strain. In today's society, people move much less in everyday life than they did 50 or 100 years ago, as most activities are carried out on a PC or there are machines to do the heavy work. This makes it all the more important to incorporate more exercise during breaks or leisure time, whether it's in the gym or on a daily walk. You don't have to be or become a marathon runner because, with 6000–8000 steps a day, you're already on the right track. Every smartwatch or smartphone can record your daily steps and will also remind you that you have yet to reach your daily target or celebrate new records.

7.3.2 Principle #2: Eat the Right Things at the Right Time

Hippocrates said about 400 B.C.: "*Just as food causes chronic diseases, it can be the most powerful cure.*" For the Greek physician, it was clear that only those who eat healthily can stay healthy. In other words: "*Your food should be your remedy, and your remedy should be your food.*"

So healthy eating has always been an issue, and not just when fast food chains were invented or fish sticks were one of the first convenience products from the freezer.

7.3.3 Principle #3: Back to Nature—Be Wild and Free

In recent centuries, humans have increasingly forgotten how to draw their energy and, thus, their resilience from nature. Industrial man has become effeminate. They fall ill quickly and take a long time to recover and without headache pills or antibiotics, nothing usually works because the natural immune system is disturbed or running on low heat.

If domestication is the problem, as with wolves and dogs, then re-wilding can be the solution. A diet close to nature in the form of less processed products and less industrial sugar is a good start. Alternating showers boost circulation and strengthen the immune system, but few people outside of wellness temples use these natural aids.

7.3.4 Principle #4: Eat Your Greens—and Less Meat

The trend towards a more plant-based diet is not only demonstrably better for the climate due to fewer greenhouse gas emissions from livestock but also better for the human body. This has been shown in various studies of twins with the same gene pool [7], and the benefits of fewer injuries and improved regeneration have also been recognized in competitive sports [8]. A purely vegan diet is not absolutely necessary, but reducing red meat and dairy products can work wonders.

7.3.5 Principle #5: Find a Spring—Drink Natural Water

As with food, we also need to drink more or more of the right thing. In addition to artificial soft drinks with chemical sweeteners, fruit juices are also unhealthy in the long term because of the fructose they contain, and every child knows that alcohol is a harmful neurotoxin. But what many also fail to realize is that water or mineral water can also be a highly processed product that has minerals removed or added and may contain chemical additives. It is therefore advisable to prefer natural mineral water without artificial carbon dioxide, which naturally contains the necessary minerals.

7.3.6 Principle #6: Breathe Easy—Breathe Air from Nature

Do we consider the air we all breathe every day to be food? When you sit in air-conditioned rooms all day, this air passes through many pathways and filters. Exercising regularly in the great outdoors in all weathers and breathing deeply through the diaphragm not only helps to relieve stress but also supplies the muscles with natural oxygen. Of course, only if you don't walk through a stuffy desert of fine dust in a big city, but if possible, in a forest or near green spaces.

7.3.7 Principle #7: Follow the Sun—Expose to Sunlight

Sunlight is part of our natural diet and produces vitamin D, the sun hormone. Artificial light indoors is no substitute for sunlight on the skin. But here, too, you have to be aware of the downsides. Without sun protection, it is also unhealthy in the long term due to skin cancer and premature skin aging. Supplementation with vitamin D is therefore necessary in most regions in Western Europe because otherwise the body produces too little.

7.4 Biohacking Is Monitoring Next Level

Progress means better than before, and therefore, data collection is necessary. Analog journals or digital apps and wearables can be used to continuously control health data like vital parameters, diet, workouts, sleep, or blood. Ideally, health experts and physicians consult this process [6].

In terms of biohacking, the basic pillows of Nutrition, Exercise, and Mindset should be established to control health and well-being, the so-called monitoring—it's like a dashboard with the main KPIs and signals to stay in control [9].

In addition, biohacking is beyond physical health because mental health and an ethical mindset could also improve for better living [9]. Not only is nutrition a main factor of longevity but also behaviors, especially in hard times, and in addition, having sex, like 80% of the people between ages 65 and 100 in the region of Ikaria without the need for enhanced drugs. Independent studies in Great Britain [10] and the USA [11] found that sex is also a verified longevity enhancer for men and women by reducing the coronary heart disease mortality risk by 50%.

Many behavioral interventions, such as kindness, optimism, and stress reduction, can impact life expectancy. This is similar to dietary and fitness behaviors that people should change for their lives not a few weeks after Christmas. These impacts can be huge. For example, optimism can add 10 years to life, or a happy marriage can lower the mortality risk more than a person quitting smoking two packs every day.

In an ideal scenario, all these things add up and work best together. Healthy plant-based eating, exercise regularly, and being kind, social, ethical, optimistic, and conscientious are the key elements of longevity [12].

7.4.1 From Blue Zones to Blue Print: Living Longer vs. Living Forever?!

Survival of the fittest has been the main issue since the beginning of humankind. In the Stone Age, humans could only survive if they were faster and smarter than the saber-toothed tiger. Later, in Egypt, Cleopatra and the Pharaohs experimented with the first Anti-Aging therapies, like bathing in honey and milk. Mummification was also intended to enable the soul to return to the body in the afterlife. To summarize the lessons learned of the people in the Blue Zones: Not only the nutrition is a main factor of longevity, but also the behaviors, and this without the need of enhanced drugs [13].

Nowadays, survival is not the main problem, but long and healthy living is an emerging trend again. Based on GARTNER's Hype Cycle for emerging technologies, the Hype Cycle of Digital Health is the adaptation for BioHacking, and Gartner said in 2018: "AI and biohacking will shape the future of tech" [14].

Today, a few years later, there are a significant number of solutions available according to this trend:

The Hype Cycle contains five key phases of a technology in the life cycle, starting with the "Innovation Trigger," when a potential technology appears for the first time and often no usable products exist and commercial viability is unproven. Over the "Peak of Inflated Expectations," when the first success stories are published and the first movers, companies take action and learn from failures. Until the bottom "Trough of Disillusionment," when experiments or implementations of products fail, and the satisfaction of early adopters is lower than expected. Slope to the "Path of Enlightenment," when second- and third-generation products appear and enterprises fund pilots because the benefits are more visible for a wider range of users. Ideally, the cycle ends with the "Plateau of Productivity," when the relevance of the technologies is clear for mainstream adopters to bring it market applicability and the criteria for assessing paying off [15]. Biohacking has reached the phases of adoption, and products are available all over the world, some are famous, and others are only discussed in experts' circles [16].

7.5 Biohacking in Practice

Biohacking differs from conventional medicine in many ways, although biohacking is based on its methods and diagnostics for self-optimization. This goes far beyond sleep monitoring or dietary changes and can sometimes go far beyond mental and physical performance or is simply outlandish.

The following table (Table 7.1) compares the main differences:

There is more than just one way to biohack yourself. Biohacking looks at all aspects of human life, including diet, exercise, sex, sleep, and mental health. In some extreme cases, what is often referred to as "true biohacking" is about more than just a healthy lifestyle but maximum performance enhancement.

More ambitious biohackers often even undergo medical interventions despite questionable success, have computer chips implanted in various parts of their bodies, and use neurofeedback to regulate their brainwaves, and these are just a few examples. Inspired by biotechnology and "transhumanism," these people want to blur the line between humans and technology [17].

Table 7.1 Comparison of conventional medicine vs. biohacking (based on source digiwell.com [1])

Criteria [1]	Conventional medicine [1]	Biohacking [1]
Center of attention?	Treat symptoms	Focus on more energy and better energy production
Orientation on what?	Disease-oriented	Health-oriented
Understanding of body as?	The body as a collection of independent organs	The body as an integrated quantifiable system
Optimization through?	Prescribing medication	Other lifestyle, science, nature, technology, nutritional supplements
Longevity because of?	Higher life expectancy	Higher health expectation
Focus on whom? [1]	DOCTOR-oriented [1]	SELF-oriented [1]

Source: Biohacking comparison by digiwell.com [1]

Whether moderate or radical, biohacking can generally be divided into four categories [1]:

7.5.1 Category #1: Nutrigenomics

This form of biohacking involves the conscious manipulation of nutrition, in contrast to classic health and mind hacking (sleep, fitness, meditation). Not only natural foods are served, but artificial substances such as hormones or steroids are often included in the diet plan. Nutrigenomic biohackers make all their nutritional decisions with the aim of improving their physical or mental performance and not necessarily living healthier or longer (e.g. BodyBuilder).

7.5.2 Category #2: 3D Bioprinting

Bioprinting is a special form of biohacking in which organic substances are artificially created in a 3D printer. This process originally comes from the research field of tissue engineering, i.e., computer-controlled techniques for creating organic structures from living tissue. Biohackers see opportunities here to print certain extensions—so-called enhancements—for their own bodies using their own tissue (e.g., flippers between the toes of extreme swimmers).

7.5.3 Category #3: DIY Biology or DNA Hacking

In the old millennium, experiments were mostly carried out on the basis of chemical or physical laboratory tests. Since the new millennium, DNA hacking has increasingly become the focus of attention and today the human genome has been fully decoded. Some protagonists only hack the DNA of bacteria and make it glow, while others carry out biological experiments on themselves or their environment. In the USA, for example, DNA hacking is already widespread in dog breeding, and it is said that "designer babies" are already possible in Asian countries (e.g., the choice of eye color among other characteristics, as in the car configurator).

In the future, it is conceivable that a DNA biohacker could use his own body cells and examine them at home or inject CRISPR DNA into his own body (in extreme cases, carry out his own fecal transplants).

7.5.4 Category #4: Grinder Biohacking or Body Hacking

By far the most extreme form of biohacking is grinder biohacking or body hacking. In this form, the human is depicted as a machine and is fixated on using technology to push the limits of the human body far beyond its limits.

Grinder biohackers are known for making their lives easier and smoother by implanting microchips, magnets, RFID transponders, data transmitters, or other aids into their bodies. The reason for this body optimization is not always a pronounced lifestyle, but these microchip implants can also help people with physical disabilities to cope better with everyday life, such as replacing the front door key with a microchip or carrying medical emergency data under the skin, always ready to hand for the emergency doctor.

Some of the microchip implants used in body hacking are no bigger than a grain of rice. They can be inserted under the first layer of skin in seconds and removed again. However, the digital possibilities can also take on more extreme forms (see Brainchip Neuralink by Elon Musk).

7.6 Project BLUEPRINT: Beyond Longevity

The most extreme example of Biohacking from Self-Experiments to ready-to-use products is the project "Blueprint" from the US-Tech Billionaire Bryan Johnson. After his lucrative exit from one of his tech companies, Bryan Johnson was looking for a new target and launched 2021 his own Blueprint project and his outcomes promises a way back to youth again:

> ***Two years and millions were spent developing Blueprint, an algorithm that takes better care of me than I can myself. Now, you can build your autonomous self as well*** [18].

Since then, he has invested 1–2 million US dollars every year in his partly experimental rejuvenation methods and swallows over 100 pills a day, following a strict protocol with special routines in the areas of nutrition and fitness. He is also the best-measured person in the world, as he is equipped with gadgets from head to toe and sometimes wears them at night (even in his private parts). Bryan measures everything and undergoes tests almost every day and has his blood values and DNA continuously monitored.

Table 7.2 Current results from 3 years with Blueprint (based on source protocol.bryanjohnson.com [18])

Top-results [18]	Other achievements [18]
Top 1%: speed of aging (epigenetic) Top 1%: muscle mass and function Top 1%: fat mass Top 1%: inflammation Top 1%: VO_2 max (cardiovascular) Top 1%: bone mass Top 1%: sleep Top 1%: combined clinical markers [18]	+ Speed of aging slower than 99% of 20-year-olds + Body inflammation is 85% below the average 18-year-old (hsCRP 0.15) + VO_2 max: 58.7 mL/(kg·min), top 1.5% of 18-year-old + Total Bone Mineral Density top 0.2% of 30-year-old + Nighttime erections 179 min, better than ave. 18-year-old + Perfect liver fat (1.36%, top 10%), iron and stiffness (MRI) + Top 99.5% muscle volume + Bottom 0.5% visceral fat, muscle fat, and subcutaneous fat volume + Top 1% sleep performance and recovery (whoop) + Possibly increased thymocyte volume to 7 years younger, further testing + Ideal whole body muscle and fat (MRI) + 50+ optimal clinical outcome biomarkers + 100+ markers < chronological age + Perfect liver markers: ALT + AST + GGT = 49 + Leg press single rep max: 800 lb. Top 1–2% of 18-year-old + Bench press single rep max: 240 lb. Top 10% of 18-year-old + 12 year age reversal in 500 day average HRV + Reduced Alpha Klotho biological age by 21 years in 5 months (from 42) + 31 year age reversal in gray hair age (80% reduction in gray hair) + Identified and corrected (w/o surgery) ticking time bomb: bilateral internal jugular vein (IJV) stenosis + 30+ organ ages quantified + Free testosterone index (FTI) biological age reduced 20 years + Improved homocysteine (hcy) by 49% (5.9 µmol/L) [18]

Source: Blueprint protocol by protocol.bryanjohnson.com [18]

Bryan says Blueprint is affordable for everyone and costs "only" 1000–1500 US dollars per month, the millions he had invested were mostly for research and development because much of his Blueprint protocols is not rocket science at first sight (1) Diet and meal preps, (2) Fitness routine, (3) Sleep protocol, (4) Oral health, (5) Skin health, (6) Supplements, (7) Tracking and monitoring. Therefore, he shares his results publicly on his blog and on social media for free, and his progress, or regression in his case, in terms of the aging process is quite remarkable (see the results in the following Table 7.2):

Based on his measurement results, Longevity Millionaire Bryan Johnson also only celebrates his birthday every 19 months, as he claims his mortality would be slower due to Blueprint.

In addition, Johnson created a "Rejuvenation Olympics" with a leaderboard of the best biohackers. Which is a global community dedicated to understanding and improving aging. The stated goal is to advance the science of biological aging through rigorous competition and collaboration [1].

7.7 Discussion About Blueprint-Biohacking by B. Johnson

What is remarkable about Bryan Johnson's Blueprint experiment is that his unconditional commitment to his health for the purpose of science evidently goes beyond the monetary aspect, even if the typical American advertising messages for his Blueprint supplements on his webshop sometimes give a different impression and sales are the main focus there.

His endeavors indicate his unwavering focus on health and longevity. He exemplifies the philosophy through his meticulous work without compromise and is certainly a role model for many imitators of a similar mindset who seek the conscious and subconscious alignment of the mind in the pursuit of well-being.

Johnson sometimes takes complex paths to a deeper understanding and commitment to his own health, and his findings benefit others directly or indirectly to some extent. His willingness to share and demystify this knowledge is invaluable.

7.8 Conclusion and Future Outlook

At Europe's largest future institute, the "2b AHEAD ThinkTank" in Germany, scientists, managers, and innovation leaders from the industry discuss possible future scenarios and strategy recommendations for the next 10 years [19].

The "future of genetics" and humanity's dream of eternal life were already the subject of controversial discussion in 2018. According to the forecast for 2030, "designer babies" and deliberate interventions in genetics are the order of the day, and the ethical question increasingly arises as to whether genetically modified ("improved") humans will still be humans in the traditional sense.

7.8.1 People Are Becoming Healthcare Consumers

Futurologists expect the biggest change between now and 2030 to be in the way people deal with illness and health. Billions are being invested in this area by technology companies and investors in innovative start-ups. The formula for success is very simple: health is already measurable, optimizable, and therefore increasingly for sale. This does not mean two-tier medicine, which is propagated by private health insurance companies, because there will be offers for every budget. The biggest trend of 2030 is, therefore, a completely different one, namely individualized medicine!

Conversely, this means that we will no longer inevitably die from genetic defects [20].

In the next decade, the focus will be on "genetic engineering," the third key enabling technology alongside artificial intelligence and quantum computing. At the beginning of the 2000s, a complete analysis of the genome was far too expensive for the masses because the computing power was too low and the costs too uneconomical. This is changing rapidly due to the exponential development of computer performance and the simultaneous disproportionate fall in prices. Complete genome analysis will then no longer cost less than 100 US dollars, but will be somewhere in the cent range. In the age of the smartphone, every modern person will soon have their genetic code literally in their hands, and if they wish, health insurance companies will be able to use big data to proactively point out potential health risks. And what will happen then?

The CRISPR technology described above could be the new panacea for diseases, bringing us a great deal closer to the human dream of eternal life. The field of biohacking is, therefore, only the peak of the iceberg of future improvements in health through the usage of modern technology from the outside and the inside of the human body [21].

So is the human being a programmed machine after all, which can be optimized by intervening in the genetic code through genetics or biohacking? Or are other technologies necessary, as the proponents of "epigenetics" suggest?

Epigenetics is a rapidly growing field of research that scientifically investigates the interactions between genes and environmental factors. In classical genetics, the focus is exclusively on the DNA sequence. In contrast, epigenetics deals with complex molecular changes without changing the DNA sequence itself and can regulate gene expression at the same time.

The research field of epigenetics offers far-reaching implications for a completely new understanding of the interactions between health and disease. For example, typical environmental factors such as nutrition, stress, or toxins can cause epigenetic changes and affect the health of living organisms. An exciting aspect of this is that some of these changes are even reversible. As a result, targeted therapies can be developed and applied in a targeted manner, e.g., through a specific dietary change or better stress management, in order to change epigenetic measures and thus prevent, treat, or even prevent potential diseases. Epigenetics thus represents an extension of our understanding of genetics and offers completely new approaches for the preventive treatment of specific diseases. It, therefore, forms the basis for personalized medicine, which takes epigenetic variables into account in addition to purely genetic factors [22].

References

1. TruDiagnostic, LLC (REJUVENATIONOLYMPICS.com). The leaderboards: where you win by never crossing the finish line. 2024. https://rejuvenationolympics.com/leaderboard. Last accessed 16 Mar 2024.
2. Heise Medien GmbH & Co. KG (HEISE.de). Warnung vor dem Biohacking. 2017. https://www.heise.de/blog/Warnung-vor-dem-Biohacking-3894885.htm. Last accessed 11 Jan 2024.
3. BIOMES NGS GmbH (BIOMES.world). Biohacking und Ernährung: Vorsicht vor Selbstoptimierungswahn. 2020. https://biomes.world/de/presseportal/biohacking-und-ernaehrung-2. Last accessed 17 Feb 2024.
4. G+J Medien GmbH (GEO.de). GESUNDHEIT - Biohacking: Was hinter dem System der Selbstoptimierung steckt. 2021. https://www.geo.de/wissen/gesundheit/23998-rtkl-gesundheit-biohacking-was-hinter-dem-system-der-selbstoptimierung. Last accessed 22 Mar 2024.
5. Memon Bionic Instruments GmbH (MEMON.eu). Was ist Biohacking? 2023. https://www.memon.eu/es-ES/blog/biohacking. Last accessed 21 Mar 2024.
6. Medium publishing platform (MEDIUM.com). The beginner's guide to biohacking. 2014. https://betterhumans.pub/the-beginners-guide-to-biohacking-5179b9967c16. Last accessed 3 Mar 2024.

7. Nat. Geographic (nationalgeographic.de). Zwillingsstudie zeigt: Wer sich vegan ernährt, lebt länger. 2023. https://www.nationalgeographic.de/wissenschaft/2023/12/zwillingsstudie-zeigt-wer-sich-vegan-ernaehrt-lebt-laenger-gesundheit-fleisch-essen?image=iss068e041225-large. Last accessed 15 Mar 2024.
8. JAMA Network Journals of the American Medical Association (jamanetwork.com). Cardiometabolic effects of omnivorous vs vegan diets in identical twins a randomized clinical trial. 2023. https://jamanetwork.com/journals/jamanetworkopen/fullarticle/2812392?resultClick=3. Last accessed 15 Mar 2024.
9. Prestige online (prestigeonline.com). What is biohacking? A look at the growing global trend for science-based health optimisation. 2021. https://www.prestigeonline.com/th/lifestyle/wellness/biohacking-is-the-growing-global-trend-for-science-based-health-optimisation. Last accessed 15 Jan 2024.
10. Smith GD, Frankel S, Yarnell J. Sex and death: are they related? Findings from the Caerphilly cohort study. BMJ. 1997;315:1641. https://doi.org/10.1136/bmj.315.7123.1641. Last accessed 8 Feb 2024.
11. Liu H, Waite LJ, Shen S, Wang DH. Is sex good for your health? A national study on partnered sexuality and cardiovascular risk among older men and women. J Health Soc Behav. 2016;57(3):276–96. https://doi.org/10.1177/0022146516661597. Last accessed 29 Feb 2024.
12. Zaraska M. Growing young: how friendship, optimism, and kindness can help you live to 100. Softcover, 2020. ISBN-13: 9780525610182.
13. Bluezones LLC (BLUEZONES.com). The Blue Zones explorations. 2024. https://www.bluezones.com/live-longer-better. Last accessed 5 Feb 2024.
14. GARTNER, Inc. (GARTNER.com). Gartner identifies five emerging technology trends that will blur the lines between human and machine. 2018. https://siliconangle.com/2018/08/20/gartner-says-ai-biohacking-will-shape-future-tech. Last accessed 8 Mar 2024.
15. Price L. UCL Global Business School for Health (HEALTHCARE.digital): "Digital Health Hype Cycle 2023". 2021. https://www.healthcare.digital/single-post/digital-health-hype-cycle-2021 and https://www.linkedin.com/pulse/digital-health-hype-cycle-2021-lloyd-price. Last accessed 12 Jan 2024.
16. Webicina Kft (MEDICALFUTURIST.com). Hype cycle of the top 50 emerging digital health trends by the medical futurist. 2023. https://medicalfuturist.com/healthcare-trends-hype-cycle. Last accessed 20 Mar 2024.
17. Upgraded Humans (DIGIWELL.com). Biohacking: Die Suche nach dem ewigen Leben. 2021. https://digiwell.com/biohacking_suche_nach_dem_ewigen_leben. Last accessed 29 Jul 2024.
18. Blueprint Labs (BLUEPRINT.BryanJohnson.com). DON'T DIE—blueprint protocol. 2024. https://protocol.bryanjohnson.com. Last accessed 17 Mar 2024.
19. 2b AHEAD ThinkTank GmbH (2bAHEAD.com). Die Zukunft der Genetik: Von Designerbabies und dem Traum ewigen Lebens. 2018. https://www.zukunft.business/foresight/trendanalysen/analyse/die-zukunft-der-genetik-von-designerbabies-und-dem-traum-ewigen-lebens. Last accessed 31 Jan 2024.
20. Jánszky SG, Absicht L. 2030: Wie viel Mensch verträgt die Zukunft? Softcover. 2018. ISBN-13: 978-3947590049.
21. 2b AHEAD ThinkTank GmbH (2bAHEAD.com). Die Zukunft von Krankheit: Der Mensch als Gesundheitskonsument. 2019. https://www.zukunft.business/foresight/trendanalysen/analyse/die-zukunft-von-krankheit-der-mensch-als-gesundheitskonsument. Last accessed 31 Jan 2024.
22. Akademie für menschliche Medizin GmbH (SPITZEN-PRAEVENTION.com). Zeit für ein neues Paradigma: Epigenetik als Grundlage einer Neuen Gesundheitskultur. 2023. https://spitzen-praevention.com/2023/11/05/epigenetik-neue-gesundheitskultur. Last accessed 29 Mar 2024.

Stefan Odenbach-Wanner (MBA) is like the Swiss army knife for digital health thanks to his many years of expertise in the healthcare sector. His main job is in the pharmaceutical world. He does a lot of sport and is also a certified personal trainer and nutritionist.

8 Futuristic Dentistry: Towards Medical–Dental Integration and Minimalistic Approaches

Andrea Lorena Basualdo Allende

8.1 Oral Microbiome and Further Applications

In the latest years, there has been growing interest in oral microbiome, in healthy and disease states. The composition of the oral microbiome is strongly associated with periodontal disease and dental caries. This condition, "dysbiosis," means a substantial detrimental alteration in the relative abundances and individual components of the microbiome and dysbiosis of the oral microbiome that is responsible for dental caries and periodontal disease. But the most important fact is that this dynamic behavior leads to bidirectional communication between the oral cavity and systemic organs [1, 2].

In fact, there is increasing evidence linking the oral microbiota to systemic diseases, such as obesity, diabetes, cardiovascular disease, inflammatory bowel disease, nonalcoholic fatty liver disease, rheumatoid arthritis, colorectal cancers, and Alzheimer's disease [2]. Oral illnesses, such as dental caries, are significantly influenced by the oral microbiome. Oral bacteria are related with disease states, such as diabetes, and various forms of cancer, such as pancreatic cancer associated with periodontitis. The presence of *Porphyromonas gingivalis* and *Fusobacterium nucleatum* cause poor prognosis in colorectal cancer patients and the decrease in *Prevotella histicola* and *Prevotella oulorum* have been seen in patients with rheumatoid arthritis and cognitive decline. But oral bacteria may also affect the dietary preferences of their human hosts, and they, as an ecosystem, interact, like for example, *Lactobacilli* can inhibit the proliferation of *S. mutans* [3, 4].

The influence of habits on the salivary microbiome are so important, for example, smokers have distinct bacteria in relation to age. Likewise, also dietary habits,

The original version of the chapter has been revised. A correction to this chapter can be found at https://doi.org/10.1007/978-3-031-77302-0_16

A. L. B. Allende (✉)
SOCCAS (Sociedad Chilena Calidad Asistencial), Chilean Society of Quality in Healthcare Institutions, Santiago, Chile
e-mail: rrii@soccas.cl

P. Plugmann, D. Portius (eds.), *Innovations in Healthcare and Outcome Measurement*, https://doi.org/10.1007/978-3-031-77302-0_8

alcoholism, and consumption of coffee can affect oral microbiome. More important, benefits of salivary microbiome in forensics, could help in the characterization of an individual's habits, like smoking, alcohol consumption, and dietary preferences [5]. In cases where sufficient human DNA can't be collected from a crime scene, microbiome analysis can provide valuable forensic insights. [6].

The growing evidence linking the oral microbiome with several systemic diseases had opened new doors, and new tests are now on the market that give personalized oral care products. Some of them use RNA technology to discover health insights and develop precise and personalized nutritional products, empowering people to take control of their health. Healthy eating has been identified as a priority area by the World Health Organization when initiating and strengthening oral health programs [7, 8].

Higher vegetable consumption is associated with lower caries incidence, and nitrates as a supplement to diet can also have important anticaries effects. The long-term intake of nitrate-rich vegetables and fruits can reduce the risk of cancer and cardiovascular disease and facilitate longevity. In the oral cavity, nitric oxide (NO) seems to inhibit sensitive species as part of the nonspecific oral immune system, and exogenous administration of nitrate can maintain a balance in the pH of saliva. A decreased concentration of nitrate is typical in the saliva of patients with dental caries compared with healthy individuals and during caries progression [9, 10]. However, the relationship between periodontitis, nitrate-rich foods, and systemic health consequences is yet to be elucidated [11].

In recent years, accumulating evidence has highlighted the beneficial roles of various foods, including fermented products, such as kombucha, yogurt, kefir, kvass, kimchi and sauerkraut, as well as other dairy-based foods like butter-milk. [3, 4]. Also, a blend of essential oils, which includes peppermint, Japanese mint, bergamot mint, and spearmint essential oils, has been suggested in a recent study to reduce the abundance of bacteria associated with halitosis and periodontal diseases, such as *Actinomyces* and *Streptococcus*. The study also found an increase in *Corynebacterium* species and a decrease in *Streptococcus* following its usage [12].

Also, genetic markers are being investigated that may allow personalizing the therapeutic approach toward various diseases, so the possibility of realizing personalized programs that can monitor the microbial environment of the oral cavity responsible for caries, periodontitis, and cancers, in addition to masticatory and respiratory function would lead to a better management of the cost-benefit of the budget of the healthcare system [3]. Secretory S IgA produced by the oral mucosa and salivary glands can bind to viruses and resident bacteria blocking their adherence to the oral mucosa and can also bind to those that have not yet caused infection. So it can be a powerful tool against novel pathogens like severe acute respiratory syndrome coronavirus 2 (SARS-CoV2) [4].

Nevertheless, all the progress made, there are still some questions remaining, like: How does a particular group of bacteria impact others within the population and the rest of the oral microbial community? Is it possible to shift to a state of dysbiosis to symbiosis by selectively targeting specific groups or subgroups of bacteria and regulate their growth? These and other emerging questions are sure to arise as research in this field advances [1].

8.2 Saliva Biomarkers and Chronic Inflammation

Human saliva is like a "body mirror" because it can reflect the physiological and pathological conditions of the whole body, including the oral cavity. Therefore, it can represent an important diagnostic and monitoring tool in many fields such as dentistry, allowing dentists to assess some medical conditions, such as in athletes, or other situations that require an oral health advisor [13].

Dentistry has been for several years a leader in analyzing gingival and crevicular fluids to detect oral disorders, medical conditions, and do monitoring, but now the groundbreaking results from salivary analysis have led to a significant paradigm shift in diagnostic analyses. Salivary glands can exchange different compounds by passive diffusion or active transport, from blood to saliva and vice versa. Saliva testing is also based on its versatility in covering genomics, proteomics, microbiomics, metabolomics, and transcriptomics [14]. For example, bacterial endotoxins that are found in saliva contain lipopolysaccharides. Quantitative evaluation of *Porphyromonas gingivalis* lipopolysaccharides has become a key measure in oral health, because the salivary presence in a high concentration suggests a chronic periodontitis disease, but also because of the implications in other important systemic diseases [15].

The diagnostic utility of saliva to detect cardiovascular diseases, systemic and local inflammation, and endocrinological and metabolic disorders seems to get more importance bidirectionally [16]. Also because, preventing periodontitis and maintaining periodontal health may contribute to the control of metabolic syndrome, as both are significantly associated. This association seems to be stronger in women [17, 18].

Chronic diseases, including cardiovascular diseases, cancer, obesity, and type 2 diabetes, are becoming increasingly prevalent and place substantial financial strains on healthcare systems. These costs arise not only from the direct expenses of treatment but also from the long-term nature of these conditions, their acute exacerbations, and the significant psychological and emotional burden they impose on patients and caregivers. Interestingly, early prevention is possible, but the culture of prevention is not well rooted in the healthcare systems, yet even that are actions helping on that matter. Most chronic diseases are preceded by a chronic low-grade inflammation, this make possible that conceivable biomarkers can be measured, acute phase proteins, cytokines and chemokines, pro-inflammatory enzymes, and oxidative stress mediators [16]. This is particularly crucial in Type 2 Diabetes Mellitus, where changes in the oral microbiome highlight the need for standardized research methods to enhance understanding of its role and develop improved diagnostic and therapeutic strategies [19].

In relation with nitric oxide (NO) levels, there is a pioneering diagnostic method to determine pathological conditions of the oral cavity in exhaled air, which suggests that the measurement of NO in exhaled air can be a complementary, noninvasive diagnostic monitoring method. So, for example, the level of NO concentration in the exhaled air turned out to be lower in patients with good oral hygiene. This approach can also be applied in the diagnosis of COVID-19, as studies have demostrated that vaccinated individuals with a history of COVID-19, as well as post-COVID-19 patients, exhibit significant higher levels of NO in exhaled air compared to vaccinated individuals without a prior history of the disease. [20].

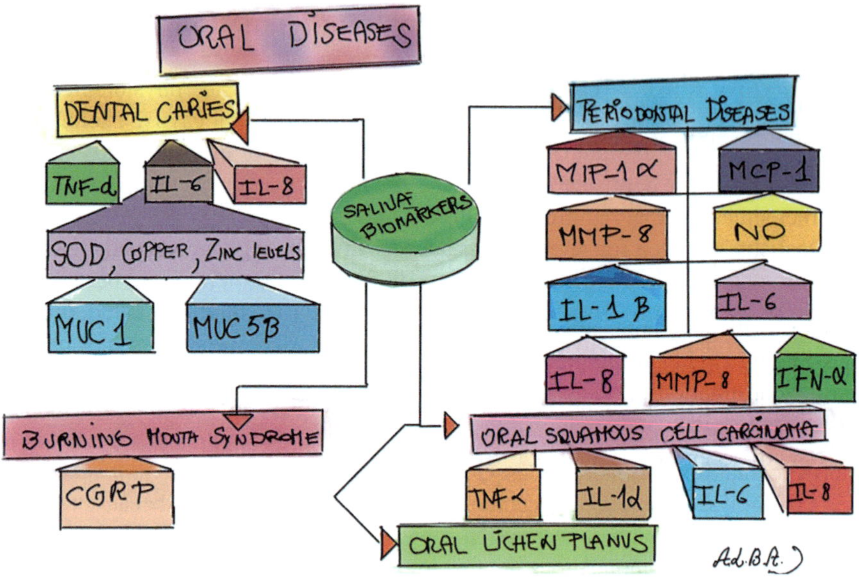

Fig. 8.1 Saliva biomarkers in oral diseases

Salivary NO is significantly higher in normotensive when compared to hypertensive subjects [21]. *Haemophilus* and *Neisseria* are essential oral nitrate-reducing bacteria that regulate systemic blood pressure (BP) via the nitrate-nitrite-NO pathway. A dysbiosis or reduction of these critical salivary bacteria that regulate BP may promote endothelial dysfunction and increase the risk of cardiovascular disease [22, 23].

The promising applications of human-derived saliva biomarker testing can be categorizedas follows:

Biomarkers for oral diseases, gastroenterological cancers, and forensic body fluid identification: These include long noncoding RNAs, microRNAs, circular RNAs and messenger RNAs, which show potential in disease identification and forensic applications. Biomarkers for disease diagnosis and prognosis: Salivary biomarkers such as DNA methylation, cell-free DNA, circulating tumor DNA and telomere length are emerging as valuable tools for the early detection and prognosis of various diseases. Diagnostic and prognostic indicators: Enzymes, hormones, immunoglobulins, glycoproteins, and C-reactive protein provide critical insights into disease diagnosis and progression. Exosomes in cancer diagnostics and aging research: Exosomes are gaining recognition for their role in cancer diagnosis and as key indicators in the study of aging processes. (Fig. 8.1). Among these potential biomarkers, salivary hormones have emerged as particularly promising candidates for clinical diagnostic applications.

So, saliva testing shows value for diagnostics in oral diseases, diabetes, renal diseases, hepatitis, neurodegenerative diseases, and immunodeficiency disease and even in psychological states. Free cortisol levels in saliva can show psychobiological states [24]. Even in dental caries, nitrite (NO_2^-) levels in saliva are a possible biomarker, showing lower NO_2^- levels in children affected by dental caries [25].

8.3 Oral Wearables and Digital Biomarkers in Saliva

Saliva, as a noninvasive diagnostic tool, can identify and quantify various biomarkers. For instance, it can detect Interleukin-6 (IL-6), which tends to increase in elderly subjects, and tumor necrosis factor alpha (TNFα), IL-1, C-reactive protein (CRP), α1-acid glycoprotein, and fibrinogen, which also exhibit age-related elevation. Additionally, elevated levels of IL-18, IL-2, IL-17, and IL-12 have been observed in the elderly, often associated with conditions like cardiovascular diseases, stroke, type 1 diabetes, Alzheimer's disease, and osteoarthritis. Overweight individuals tend to have increased C-reactive protein levels [16, 26].

The incorporation of oral wearable biosensors to measure saliva biomarkers has been made possible through recent advancements in microelectronics, nanotechnology, and the Internet of Things. The oral cavity's exceptional adaptability, physiological significance, and abundance of biomarkers have positioned it as an optimal site for health monitoring using wearable sensors, with diverse applications in the biomedical field. Wearable devices, when paired with smartphone apps, are gaining popularity for monitoring various health aspects, such as pain levels, postoperative symptoms, wound healing progress, and even home oral health habits [14]. What distinguishes oral wearable sensors is their capability to continuously track the physical and chemical parameters within the oral cavity to manage health, all the while enabling users to move freely without disruption. Notably, oral sensors offer unique advantages over devices applied to the skin or eyes, owing to the oral cavity's natural tolerance for foreign substances [27].

These biosensors can communicate wirelessly with computers and smartphones, allowing for online data analysis and data transfer via Wi-Fi and Bluetooth low energy [27].

Oral wearable sensors are based on wearable sensor technology and can be used for dental disease monitoring, salivary biochemical monitoring, and food-intake monitoring. This tool holds significant importance as a novel diagnostic and prognostic tool for chronic disorders, aligning with the broader quest for personalized medicine and dentistry. Once saliva biomarkers are detected, they can be combined with the genetic and anthropometric characteristics of patients [9].

An optimal salivary sensor must have a seamless integration with the oral anatomy, ensuring minimal discomfort for prolonged wear. It should be mechanically robust and securely fixed in the oral cavity, to prevent accidental ingestion. Therefore, various sensor formats like flexible polymer foils on mouthguards, pacifier, dentures, vacuum-formed oral appliances, or silk-based dental tattoos have been innovatively developed to address these requirements [28]. The detected data can be transmitted wirelessly to nearby smart phones and networks. Oral wearable sensors for food intake monitoring are supposed to prevent diseases and aid in treatment via formulating personalized dietary interventions to individuals based on their personal condition. With the help of oral wearable sensors, people can achieve healthy diets as well as healthy lifestyles more easily than before.

It is well known that higher vegetable consumption is associated with lower caries incidence. Long-term intake of nitrate-rich vegetables and fruits can reduce the risk of cancer and cardiovascular disease and facilitate longevity. A decreased concentration of nitrate is typical in the saliva of patients with dental caries [9, 10]. The appearance and development of diet sensors can indeed reduce the risk of disease and improve general health and lifetime of humans to some extent [29]. Furthermore, the monitoring of food intake can be executed by physical sensors that precisely capture oral motion [27, 29, 30].

When it comes to oral health, predicting the risk of caries involves assessing various factors, including the presence of cariogenic bacteria, histatin peptides, IgA, and IgG. Additionally, hidden dental caries has been linked to the local release of volatile sulfur compounds, stemming from the breakdown of sulfur-containing proteins by anaerobic bacteria. Consequently, the preliminary diagnosis of the hidden dental caries could be confirmed via monitoring the local release of volatile sulfur compounds [31].

To assess susceptibility to develop periodontal diseases are many salivary biomarkers, such as salivary IgA and IgG against the pathogens *Porphyromonas gingivalis* and *Treponema Denticola*, IL-6, Matrix metalloproteinase-8 (MMP-8), and Prostaglandin E2 (PGE2). Salivary biopsy has also been explored for the early detection of head and neck cancer, with cell-free DNA (cfDNA) and cell-free mitochondrial DNA (cf mtDNA) from saliva serving as reliable indicators of cancer severity, prognosis, and the risk of oral mucositis associated with radiotherapy. Proteomics has revealed that specific protein concentrations are associated with a predisposition to mucositis as a side effect of radiotherapy. Interestingly, salivary lactate dehydrogenase can be employed for the diagnosis, prognosis, and monitoring of oral cancer, as well as for tracking tobacco users and oral potentially malignant disorders [3, 32].

In Orthodontics, Smart brackets allow dentists to learn the exact force applied to teeth rather than estimate by experience, so that risks of orthodontic treatment caused by excessive force can be greatly reduced. However, there remain challenges when applying dental sensors to multiple teeth simultaneously, resulting in a significant volume of data [14, 33].

In implantology, oral wearables can help as an important indicator to monitor peri-implant diseases, given that temperature can be a targeting parameter of inflammation with the measure of the local temperature near the implant [27].

Currently, there is no consensus on which biomarkers should be used for what specific targets and with which intention. But metalloproteinases and interleukins seem to be the most promising ones, at least in periodontology, where personalized workflows are easier to implement. Additionally, implantology presents an intriguing field for exploring biomarker utilization, especially in cases of peri-implantitis [34].

Early diagnosis holds paramount significance in public health. Dentistry has the potential to serve as a gateway for routine diagnostic practices in medicine, thereby contributing to medical-dental integration. This approach seeks to promote a more holistic model of healthcare, where dentists are not solely focused on oral rehabilitation but are also aware of the intricate relationship between oral health and systemic health. [3, 20, 34]. Maintaining a good oral health and engaging in social interactions are factors related to a better cognitive function. Early monitoring of these biomarkers can prevent disease burden in the future [33]. However, the use of salivary biomarkers for diagnostics is challenged by the natural variability in saliva composition, influenced by factors such as age, gender, diet, circadian rhythms, and health status. Hormonal fluctuations, dehydration, and salivary gland dysfunction further complicate biomarker levels. Additionally, stability during collection, storage, and transport is also critical, as enzymatic activity and biochemical processes can alter biomarker profiles. Addressing these challenges is vital to ensure the reliability of saliva as a diagnostic tool in clinical settings [35].

Efforts to better integrate dental and medical Electronic Health Records (EHRs), establish consistent methods for incorporating patient genetics, enhance natural language processing capabilities, and provide additional training to dentists in data science and vice versa [14].

8.4 Teledentistry, AI, and Metaverse: The Golden Team

Oral health is based on the United Nations 2030 Agenda for Sustainable Development and its 17 goals. The World Health Organization's Global Strategy on Oral Health calls for prioritizing sustainable and less invasive care. Clinical disciplines in dentistry urgently require advancements in diagnostic methodologies, treatment planning, leadership strategies, and teledentistry-based monitoring systems.require urgently, update, for diagnosis, treatment scheduling, leadership, and telemedicine surveillance. AI is currently mostly used in dentistry to evaluate digital diagnostic techniques, particularly radiology. AI also has several applications in endodontics, such as the anatomy of the root canal system, detecting periapical lesions and root fractures, determining working length measurements, predicting the viability of dental pulp stem cells, and predicting the success of retreatment procedures. In maxillofacial surgery, applications include predicting outcomes and planning orthognathic and craniofacial surgical procedures. In therapeutic dentistry, the detection of dental caries on periapical radiographs can be performed with the help of a deep learning-based convolutional neural network algorithm [36–40].

Teledentistry offers enhanced access to dental care, particularly benefitting people with special needs, like the elderly, patients with health disparities, and those in remote areas that lack dental services. It proves value by reducing the necessity for in-person dental visits, saving time, improving treatment adherence and telemonitoring. It has an undiscovered worldwide value in managing dental emergencies. Uses of teledentistry are in cariology, oral pathology and oral medicine, endodontics, and oral radiology, as well as in dental education. In the field of oral pathology, teledentistry highly proves value, contributing to precise diagnosis and early detection of oral cancer. Moreover, when integrated with intraoral and high-resolution extraoral cameras, it extends the reach of specialized care to patients in rural communities, thereby substantially improving access to dental services [41, 42].

The use of teledentistry in schools, for early detection of dental caries and oral diseases for non-dental and dental personnel is believed to be cost-effective and it can also help in detecting child abuse [43].

However, the global implementation of teledentistry faces challenges, as it depends on country-specific policies and laws that may facilitate or not. Some countries mistakenly adapt telemedicine policies for teledentistry, despite differences in scope and treatment end points. Teledentistry's capacity to provide care is more constrained than telemedicine, due to its focus on surgical aspects in dental care. Nonetheless, future developments in the field of robotics, may introduce a second generation of teledentistry, allowing indirect interventions via the internet [41, 42].

One of the primary challenges encountered in teledentistry is the resistance to change. This resistance largely stems from the perceived limitations, notably the empirical nature of diagnosis and the continued reliance on dental radiography as the gold standard for accuracy. So, how can this challenge be effectively addressed? One promising solution involves the incorporation of ultrasound technology in conjunction with intraoral cameras. These cameras can be employed for tasks such as detecting occlusal caries, diagnosing plaque, calculus, and gingival inflammation. The beauty of this approach lies in its remote application through teledentistry, coupled with augmented reality to guide another clinician, that can tele-assist another one, in this modality of telepresence, enhancing the value of teledentistry, like for example, in the remote diagnosis of root canal orifices (Fig. 8.2) This, in turn, can streamline referrals to appropriate dental providers, spanning fields like orthodontics and oral surgery, among others [24].

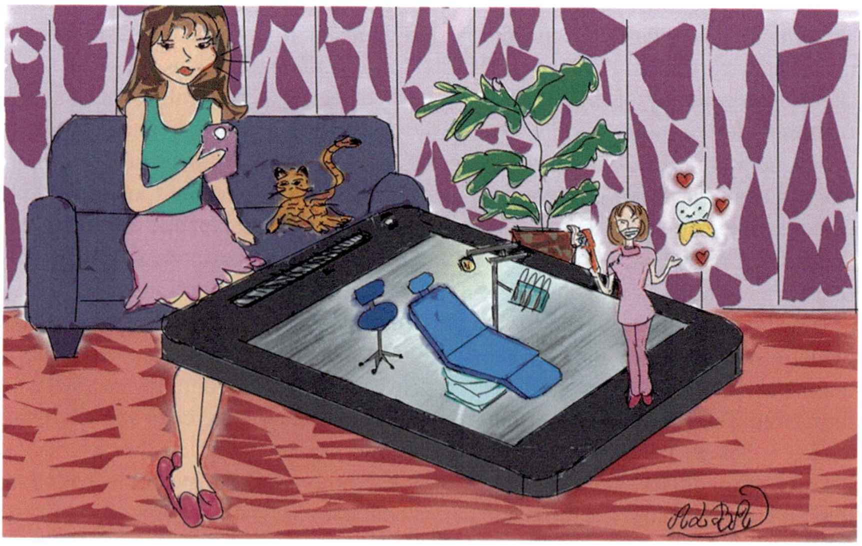

Fig. 8.2 Teledentistry.Illustration of a patient with a submucosal abscess undergoing remote evaluation via teledentistry, highlighting its role in early diagnosis and clinical management.

Furthermore, patient compliance plays a crucial role in this context. The ability for patients to directly observe their treatment in real-time enhances their understanding, which is especially beneficial for children and anxious patients. Moreover, if employed at home, teledentistry empowers patients to monitor their own oral health more effectively, promoting better oral hygiene practices. Teledentistry can enhance the quality of oral healthcare and enhance oral health equity [24, 44].

Dentistry is currently exploring a range of imaging techniques, including ultrasound or ultrasonography. These methods utilize ultrasound signals, which bounce off tissues to create images. Ultrasound imaging offers several notable advantages, including the use of non-ionizing radiation, ease of deployment, and portability. Recent studies have demonstrated its effectiveness in assessing conditions like peri-implantitis and aiding in implant placement planning. For example, Doppler ultrasonography can evaluate blood flow to estimate tissue perfusion at implant and palatal donor sites following soft tissue augmentation using a connective tissue graft [45, 46].

As technology advances, it is likely that one day, these ultrasound methods will become sensitive enough to provide accurate and time-efficient 3D mapping of the entire sulcus or periodontal pocket around teeth. This potential development could revolutionize the field by enabling comprehensive imaging of periodontium architecture and assisting in assessing periodontal depth without the need for traditional probing [45, 46].

The rapid integration of Artificial Intelligence (AI) into oral health services and dentistry highlights the crucial role of dental professionals in ensuring the quality of AI applications. To effectively navigate this technological shift, dental professionals must acquire fundamental knowledge and skills to assess dental AI [47]. AI will bring a lot of changes in dentistry and challenges, not only in the clinical field but also in the interaction with patients, dental education, and inside the dental team. Digital dental assistants powered by AI can carry out several duties more accurately, with fewer mistakes [40].

AI not only introduces changes and challenges in the clinical domain but also fosters a more participatory healthcare approach, particularly when patients actively contribute their data. Empowering patients through self-monitoring and self-management, along with continuous utilization of collected data, addresses the limitations of brief on-off medical encounters. This is particularly pertinent for health conditions like periodontal disease, which develop over years and manifest intermittently. Continuous, noninvasive health and behavior monitoring enables a deeper understanding of individual drivers and processes related to health and disease. The potential reduction in diagnostic and treatment costs can alleviate the burden on healthcare systems grappling with an aging population and an increasing number of complexes, chronic cases [2, 48].

AI technology is starting to be applied in dental radiology and has been widely applied in endodontics. According to research on the use of AI in endodontics, the neural networks performed similarly to the dental experts with more accuracy and precision. The applications of AI in endodontics are several: Dental caries, locating minor apical foramen, periapical lesions, root fractures, success of retreatment, difficulty level, root caries, working length, stem cell viability, root fractures, and root canal system anatomy [49].

The need for updates in dental university curriculums is evident considering the paradigm shift driven by AI. The incorporation of AI into dentistry is an evolving area, and its integration into dental education relies on the availability and effectiveness of AI technology, as well as the willingness of universities to embrace these advancements [47]. It is also essential to consider the potential ethical implications of using AI in dentistry and the need for dental professionals to be properly trained in its use [50].

ChatGPT, a large language model-based chatbot is another form of generative AI and has demonstrated its effectiveness in helping with the authoring of scientific research and dental studies. Researchers can summarize, interpret, and rephrase scientific data by using ChatGPT. However, the scientific writing produced by the chatbot is still not thoroughly reviewed, and additional research is needed to examine the ethical issues and unfavorable effects of this program, but proper rules and norms of conduct are urgent [40].

ChatGPT has proven its ability in assisting researchers with medical and dental research writing, as reported by previously published papers. Its use enables researchers to efficiently summarize, translate, and paraphrase scientific information. However, reliance solely on ChatGPT for research writing is cautioned, as the scientific output generated by this chatbot has not yet been fully evaluated and more studies are required to investigate the ethical concerns and negative impacts of this program [51].

AI can complement and enhance human tasks and have a far-reaching impact in academia and healthcare. Its adoption holds the promise of improving educational experiences and transforming the delivery of care, supporting existing functions, and paving the way for future innovations [52].

However, AI solutions have not entered routine dental practice fully, basically because the limited data availability, the lack of methodological rigor, standards, and practical questions about the usefulness of these solutions, with the implications of ethical aspects [36–39]. We must be concerned and aware about the potential negative consequences of AI, such as AI plagiarism, lack of quality standards and bias. Regulations of ethics, laws, and quality performance should be done as soon as possible, so healthcare providers can offer safety treatment to patients [50].

Finally, the last member of this golden team: Augmented reality (AR) and virtual reality (VR) have emerged as powerful educational tools for dental students and hold significant promise for ongoing professional development among healthcare providers. In the realm of Dentistry, AR facilitates real-time communication between patients and dentists, enhancing the patient's understanding through video sharing, image presentations, and 3D models. On the other hand, VR employs advanced software and hardware to create immersive 3D digital environments, which find primary application in dental student training. Furthermore, the concept of mixed reality combines elements of both AR and VR, primarily employed in oral and maxillofacial surgery, dental implant placement, and orthognathic surgery. This last one, stands out as a prominent field of AR application in dentistry. It employs computer-generated VR environments to gradually expose patients to potentially anxiety-inducing situations, serving as a non-pharmacological analgesic for dental pain. Numerous studies have reported that VR significantly reduces patients' perception of dental pain and keeps them deeply engaged during treatment [53].

AR and VR, offer substantial benefits for educating patients of all ages. In oral home care, they serve as digital tools to enhance oral hygiene practices in both children and adults, fostering the prevention of oral diseases while making educational experiences more engaging with 3D digital images. The application of AR and VR in healthcare has even extended to innovative methods for objective pain detection and localization through portable neuroimaging-based frameworks, incorporating clinical AR and AI (known as CLARAi), enabling direct assessment of pain from the patient's brain [14].

The use of an AR tool in an art-therapy setting on individuals with autism, has shown to be very effective, in this population. Patients in the autism spectrum disorder tend to have a more significant caries prevalence index, for several reasons like, lack of manual dexterity to brush their teeth, more chewing time, sensory aversion to the taste of toothpaste or a cariogenic diet. Also because of the use of xerostomic drugs to manage the symptoms. Using AR, can help the child or an adult to immerse himself inside the dental office, and get to know in advance the setting before the visit take place, so it can familiarize with the characteristic noises of the environment, meet the operators and the instruments, and have some control over a stressing environment, so there are no surprises, and broke of the routines, which normally makes them more comfortable and less anxious [54].

The integration of the metaverse into dentistry marks a transformative shift, redefining education, research, patient care, and professional collaboration. Although metaverse technologies are advancing in medical fields, a significant research gap remains in identifying and classifying the specific needs of dentists within this virtual domain [55, 56]

8.5 Robotics and Regenerative Dentistry: The Next Step

While science and technology have significantly advanced medical innovations, progress in dentistry has been comparatively slower. However, the integration of robotic technologies is driving the development of precision-based and minimally invasive dental interventions. New development in specialized dentistry fields is being used with the help of tooth-crown-preparation robots, tooth-arrangement robots, drilling robots, and orthodontic arch wire-bending robots [57].

Robot-assisted surgery has revolutionized many aspects of oral-facial surgery [58]. In implantology, there are assisted robots or fully automated robots for implants, which have shown very impressive results. The help of the intelligent robots in oral implantology is focused on preoperative digital 3D scanning of the implant site, analysis diagnosis, digital plan design of the implant surgery, and automatic drilling, to improve the accuracy of dental implant surgery, reduce surgical trauma, and shorten the operation time (Fig. 8.3) The help of intelligent robots in oral implantology is focused on preoperative digital 3D scanning of the implant site,

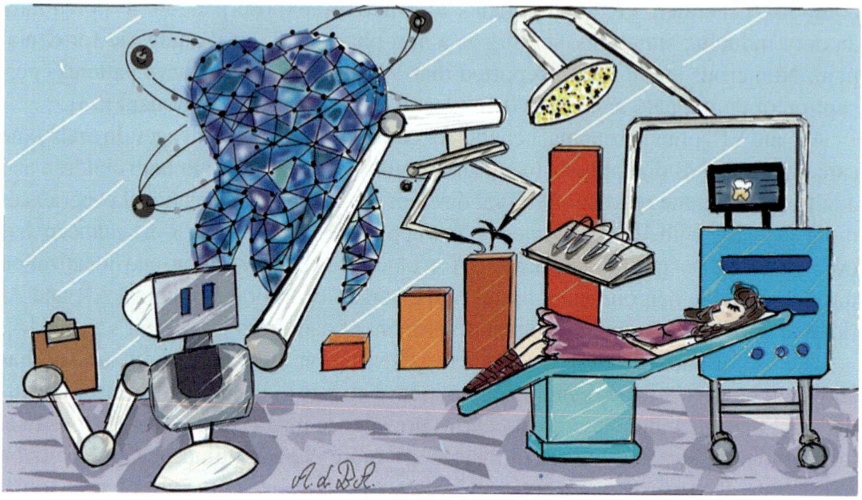

Fig. 8.3 Dental robotics. As an emergent technology can improve oral health, giving quality, safety, accuracy, and precision to dental procedures in mostly all dental specialties

analysis, diagnosis, digital plan design of the implant surgery, and automatic drilling. Some robotic solutions, such as the robot "Yomi" (Neocis), have become commercially available and received 510(k) clearance from the FDA for implant placement, especially in edentulous patients [14].

Robotically assisted surgery, outfitted with haptic feedback technology that simulates touch and sensation, has improved the sensibility for surgeons and precision of the oral surgery [58]. In endodontics, there are also robots to help in the training of root canal treatment, to be able to calculate the feedback force, during endodontic procedures. The development of robotic systems, including the "Omin Phantom," and intelligent micro-robots is designed to enhance training efficacy in endodontic procedures, while mitigating complications such as instrument breakage and root perforation. Additionally, the use of robotics can overcome limitations in traditional treatments, particularly in individuals with limited mouth opening, and is also being utilized to assist patients with special needs, such as the elderly and handicapped individuals, with automatic tooth-cleaning mouthpiece robots [57, 59]. Magnetic microrobots are being designed to improve disinfection by targeting biofilms. However, the high costs of setup, maintenance, and patient reluctance hinder the widespread adoption of robotic systems in endodontics and other dental specialties, particularly when compared to traditional methods [59, 60].

Dental robotics is currently undergoing a transition from computer-assisted operations to fully autonomous technology, with the aim of enabling virtual robotic surgery in the future. This will enable surgeons to operate on patients from a remote location, sooner than we expected [53]. However, it is important to mention that an in vitro study, this year, compared the accuracy of freehand, static computer-assisted and robot-assisted dental implant placements, but no significant differences were observed, between the last two [61].

The more preventive and minimalistic approach, with growing emphasis on quantitative and regenerative dentistry is gaining prominence as it explores innovative materials aimed at conserving or reconstructing dental tissues. Those advances are mainly focused on stem cells, bioactive molecules, and biomaterials. Regeneration of damaged periodontal tissues is a promising stem cell therapy; using specific dental progenitor cells in periodontitis treatment showed a better efficacy in the regeneration process [23].

In the domain of endodontics, the recognition of the significance of preserving the pulp nerve in teeth has prompted increased efforts and guidelines. The objective is to restore normal pulp function in teeth with reversible pulpitis and achieve the regeneration of the pulp-dentinal complex in necrotic teeth. The goal is to recover normal pulp function in teeth with reversible pulpitis and the regeneration of pulp-dentinal complex in necrotic teeth. Notably, promising outcomes have been observed in the transplantation of autologous dental pulp stem cells, extracted from third molars, and subsequently transplanted into pulpectomized teeth with granulocyte colony-stimulating factor in atelocollagen. Additionally, the use of human umbilical cord mesenchymal stem cells in mature permanent teeth with apical lesions has shown encouraging results. Even dental stem cell-based therapy has been considered as promising for treating diabetes [22].

In periodontics, the guided tissue regeneration is the gold standard for periodontal tissue regeneration, but new biomaterials like composite membranes of polycaprolactone and gelatin loaded with zinc oxide nanoparticles have demonstrated efficacy in inhibiting the growth of *Staphylococcus aureus*. Furthermore, the application of bone marrow mesenchymal stem cells in osteoarthritic temporomandibular joints has shown promise. Despite these advancements, stem cell therapy in clinical dentistry has encountered challenges, including poor cell retention and viability [62].

The use of hydrogel systems would help with a more personalized treatment in mandibular reconstruction. This biopolymer can be made from natural or artificial materials, are more flexible, integrate well with tissues, so inflammatory reactions are rare [23]. The hydrogel applications involve tooth fluoride, cavity filling, direct pulp capping, and root canal treatment or revascularization. The drawback is swelling of the hydrogel and insufficient adhesion [63].

Hydrogels composed of antimicrobial peptides have been also in the radar of dentistry due to their biocompatibility, biodegradability, self-assembly, and antimicrobial properties. Recently, DNA hydrogels have shown long-term release of cytokine interleukin-10 for immunomodulation, making them promising materials for treating periodontal diseases, but their antimicrobial performance in endodontics and periodontics, still need to be evaluated [64].

Lately photo biomodulation therapy (laser or broad-spectrum light, like light-emitting diode), formerly known as low-level laser therapy, has shown promising effects on the proliferation, viability, and differentiation. Immunomodulatory approaches based on molecular, epigenetic technologies could also revolutionize endodontic therapy, especially in postoperative pain management [65]. Also, to treat periodontal disease and periimplantitis, by modifying host immune responses, still there is not enough data to give definitive conclusions [66–68]. It also, appears to be effective for tissue repair in the treatment of avulsed teeth, depending on the means of conservation of the avulsed tooth and the laser application protocol [69].

Conventional treatments like Guided Tissue Regeneration (GTR) and Guided Bone Regeneration (GBR) have limitations in fully restoring periodontal tissues, particularly the periodontal ligament, alveolar bone, and cementum. Stem cell therapy has shown promise in improving periodontal regeneration, with recent advancements focusing on endogenous stem cells and tissue engineering to address these challenges [70].

Consequently, current trends and future perspectives in regenerative dentistry are shifting towards the utilization of cell sheets, spheroids, and organoids. These innovative approaches not only aim to recover lost tissues but also strive to restore optimal functionality [62].

8.6 Space Dentistry: The Next Future

Emerging as a field of increasing interest, space dentistry addresses the challenges posed by microgravity and radiation conditions during space travel. The unique environment of space, characterized by microgravity, has been identified to induce muscle atrophy and compromise essential oral functions such as speaking and maintaining proper oral hygiene. These alterations share similarities with age-related diseases [71]. NASA has identified six dental problems such as "Abscess," "Avulsion/Tooth Loss," "Caries," "Crown Replacement," "Exposed Pulp/Pulpitis," and "Filling Replacement" in Design Reference Missions. Simulated space environments have revealed the deterioration of oral defensive functions, emphasizing the necessity for targeted interventions to address these challenges [72–74]. Simulated microgravity has been linked to increased pathogen virulence, gene expression, and antibiotic resistance, which are critical for astronauts' health and offer insights into disease progression mechanisms applicable to Earth-based clinical practice [75].

Microgravity can negatively impact on oral health by reducing salivary flow, causing osteoporosis in the maxilla and mandible, increasing the risk of dental caries, periodontal diseases, pathogenic bacterial growth, and odontocrexis (occurs when dental restorations, like fillings or crowns, fail at high altitudes due to trapped gases expanding, causing restorations to dislodge forcefully). Microgravity also compromises oral immunity and leads to degenerative changes in the temporomandibular joint (TMJ) [74].

Space missions, with their unique conditions, may lead to unexpected changes in craniofacial bones, increasing the risk of dental issues in space. Given the isolated nature of space missions, preventing dental emergencies becomes paramount. However, reports indicate the occurrence of dental issues during space travel, ranging from the loss of restorations to more severe complications like pulpitis. Furthermore, the impact of microgravity on mineral bone density, sleep patterns, and temporomandibular joint stress adds complexity to the multifaceted challenges faced by astronauts [71, 76].

It is estimated that bone mass decreases by approximately 1–2% monthly, resulting in the loss of calcium from bones, which can contribute to conditions such as osteoporosis. Factors such as sleep deprivation, increased liver blood flow, and heightened liver metabolism at high altitudes can induce changes in drug metabolism, warranting careful consideration. Exposure to radiation can disrupt immunity and increase the risk of developing cancers. Space flights may impact dentition, with studies showing increased pulp size, indicating deficient dentin formation, and conflicting results on calcium and phosphorus content in dentin. While no studies have explored cosmic radiation's effects on dental tissues, it is hypothesized that prolonged exposure could degrade their structure and composition, like radiation caries observed in cancer therapy [75]. Additionally, phenomena such as barodontalgia and dental barotrauma can be explained in terms of Boyle's law, potentially leading to the fracturing of dental restorations [73, 77].

Long-term space missions have been associated with notable alterations in oral health parameters (Jaw pain, weakened mastication muscles, and altered occlusion due to muscle tone loss), as evidenced by lower levels of salivary IgA, IgM, and IgG. Additionally, oral mucosal issues, including sarcopenia, neuromotor dysfunction, nociplastic pain, and chewing-related pathologies, are common. Noninvasive brain stimulation techniques like transcranial electrical and magnetic stimulation show promise in managing spaceflight-induced pain. Changes in the oral microbiome characterized by an increase in the anaerobic components of dental plaque, like for example, it has been reported that in conditions of microgravity, acid resistance of *S. mutans* is enhanced [75, 77].

In contrast, short-duration space missions (10–16 days) and simulated gravity conditions have reported heightened concentrations of metalloproteinases, amylase, and cortisol in saliva [71, 73, 76, 78]. Studies have reported incidences of dental cavities, periodontal diseases, oro-maxillofacial fractures, pain, sensory abnormalities in the teeth and oral mucosa, salivary gland stone formation (sialoliths), craniomandibular joint disorders, masticatory muscle atrophy, and oral cancer in astronauts [73].

It has been seen that pure oxygen inhalation may cause corrosion of dental amalgam restorations in space, so in long duration space missions, could become an issue. Crowns cemented with resin cement demonstrated better retention and no microleakage, compared with performance of zinc phosphate and glass ionomer cements. That can be attributed to the porosities incorporated at the time of their manipulation [77].

Dental emergencies are one of many important risks to be assessed in preparation for future long-term exploration missions. In addition to intensive preflight examinations and evaluations, as well as strategies for in-flight-prevention, it will be necessary to introduce guidelines and procedures for the treatment of dental emergencies. Astronauts will have to be trained accordingly and equipment and procedures must be developed and tested. Notably, there currently exists no procedure or technology capable of sustaining and restoring teeth for extended durations during space missions [79, 80].

Innovative approaches are being explored for future space missions, where astronauts would autonomously conduct intraoral scanning to generate individualized

3D scans of their teeth and surrounding tissues. Subsequently, these 3D scans would be transmitted to Earth, where a team of dental experts would assess the data. A dental technician would then design a virtual 3D model for the required dental splint, crown, or dental prosthesis tailored to the crew member's needs. The resulting data sets would be transmitted back to the Mars habitat, where an onboard 3D printer or milling machine could automatically manufacture the restoration using ceramics, resin, or other suitable materials [73, 79].

New innovative dental materials will come with the help of nanotechnology, which can challenge the space environment conditions. The use of teledentistry, with AI algorithms and wearable devices to monitor astronauts will allow real-time consultation with dental professionals on Earth.

NASA's Mars missions emphasize the importance of microbial screening, infection prevention, and extensive preflight dental care. However, prolonged space conditions may lead to microbial evolution and unique oral health challenges. The presence of a dentist during long-term missions is crucial, as advanced dental care, such as radiographs and root canals, is unavailable in space. With extended mission durations, both preflight and in-flight prevention must be prioritized. Crew members should be trained to manage dental emergencies, including caries, pulpitis, abscesses, fractures, and crown displacement, to ensure mission success [75, 81].

References

1. Moon JH, Roh DH, Kwack KH, Lee JH. Bacterial single-cell transcriptomics: recent technical advances and future applications in dentistry. J Dent Sci Rev. 2023;59:253–62. https://doi.org/10.1016/j.jdsr.2023.08.001.
2. Baker JL. Illuminating the oral microbiome and its host interactions: recent advancements in omics and bioinformatics technologies in the context of oral microbiome research. FEMS Microbiol Rev. 2023;47(5):fuad051. https://doi.org/10.1093/femsre/fuad051.
3. Malcangi G, Patano A, Guglielmo M, Sardano R, Palmieri G, Di Pede C, de Ruvo E, Inchingolo AD, Mancini A, Inchingolo F, Bordea IR, Dipalma G, Inchingolo AM. Precision medicine in oral health and diseases: a systematic review. J Pers Med. 2023;13(5):725. https://doi.org/10.3390/jpm13050725.
4. Nagakubo D, Kaibori Y. Oral microbiota: the influences and interactions of saliva, IgA, and dietary factors in health and disease. Microorganisms. 2023;11(9):2307. https://doi.org/10.3390/microorganisms11092307.
5. Yadav S, Kumari P, Sinha A, et al. Salivary microbiomes: a potent evidence in forensic investigations. Forensic Sci Med Pathol. 2024;20(3):1058–65. https://doi.org/10.1007/s12024-023-00759-3.
6. Yu KM, Cho HS, Lee AM, Lee JW, Lim SK. Analysis of the influence of host lifestyle (coffee consumption, drinking, and smoking) on Korean oral microbiome. Forensic Sci Int Genet. 2024;68:102942. https://doi.org/10.1016/j.fsigen.2023.102942.
7. Lieffers JRL, Vanzan AGT, Rover de Mello J, Cammer A. Nutrition care practices of dietitians and oral health professionals for oral health conditions: a scoping review. Nutrients. 2021;13(10):3588. https://doi.org/10.3390/nu13103588.
8. Antoniadou M, Varzakas T. Breaking the vicious circle of diet, malnutrition and oral health for the independent elderly. Crit Rev Food Sci Nutr. 2021;61(19):3233–55. https://doi.org/10.1080/10408398.2020.1793729.

9. Feng J, Liu J, Jiang M, Chen Q, Zhang Y, Yang M, Zhai Y. The role of oral nitrate-reducing bacteria in the prevention of caries: a review related to caries and nitrate metabolism. Caries Res. 2023;57(2):119–32. https://doi.org/10.1159/000529162.
10. Tenelanda-López D, Valdivia-Moral P, Castro-Sánchez M. Eating habits and their relationship to oral health. Nutrients. 2020;12(9):2619. https://doi.org/10.3390/nu12092619.
11. Rosier BT, Johnston W, Carda-Diéguez M, et al. Nitrate reduction capacity of the oral microbiota is impaired in periodontitis: potential implications for systemic nitric oxide availability. Int J Oral Sci. 2024;16(1):1. https://doi.org/10.1038/s41368-023-00266-9.
12. Abdelrahman SM, El Samak M, El-Baz LM, Hanora AM, Satyal P, Dosoky NS. Effects of mint oils on the human oral microbiome: a pilot study. Microorganisms. 2024;12(8):1538.
13. Tripodi D, Cosi A, Fulco D, D'Ercole S. The impact of sport training on oral health in athletes. Dent J (Basel). 2021;9(5):51. https://doi.org/10.3390/dj9050051.
14. DaSilva AF, Robinson MA, Shi W, McCauley LK. The forefront of dentistry-promising tech-innovations and new treatments. JDR Clin Trans Res. 2022;7(1 Suppl):16S–24S. https://doi.org/10.1177/23800844221116850.
15. Han D, Xie S, Steckl AJ. Salivary endotoxin detection using combined mono/polyclonal antibody-based sandwich-type lateral flow immunoassay device. Sens Diagn. 2023;2:1460–8. https://doi.org/10.1039/D3SD00158J.
16. Dongiovanni P, Meroni M, Casati S, Goldoni R, Thomaz DV, Kehr NS, Galimberti D, Del Fabbro M, Tartaglia GM. Salivary biomarkers: novel noninvasive tools to diagnose chronic inflammation. Int J Oral Sci. 2023;15(1):27. https://doi.org/10.1038/s41368-023-00231-6.
17. Saito M, Shimazaki Y, Yoshii S, Takeyama H. Periodontitis and the incidence of metabolic syndrome: an 8-year longitudinal study of an adult Japanese cohort. J Clin Periodontol. 2024;51(1):54–62. https://doi.org/10.1111/jcpe.13881.
18. Montero E, Molina A, Carasol M, Fernández-Meseguer A, Calvo-Bonacho E, Teresa García-Margallo M, Sanz M, Herrera D. The association between metabolic syndrome and periodontitis in Spain: results from the WORALTH (Workers' ORAL healTH) Study. J Clin Periodontol. 2021;48(1):37–49. https://doi.org/10.1111/jcpe.13391.
19. Guan H, Zhao S, Tan Y, Zhang Y, Zhang Y, Xinyi F, et al. Microbiomic insights into the oral microbiome's role in type 2 diabetes mellitus: standardizing approaches for future advancements. Front Endocrinol. 2023;15:1416611.
20. Wyszyńska M, Czelakowska A, Rosak P, Kasperski J, Łopacińska M, Ghanem A, Mertas A, Skucha-Nowak M. The impact of COVID-19 on the oral bacterial flora in patients wearing complete dentures and on the level of exhaled nitric oxide as a marker of inflammation. J Clin Med. 2023;12(17):5556. https://doi.org/10.3390/jcm12175556.
21. Murugesan S, Al Khodor S. Salivary microbiome and hypertension in the Qatari population. J Transl Med. 2023;21(1):454. https://doi.org/10.1186/s12967-023-04247-8.
22. Kanafi MM, Bhonde RR. Diverse approaches toward application of dental pulp stem cells from human permanent and deciduous teeth in the treatment of diabetes. Curr Diabetes Rev. 2024;20(1):19–26.
23. Budi HS, Jameel MF, Al-Dolaimy F, Alahmari MM, Abullais SS, Ebrahimi S, et al. Injectable and 3D-printed hydrogels: state-of-the-art platform for bone regeneration in dentistry. Inorg Chem Commun. 2024;161:112026.
24. Pentapati KC, Siddiq H. Clinical applications of intraoral camera to increase patient compliance—current perspectives. Clin Cosmet Investig Dent. 2019;11:267–78. https://doi.org/10.2147/CCIDE.S192847.
25. Díaz-Fabregat B, Ramírez-Carmona W, Cannon ML, Monteiro DR, Pessan JP, Antoniali C. Are salivary NO2−/NO2− and NO3− levels biomarkers for dental caries in children? Systematic review and meta-analysis. Nitric Oxide. 2024;144:11–9. https://doi.org/10.1016/j.niox.2024.01.001.
26. Huang M, Chen W, Nakamura T, Kimura Y. Editorial: discovery of digital biomarkers in the background of big data and advanced machine learning. Front Physiol. 2023;14:1239219. https://doi.org/10.3389/fphys.2023.1239219.

27. Li Y, Tang H, Liu Y, Qiao Y, Xia H, Zhou J. Oral wearable sensors: health management based on the oral cavity. Biosens Bioelectron X. 2022;10:100135. https://doi.org/10.1016/j.biosx.2022.100135.
28. Timpel J, Klinghammer S, Riemenschneider L, Ibarlucea B, Cuniberti G, Hannig C, Sterzenbach T. Sensors for in situ monitoring of oral and dental health parameters in saliva. Clin Oral Investig. 2023;27(10):5719–36. https://doi.org/10.1007/s00784-023.
29. Sempionatto JR, Montiel VR, Vargas E, Teymourian H, Wang J. Wearable and mobile sensors for personalized nutrition. ACS Sensors. 2021;6(5):1745–60. https://doi.org/10.1021/acssensors.1c00553.
30. Hong W, Lee WG. Wearable sensors for continuous oral cavity and dietary monitoring toward personalized healthcare and digital medicine. Analyst. 2021;145(24):7796–808. https://doi.org/10.1039/d0an01484b.
31. Lee SH, Baek DH. Effects of Streptococcus thermophilus on volatile sulfur compounds produced by Porphyromonas gingivalis. Arch Oral Biol. 2014;59(11):1205–10. https://doi.org/10.1016/j.archoralbio.2014.07.006.
32. Shah FY, Shetty DC, Kaur G, Gupta S, Pathak A, Aggarwal V. Serum and saliva LDH levels in patients with habit, oral potentially malignant disorders (OPMDs), and oral squamous cell carcinoma (OSCC): a spectrophotometry study. J Pharm Bioallied Sci. 2023;15(Suppl 2):S881–4. https://doi.org/10.4103/jpbs.jpbs_90_23.
33. Chung PC, Chan TC. Digital oral health biomarkers for early detection of cognitive decline. BMC Public Health. 2023;23(1):1952. https://doi.org/10.1186/s12889-023-16897-w.
34. Paqué PN, Hjerppe J, Zuercher AN, Jung RE, Joda T. Salivary biomarkers as key to monitor personalized oral healthcare and precision dentistry: a scoping review. Front Oral Health. 2022;3:1003679. https://doi.org/10.3389/froh.2022.1003679.
35. Alotaiby F. Salivary biomarkers: a new wave in early disease detection and diagnosis. Natl Editorial Advis Board. 2024;35(3):91–6.
36. Ducret M, Mörch CM, Karteva T, Fisher J, Schwendicke F. Artificial intelligence for sustainable oral healthcare. J Dent. 2022;127:104344. https://doi.org/10.1016/j.jdent.2022.104344.
37. Alqahtani T, Badreldin HA, Alrashed M, Alshaya AI, Alghamdi SS, Bin Saleh K, et al. The emergent role of artificial intelligence, natural learning processing, and large language models in higher education and research. Res Social Adm Pharm. 2023;19(8):1236–42. https://doi.org/10.1016/j.sapharm.2023.05.016.
38. Schwendicke F, Samek W, Krois J. Artificial intelligence in dentistry: chances and challenges. J Dent Res. 2020;99(7):769–74. https://doi.org/10.1177/0022034520915714.
39. Thurzo A, Urbanová W, Novák B, Czako L, Siebert T, Stano P, et al. Where is the artificial intelligence applied in dentistry? Systematic review and literature analysis. Healthcare (Basel). 2022;10(7):1269–328. https://doi.org/10.3390/healthcare10071269.
40. Tiwari A, Kumar A, Jain S, Dhull KS, Sajjanar A, Puthenkandathil R, Paiwal K, Singh R. Implications of ChatGPT in public health dentistry: a systematic review. Cureus. 2023;15(6):e40367. https://doi.org/10.7759/cureus.40367.
41. El Tantawi M, Lam WYH, Giraudeau N, Virtanen JI, Matanhire C, Chifamba T, Sabbah W, Gomaa N, Al-Maweri SA, Uribe SE, Mohebbi SZ, Hasmun N, Guan G, Polonowita A, Khan SB, Pisano M, Ellakany P, Baraka MM, Ali AA, Orellana Centeno JE, et al. Teledentistry from research to practice: a tale of nineteen countries. Front Oral Health. 2023;4:1188557. https://doi.org/10.3389/froh.2023.1188557.
42. Flores-Hidalgo A, Collie J, King S, Grant FT, Beasley NE, Moss ME, Tempel TR Jr. The use of teledentistry in clinical oral and maxillofacial pathology practice: an institutional experience. Front Oral Health. 2023;4:1063973. https://doi.org/10.3389/froh.2023.1063973.
43. Qari A, Almashhadani SS, Balbaid MA, et al. Perceptions of schoolteachers about teledentistry use in Makkah City. Cureus. 2024;16(1):e51927. https://doi.org/10.7759/cureus.51927.
44. Kengne Talla P, Allison P, Bussières A, Giraudeau N, Komarova S, Basiren Q, Bergeron F, Emami E. Teledentistry for improving access to, and quality of oral health care: a protocol for an overview of systematic reviews and meta-analyses. PLoS One. 2024;19(1):e0288677. https://doi.org/10.1371/journal.pone.0288677.

45. Barootchi S, Tavelli L, Majzoub J, Chan HL, Wang HL, Kripfgans OD. Ultrasonographic tissue perfusion in peri-implant health and disease. J Dent Res. 2022;101(3):278–85. https://doi.org/10.1177/00220345211035684g.
46. Tavelli L, Kripfgans OD, Chan HL, Vera Rodriguez M, Sabri H, Mancini L, Wang HL, Giannobile WV, Barootchi S. Doppler ultrasonographic evaluation of tissue revascularization following connective tissue graft at implant sites. J Clin Periodontol. 2025;52(1):68–79. https://doi.org/10.1111/jcpe.13889.
47. Schwendicke F, Chaurasia A, Wiegand T, Uribe SE, Fontana M, Akota I, Tryfonos O, Krois J. IADR e-oral health network and the ITU/WHO focus group AI for health. Artificial intelligence for oral and dental healthcare: core education curriculum. J Dent. 2023;128:104363. https://doi.org/10.1016/j.jdent.2022.104363.
48. Tariq S, Gupta N, Gupta P, Sharma A. Artificial intelligence in public health dentistry. Int Healthcare Res J. 2021;5(9):RV1–5. https://ihrjournal.com/ihrj/article/view/489.
49. Agrawal P, Nikhade P. Artificial intelligence in dentistry: past, present, and future. Cureus. 2022;14(7):e27405. https://doi.org/10.7759/cureus.27405.
50. Thurzo A, Strunga M, Urban R, Surovková J, Afrashtehfar KI. Impact of artificial intelligence on dental education: a review and guide for curriculum update. Educ Sci. 2023;13:150. https://doi.org/10.3390/educsci13020150.
51. Fatani B. ChatGPT for future medical and dental research. Cureus. 2023;15(4):e37285. https://doi.org/10.7759/cureus.37285.
52. Islam NM, Laughter L, Sadid-Zadeh R, Smith C, Dolan TA, Crain G, Squarize CH. Adopting artificial intelligence in dental education: a model for academic leadership and innovation. J Dent Educ. 2022;86:1545–51. https://doi.org/10.1002/jdd.13010.
53. Monterubbianesi R, Tosco V, Vitiello F, Orilisi G, Fraccastoro F, Putignano A, Orsini G. Augmented, virtual and mixed reality in dentistry: a narrative review on the existing platforms and future challenges. Appl Sci. 2022;12(2):877. https://doi.org/10.3390/app12020877.
54. Pagano S, Lombardo G, Coniglio M, Donnari S, Canonico V, Antonini C, Lomurno G, Cianetti S. Autism spectrum disorder and paediatric dentistry: a narrative overview of intervention strategy and introduction of an innovative technological intervention method. Eur J Paediatr Dent. 2022;23(1):54–60. https://doi.org/10.23804/ejpd.2022.23.01.10.
55. Odeh Y, Odeh R. Towards a comprehensive classification of dentist-centered needs in the metaverse. In: International conference on information management. Cham: Springer Nature Switzerland; 2024. p. 52–68.
56. Garavand A, Aslani N. Metaverse phenomenon and its impact on health: a scoping review. Inform Med Unlocked. 2022;32:101029. ISSN 2352-9148. https://doi.org/10.1016/j.imu.2022.101029.
57. Liu L, Watanabe M, Ichikawa T. Robotics in dentistry: a narrative review. Dent J (Basel). 2023;11(3):62. https://doi.org/10.3390/dj11030062.
58. Negi S, Kharat P, Mathur A, Tripathy S, Mehta V. Robotic oral-facial surgery with haptic feedback: a new frontier in dental surgery. Oral Oncol Rep. 2024;9:100159.
59. Nagaveni NB, Mahanthesh SP, Chiranjeevi H. Robotics in the contemporary era of conservative dentistry and endodontics. Adv Sci Technol. 2024;1:1–5.
60. Babeer A, Bukhari S, Alrehaili R, Karabucak B, Koo H. Microrobotics in endodontics: a perspective. Int Endod J. 2024;57(7):861–71.
61. Su T, Teng W, Chu M, Su Y, Zhou L. Comparing the accuracies of freehand, static computer-assisted and robot-assisted dental implant placements: an in vitro study. Int J Comput Dent. 2024.
62. Thalakiriyawa DS, Dissanayaka WL. Advances in regenerative dentistry approaches: an update. Int Dent J. 2024;74(1):25–34. https://doi.org/10.1016/j.identj.2023.07.008.
63. Song C, Liu R, Kong B, Gu Z, Chen G. Functional hydrogels for treatment of dental caries. Biomed Tech. 2024;5:73–81.
64. Atila D, Kumaravel V. Advances in antimicrobial hydrogels for dental tissue engineering: regenerative strategies for endodontics and periodontics. Biomater Sci. 2023;11:6711–47. https://doi.org/10.1039/D3BM00719G.

65. Kadam AS, Merwade S, Kumar Neelakantappa K, Naik SB, Brigit B, Bhumralkar SS, Naik BH. Effect of laser photobiomodulation on postoperative pain in endodontics: a systematic review. Photobiomodul Photomed Laser Surg. 2024;42(1):11–9.
66. Firoozi P, Amiri MA, Soghli N, Farshidfar N, Hakimiha N, Fekrazad R. The role of photobiomodulation on dental-derived stem cells in regenerative dentistry: a comprehensive systematic review. Curr Stem Cell Res Ther. 2024;19(4):559–86. https://doi.org/10.2174/1574888X17666220810141411.
67. Deschner J, Schröder A, Weber M, et al. Advancing oral immunology for improving oral health. J Orofac Orthop. 2023. https://doi.org/10.1007/s00056-023-00473-3.
68. Cronshaw M, Mylona V. Photobiomodulation therapy within clinical dentistry: theoretical and applied concepts. In: Lasers in dentistry—current concepts. Cham: Springer International Publishing; 2024. p. 173–236.
69. Figueiredo LR, Bento VAA, Sonoda CK, Pellizzer EP. Efficacy of photobiomodulation in the treatment of avulsed teeth: a systematic review of animal studies. Lasers Med Sci. 2024;39(1):50.
70. Abdelrahman MRA. Unlocking regenerative potential: stem cell and tissue engineering innovations for permanent dental restoration. Discov Med. 2024;1(1):113.
71. Dugan C, Parlatescu I, Popescu BO, Pop CS, Marin M, Dinculescu A, Nistorescu AI, Vizitiu C, Varlas VN. Applications for oral research in microgravity—lessons learned from burning mouth syndrome and ageing studies. J Med Life. 2023;16(3):381–6. https://doi.org/10.25122/jml-2022-0285.
72. Zaitsu T, Ohta T, Ohshima H, Mukai C. The importance and necessity of space dentistry. Trans Japan Soc Aeronaut Space Sci Aerospace Technol J. 2014;12:Tp_7–9. https://doi.org/10.2322/tastj.12.Tp_7.
73. Harika PD, Mehta KH, Pulluri SS, Rana P, Rajani H, Aiman A, Pulluri SS. Oral health in zero gravity: a comprehensive review of orofacial effects and countermeasures in spaceflights. Cureus. 2023;15(11):e49035.
74. Samathu JHA, Mani R, Venkatesh V, Vaishnavi A, Sacrapani L. Smile beyond the stars: a narrative review exploring the challenges for dentistry in space. Cureus. 2024;16(8):e66591.
75. Bakr MM, Caswell GM, Hussein H, Shamel M, Al-Ankily MM. Considerations for oral and dental tissues in holistic care during long-haul space flights. Front Physiol. 2024;15:1406631. https://doi.org/10.3389/fphys.2024.1406631.
76. Chitkara N, Garg A, Mittal R. Exploring astronautical dentistry: a review. Int Healthc Res J. 2017;1(4):5–8.
77. Goyal A, Malhotra P, Bansal P, Arora V, Arora P, Singh R. Mission Mars: a dentist's perspective. J Br Interplanet Soc. 2015;68:393–9.
78. Kronstadt KL. Strategic development of novel approaches to the oral health of astronauts in long-term microgravity [dissertation]. Houston: The University of Texas School of Dentistry; 2020.
79. Häuplik-Meusburger S, Meusburger H, Lotzmann U. Dental treatment during a human Mars mission with remote support and advanced technology. In: 46th international conference on environmental systems; July 2016.
80. Review of spaceflight dental emergencies. 2012. https://ntrs.nasa.gov/citations/20120002807/. Accessed 25 Aug 2013.
81. Menon A. Review of spaceflight dental emergencies (no. JSC-CN-25693); 2012.

Participation-Oriented and Health-Related Social Work

9

Ute Kahle

9.1 Introduction

Participation-oriented and health-related Social Work focuses on the cross-sectional task in the context of the discipline and profession of Social Work and Health ([1], 4). Social Work is „a practice-based profession and academic discipline that promotes social change and development, social cohesion, and the empowerment and liberation of people "[2, 3]. In addition, the Principles of social justice, human rights, collective responsibility, and respect for diversities are central… "[2, 3]. In many fields of action and practice, Social Work is oriented on the health and well-being of their addressees and makes a decisive contribution to health care and prevention.

Dimensions of social coexistence are significantly more difficult, e.g., due to the coronavirus pandemic with serious consequences for psychosocial health, supposed life safety, and professional existence ([4], 13). In this regard, the fields of Social Work and health should be strengthened, which will include the fields of activity in the institutions of health care as well as activities in other working fields which are health related ([5], 5).

This essay will give an overview of theoretical and methodical aspects, legal and political parameters and fields of action of health-related Social Work. The human rights–based approach discusses, in particular, participation orientation [6], person-centeredness, self-determination, and autonomy of vulnerable groups. On the one hand, theoretical references are provided through original theories of Social Work like "relevance for every day life" [7], the Theory of Social Justice [8] in combination with UN CRPD (UN 2006) and Basic Law (1949) and theory-based thoughts about Participation [9]. On the other hand, reference sciences and health-relevant

U. Kahle (✉)
Department of Social Work, SRH University of Applied Sciences Campus Dresden, Dresden, Germany
e-mail: ute.kahle@srh.de

P. Plugmann, D. Portius (eds.), *Innovations in Healthcare and Outcome Measurement*, https://doi.org/10.1007/978-3-031-77302-0_9

disciplines are helpful for clarifying essential aspects and influences. Social Work in the health sector is a special and obviously relevant field, which cannot be taken into account in detail here. Nevertheless, it will be named and addressed in this context.

In addition, several challenges of social injustice, which refer to digital participation, will be cited like the phenomenon called the Digital Gap [10] and the first (access), second (use/skills), and third (outcomes) level of Digital Divide [11]. Finally, the essay summarizes some important findings referring to interventions that help to strengthen participation-oriented and health-related Social Work.

9.2 Classification Attempt: Social Work—Health Related

Social Work pursues inter-alia-normative objectives while influencing the improvement of social framework conditions and individual opportunities for development (Deutscher Berufsverband Soziale Arbeit). Social Work wants to modify individual behavior and circumstances. The fields of Social Work and Health Care Social Work are differentiated in several specialized directions [12] with a wide range and diverse practices, specific requirements, legal basis, forms of organizations, and interests. Furthermore, Social Work deals with broad cross-sectional tasks e.g., health, diversity, migration, age, and gender ([4], 18). In the opinion of the Deutsche Vereinigung für Soziale Arbeit im Gesundheitswesen e. V [5]., the following workspaces provide relevant tasks for health-related Social Work:

- Medical acute care.
- Public health service.
- Health promotion and prevention.
- Medical and social rehabilitation.
- Social and Community Psychiatry.
- Addiction treatment.
- Geriatrics.
- Oncology.
- Care Facilities.
- Sociotherapy/social therapy.
- Child and Adolescent Psychotherapy.
- Health-Based Social Work within Social Services (children, adolescents…).
- Self-help and self-help support.
- Governmental and NGO Institutions.
- Universities and Research Institutes.

Health-based Social Work is oriented on the social and natural environment of people who are endangered in their autonomy by health restrictions, which results in fewer options for social participation. Both challenges are tasks for Social Work: On one side, health restrictions as the effects of socially problematic situations and social inequality, and on the other side, socially problematic situations, which are affected by health-related restrictions. Health-related Social Work has the task of supporting vulnerable people to help them get back their self-determination and social participation [13].

The two-part definition of the WHO underlines these tasks, formulating the demand and implementation of health as a human right for everyone [14]:

(a) "Health is a state of complete physical, mental, and social well-being and not merely the absence of disease or infirmity.
(b) The reduction of apparent disease and disorder due to mortality, morbidity, and disabilities and the improvement of the subjective feeling of health status."

Schlichting and Heusner [15], 29) determined that "health…is a fundamental requirement to enable someone to participate." They refer to the Ottawa-Charta, which was established in 1986, codifying statements in connection with health promotion: "Health promotion aims at a process, to enable all people a higher amount of self-estimation over their life circumstances and environment and empower them to increase their health. To attain an essential physical, mental, and social well-being, it is necessary to satisfy individual and group necessities, to perceive and realize wishes and hopes as well as cope with circumstances or change them" [16]. The development of the Ottawa-Charta led to the Setting Approach, which focuses on permanent social contexts, concrete areas of life in which people spend much time, like school, work, or district. The Setting Approach offers low-threshold interventions, not only informing or training but including and empowering conditions and structures in a health-promoting way ([17], 20). Its aim is a healthy school, healthy company, and healthy sociospatial reconfiguration (cf. Chap. 4) [18].

Dettmers [19] postulates the aspiration of health-related Social Work "to establish optimal interventions for social security, social support, and individual development for people with disabilities and chronic disease and their relatives … to justify and guarantee empirically." He points to the *Triplemandat* of Staub-Bernasconi [20] which goes beyond the demands of state and addressees, as control and help. Social Work, therefore is a "human rights profession," which is as science only liable for itself, its knowledge, and ethic. Over its dual mandate, it refers to and invokes its high professional standards. The *Triplemandat* also expresses that health-related Social Work can't have just a unilateral mandate. Rather, the *Triplemandat* focuses on sociopolitical intervention, assumes the mandate of affected persons, and stands up for a better society [21, 22].

With regard to offers in a multiprofessional structured health system, which is medically dominated, health-related Social Work has hardly any institutional roots. The competencies for health-related Social Work defined by the World Health Organization focus on health through the lens of holistic well-being, taking into consideration physical, mental, and social aspects [16].

In connection with health-oriented Social Work, the question arises as to how and which factors influence the start of illness and what bio-psycho-social results will emerge [23]. developed a model of health determinants that is compatible with the understanding of the International Federation of Social Work Dahlgren and Whitehead Dahlgren and Whitehead ([2]; see Fig. 9.1).

In the continuation of the bio-psycho-social model, the model of the International Classification of Functioning, Disability, and Health (ICF) is very fruitful in referring to participation orientation (see Fig. 9.2). It constitutes the complex

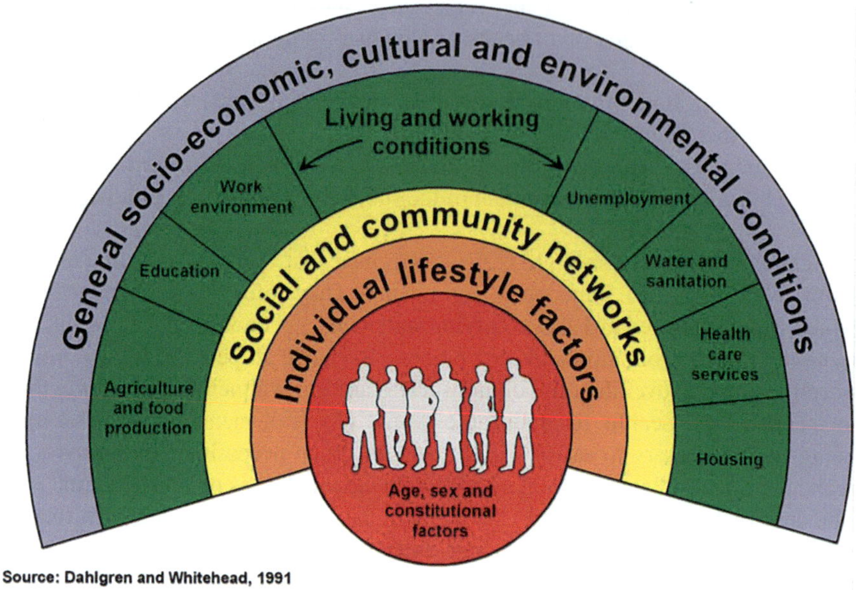

Fig. 9.1 Health-relevant factors (HAGE e.V., 2020; after [23])

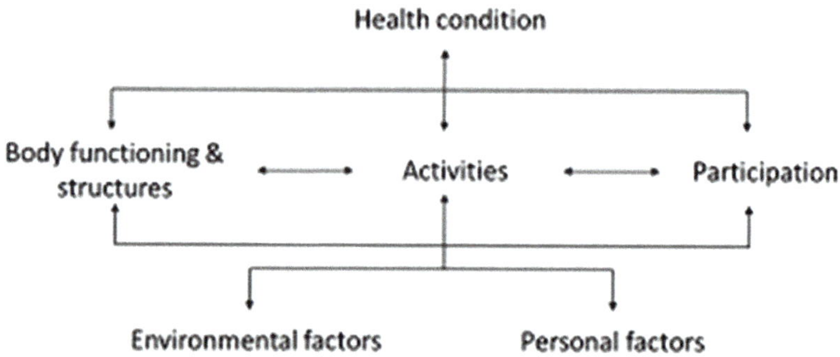

Fig. 9.2 ICF Classification–interaction between the components

interactions between body functions and structures, environmental factors, and personal factors with regard to activities and participation in order to describe health problems and derive options for participation and social life ([4], 22).

The model focuses primarily not on the consequences of illnesses but rather on "components of health" and, thus, on individual resources.

The ICF especially emphasizes the complex interactions of the individual components and sections. Even the legislator of German Social Code IX, 'Rehabilitation and Participation of Disabled Persons' from 2001, takes up the interaction in its definition in Section 2, Subsection 1:

1. People with disabilities are those who have physical, psychological, spiritual, or sensory impairments that, in interaction with barriers related to their settings and

environment, hinder their equal participation in society, with a high probability of lasting more than six months. An impairment, as per sentence 1, exists if a person's body condition and health status deviate from what is typical for their age. People are at risk of disability if an impairment, as defined by sentence 1, is to be expected.

Dettmers [4] derived six dimensions for the practice of health-oriented Social Work, which should receive attention when working with health disorders, along with their consequences for affected persons, on an individual, professional, and health-policy level:

1. Psychosocial consequences of medical restriction.
2. Social participation linked to inclusion and integration.
3. Case-related and social consequences of social inequality referring to health status.
4. Guarantee of psychosocial care.
5. Offensive professionalisation.
6. Shared access to all health-related fields of work ([4], 25).

Beyond that, the salutogenic concept [24, 25] will be given priority according to prevention, with the help-those-who-help-themselves concept as a guiding principle. In the following section, the article will especially highlight participation orientation, which is essential for the resources approach ([26], 7) and, consequently, the capability to connect with innovation in health care [27].

9.3 Participation Orientation and Participation in Society

9.3.1 Participation in Different Fields of Action in Social Policy and Social Work

Social participation, participation, and person-centeredness are guiding concepts and principles in many sociopolitical fields of action ([28], 14). As sociopolitical guiding principles, they change the view on health-oriented Social Work, rehabilitation, habilitation, rehabilitation, and participation research, one new and younger research field in progress ([29], 1).

The construct participation will not be used consistently in the different discourses and is not governed by a standardized logic why it is essential to approximate the uncertain term *interdisciplinary*. *Teilhabe* in German will be equated not seldom with the terms *participation*, *integration*, and *inclusion*. But all these terms and concepts have different meanings, which will be presented in this chapter.

As a sociopolitical guiding principle, participation stands for equal opportunities and a life in accordance with one's own visions, codetermination, and active role in society ([30], VII). In different action fields—such as rehabilitation and disability, basic income and employment promotion under Sozialgesetzbuch Zweites Buch (SGB II), child and youth welfare, assistance to the homeless, help to overcome particular difficulties, flight and migration, as well as the crossdisciplinary functions of health-related Social Work—terms and phenomena can be reconstructed differently ([9], 5).

Multidimensionality is characteristic of the term *participation* ([9], 15). In the different fields of action, various components are addressed differently according to the areas of life in which participation is considered a "positive form of participation referring to a social event" ([31], 236). While the legal sphere of SGB II aims at the general implementation of additional areas, apart from integration into gainful employment, the entitlement to participation under SGB IX extends to broad aspects of life, like education, work, and daily community life. In addition, an equality requirement is scheduled with the goal of achieving complete and effective participation ([9], 15).

At present, the common reference for participation targets is codified in the fields of rehabilitation and disability, as well as in the new Child and Youth Welfare law, which is the so-called "Big Solution" (*große Lösung*), because it will be developed into an *inclusive* Child and Youth Welfare law until the year 2028, when it will be entered into force totally (cf. *Gesetz zur Stärkung von Kindern und Jugendlichen—Kinder- und Jugendstärkungsgesetz (KJSG), Bundesgesetzesblatt* from June 6, 2021).

9.3.2 Participation as Guideline and General Target

Since the year 2001, the concept of social participation has already been linked with the new and comprehensive rehabilitation law in the *Sozialgesetzbuch Neuntes Buch—Rehabilitation und Teilhabe (SGB IX)* of the German Social Code concerning the rehabilitation and participation of people with disabilities. The development of a joint understanding causes more attention to rehabilitative issues at the public health level. Social and rehabilitative services have also been strengthened through the adoption of the UN Convention on the Rights of Persons with Disabilities (CRPD) in 2006, its ratification in Germany in the year 2009, and additionally through the WHO publication "World Report on Disability" [32].

Participation is used as a guideline of modern society for general targets and activity orientation ([33], 122), and German-speaking regions have extended the term *Teilhabe* to the political dimension ([33], 122 after [34], 4). In the CRPD, participation is a universal issue.

As a legal document, the Convention obligated the Federal Republic of Germany to put it into practice, which means to enable people with disabilities or impairments to take participation options in pursuit of a self-determined life ([35], 1). Article 1 of the UN Convention defines the primary objective—"…to promote, protect and ensure the full and equal enjoyment of all human rights and fundamental freedoms by all persons with disabilities, and to promote respect for their inherent dignity" (Article 1 UN CRPD). The UN Convention will reach "their full and effective participation in society on an equal basis with others." The principle of participation is closely connected with inclusion and nondiscrimination (cf. chapter 3.3). Participation is a human right and can also be read as an antonym to exclusion and marginalization. A positive idea of welfare participation and participation orientation is connected with the concept of quality of life and "a good life."

In March 2024, the UN CRPD was legalized for 15 years and integrated into German legislation. In the so-called UN State Report, every 4 years, Germany has to document which kind of progress politics make in converting the rights for people with disabilities (Bundesministerium für Arbeit und Soziales, 2023). Furthermore, options and offers referring the implementation of accessibility in general and especially accessibility to the education system, the labor market, the health system, sports, culture, barrier-free travel, politics, and many other areas of society and functional systems. In the year 2021 (after 12 years of enactment of the UN CRPD), the so-called "Accessibility Requirements for Products and Services enacted" law (Barrierefreiheitsstärkungsgesetz, BFSG) was adopted. With this law, the European Accessibility Act (EAA) was implemented in the German legislature. The law obliges, from the middle of the year 2025, providers of special products and services, especially from information and communication technology, to design this barrier-free. A legal regulation defines concrete access-free requirements for products and services. In many other areas, participation is not reached yet, e.g., Inclusive Education (article 24 UN CRPD), Inclusive Labor (article 27 UN CRPD), Living and Being Included in the Community (article 19 UN CRPD), or Health (article 25 UN CRPD): "…persons with disabilities have the right to the enjoyment of the highest attainable standard of health without discrimination on the basis of disability."

Participation and orientation on participation is a relational term between individuum and societal conditions ([9], 43). It means a positive norm of belonging to society ([31], 236), and it describes an extended space of possibilities, which happens through interaction between individuals and society ([9], 43). Furthermore, participation will be seen from the individual point of view instead of focusing on the system. Social structures, welfare state benefits, and offers are evaluated based on the options they provide for the individual.

From a sociological perspective, participation is connected on a micro and macro level and is a result of normative individualism, which is subject oriented. Subject orientation is described as person orientation in the reformed German Participation law (Bundesteilhabegesetz), which is also a response to the institution's criticism ([33], 324). Referring to a self-determined lifestyle (article 19 UN CRPD), participation emphasizes that people are not only exposed to structural conditions. Rather, through recognition, taking on a social role, and practicing it, they can participate actively in society. Self-determined participation is, in this respect, preconditionally dependent, as subjective actions are neither "vicariously [through] actions of others nor through other-directed predetermined actions reachable" ([36], 50; [9], 44). Participation is combined with self-determination, a self-determined lifestyle, and autonomy ([33], 104 after [37], 183). This interpretation means that people have the choice to follow their own interests. Participation could also be manifested by the decision not to participate. In addition, participation can be characterized as the "currency of social equity" ([9], 46) because equal participation, or equitability, focuses on the right to choose the service provider and their offers freely (cf. *SGB*

IX). The extent to which participation or participation orientation takes place in health-related Social Work is a permanent subject matter for sociopolitical negotiations.

9.3.3 Human Rights, Political Participation, and Quality of Life

As a cross-cutting issue, participation has played an important role in the human rights discussion for a long time ([38], 1). Already, in the Women's Rights Convention ratified in the year 1979 or the UN Convention on Children's Rights, statements referring to participation can be found. In the UN Convention on the Rights of Persons with Disabilities, participation receives even greater weight. People with disabilities or impairments especially have been excluded from political codetermination in the past because society thought that they were not capable of self-determined actions. Options for political participation are necessary for people with disabilities and impairments to lead independent lives. Participation can be described as the consideration of the living conditions of all people from the beginning of their lives, as well as integration into society ([38], 2).

Participation is a diverse proposal based on five pillars. According to international law, the English version of the CRPD is obligatory and contains, in 25 cases, the term *participation* or *participate*, while the term in the German version does not occur. Here, we find the term *Teilhabe* or *Teilnahme*. Unfortunately, significant aspects related to codetermination get lost if only the German version is examined ([38], 2). Therefore, the term *participation* was adopted in the German discussion and will be announced in this article:

1. Participation can be described as the overarching goal to open up all people to full and equal options "to promote, to protect and to ensure the full and equal enjoyment of all human rights and fundamental freedoms by all persons with disabilities, and to promote the respect for their inherent dignity" (article 1 UN CRPD). Its aim is "full, effective, and equal participation in society." All State activities are committed to this aim, as it is the responsibility of civil society.
2. Participation is a general principle of human rights (Article 3 UN CRPD) guiding the entire convention and means for the development of an inclusive education system in which people with disabilities and impairments and their organizations must be involved. This principle is, therefore, closely connected to the principles of inclusion and nondiscrimination. For example, it disallows disadvantages for people with disabilities within political processes or health care (cf. article 25 UN CRPD) and prevents discrimination or loss of privileges based on gender or other characteristics. In addition, persons with disabilities have the same range, quality, and standard of free or affordable health care and programs as provided to other persons, including in the area of sexual and reproductive health and populationbased public health programs (article 25a UN-CRPD) and that these health services are provided as close as possible to people's own communities, including in rural areas (article 25c UN-CRPD.). Furthermore,

discrimination is prohibited against persons with disabilities in the provision of health insurance and life insurance when such insurance is permitted by national law, which shall be provided in a fair and reasonable manner.

3. Participation as a specific individual right is guaranteed, e.g., the right for access to justice (Article 13 UN CRPD), the active and passive right to vote (Article 29 UN CRPD), and the right to participate and take part in cultural events or services (Article 30 UN CRPD).
4. Participation is also considered a state obligation due to the organization and implementation of the UN Convention—legislative procedure and empowerment programs have to be initialized and implemented in consideration of people with disabilities—whereby acceptance and sustainability are promoted, and useful and appropriate actions will be planned and put into practice.
5. Participation is at least anchored on the monitoring process referring to the implementation of UN CRDP. As part of civil society, people with disabilities and impairments, along with their organizations, are participants in the monitoring process and actively manage the construction and control of actions ([38], 3). All in all, participation is a necessity for people with disabilities and impairments to lead a self-conducted life [35].

Sensibly designed participation rests on the respect of people as legal entities and carriers of human dignity. Participation from people with disadvantages and disabilities or people in precarious circumstances leads political processes to qualitatively better results as more attention to the opinions of these groups is paid. The acceptance of concerned persons rises if they are involved in the processes.

Participation and participation orientation are not without preconditions but rather up for discussion by people with different conceptual considerations. Beyond the bio-psycho-social theories introduced before, the Livelihood Approach, the Capability Approach, and the Empowerment Concept are also helpful in describing the term *participation* in more detail. Regarding every concept, we can ask the following questions: "How can health participation be measured?" "How can health participation be achieved? " and "What defines quality of life?"

A gradual classification from nonparticipation to full and comprehensive participation is shown by Arnstedt's Ladder of Participation (see Fig. 9.3). Arnstedt defines three main areas of participation: manipulation and therapy are activities of nonparticipation; informing, consultation, and placation are degrees of tokenism and partnership; delegated power and citizen control represent different forms and phenomena of full participation.

His considerations are also part of the concept of dimensions of participation developed by the *Bundesverband Evangelische Behindertenhilfe* [40]. Participation qualifies the phenomenon of *Teilhabe* and is, therefore, preconditional because attitude, values, everyday acting, and structures are represented through their intersections. This is, e.g., the reason why intersectional approaches are adaptable to the discussion.

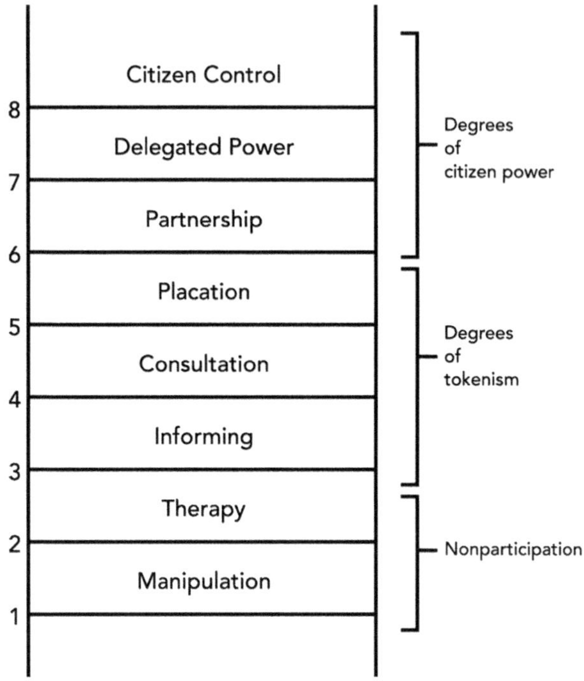

Fig. 9.3 A Ladder of Participation [39]

9.4 Sociospatial Practice and Person-Centeredness of Health-Related Social Work

Another aspect of participation-oriented and health care–related Social Work is the role of the sociospatial practice of the municipality. Communities should provide an autonomous local social policy through their comprehensive self-administration law (Article 28 German Basic Law). Against the background of participation, the sociospatial orientation has the challenge of becoming inclusive.

Here, inclusive sociospatial planning and inclusive health-related sociospatial work are used to manage tasks, which comprise both cooperation and conflict (*coopetition*; [41]). A sociospatial perspective changes the social and healthcare political focus, which leads from "the case to the field." The sociopolitical guiding principle of inclusion is characterized by a diverse society, which will be arranged by responsible citizens.

Community social policy has changed to sociospatial policy ([42], 185), which should be sensible for health care, social, cultural and economic differences. In the service provision rights, the tasks are located in the field of corporatism and competition. Instead of a commonwealth economy, the inclusive policy of sociospatial practice shows a fiscal-oriented welfare policy, which cares for users who utilize health care services and, in addition, integrates the participative engagement of stakeholders as protagonists.

The legal relationship, which is given between service providers, the public sector, social organizations, and a person who is entitled to benefits is called *the social right triangle*. The following figure shows that the person who is entitled to benefits and help has a legal claim against the service provider (see Fig. 9.4). The service procurement occurs on the basis of performance agreements, consideration arrangements, and quality agreements through so-called supply contracts.

This case-specific form of service provision will be extended through sociospatial budgets to make room for modification of the communal social policy, which should even be realized case independently. Taking into consideration that many municipalities show a strained budgetary situation, inclusive sociospatial and health-related Social Work could not be realized. However, non–community-based healthcare services violate the UN CRPD (cf. 3.3, no. 2).

Besides individual cases, controlling sociospatial and participation-oriented practice poses a challenge to the guiding principle of responsible citizenship within the community. People who are recipients of healthcare-related Social Work are often limited in their options to participate. In addition, they have mostly less influence on the offers and the development of social services. User autonomy is restricted because the transparency of offers is mostly nonexistent. The triangular relationship in social law is driven by person-centeredness, which is action guided by the so-called Federal Participation Act/SGB IX. Nonetheless, institutional system-supporting forces are effective and preserve old patterns and attitudes [33]. An inclusive sociospatial policy comes from responsible citizens who care for others and themselves and, on the other hand, are integrated into community social contexts. A new solidarity ([44], 701) will be reflected by new types of services like "Personal Budget," "Budget for Work," and "Budget for Vocational Training," which overcome the legal relationship between service providers, the social sector,

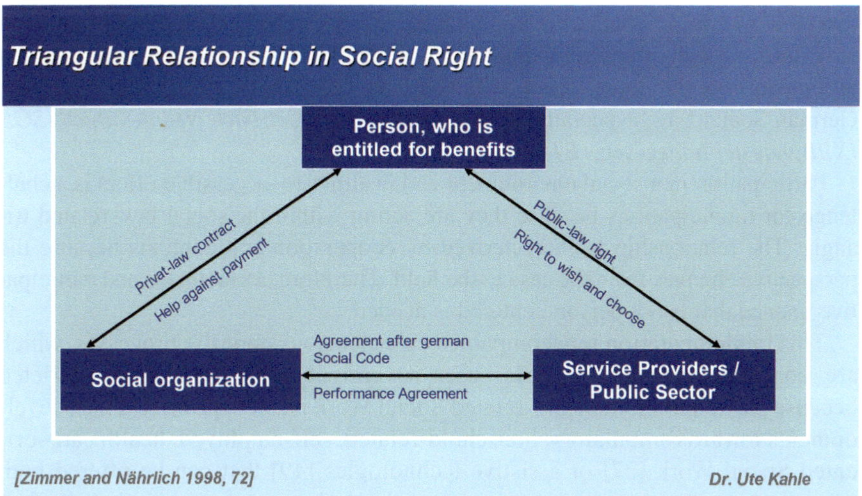

Fig. 9.4 The triangular relationship in social law ([33], after [43])

and social organizations. In this way, health care–oriented Social Work can result in more customer sovereignty through ambulatory, household-related services and probably self-employed health care–oriented Social Work.

The detailed concept of sociospatial orientation from Hinte [45] makes it clear that health care–oriented Social Work as part of an inclusive sociospatial policy focuses on case and field as well as professional attitude and action to initiate and implement participative, local, and subsidiary health-related activities. The person-centered and socioecological approach is related to participation, self-determination, solidarity, and maturity [46], especially for people in precarious situations.

9.5 A First Interim Conclusion

In the self-image of health care–related Social Work, "human beings … can easily identify in every phase of the care process of health care–related Social Work where he is, which resources professionals in Social Work use, and which targets are pursued" ([47], 26). "Health … is a basic requirement for enabling participation" ([15], 29). Social Work is in many fields oriented towards the health and well-being of its addressees and, therefore, makes essential contributions to health care. Theoretical and methodical references will be established on the basis of human rights and adapted to different concepts like participation, person-centeredness, self-determination, and autonomy of vulnerable groups of people.

On the one hand, orientation on daily life and social justice, as well as digitalization, community work, or sociospatial references, are different bases for health-related Social Work [48].

The Association for Social Work in Health Care (2015) developed a comprehensive catalog that contains relevant topics for health-related Social Work. The ICF is essential, as it highlights the complex interaction between body functions and body structures, as well as environmental and personal factors, to describe activities and participation possibilities. These statements are connectable to UN CRPD and the German Social Law, especially the so-called *Sozialgesetzbuch Neuntes Buch (SGB IX)/Bundesteilhabegesetz (BTHG)*.

Participation in a social environment and health care–accessible offers is a challenge for municipalities because they are acting within the social law–related triangle. The relationship is characterized by cooperation and conflicts because the perspective changes from the case to the field. Therefore, an inclusive and participative finance that is not person-centered is needed.

This implementation is accompanied by efficacious opposite processes, which are contradictory. For example, user sovereignty is significantly restricted because participation in health-related Social Work has less priority. Thus, developments towards ambulatory, household-related, self-employed, health care–oriented Social Work [27] or assistive technologies [49] that can be offered both person-centered and community-based might be the answer to actual challenges and problem areas.

Laws and Conventions

European Accessibility Act (EAA).

Grundgesetz (GG).

Kinder- und Jugendstärkungsgesetz (KJSG).

Sozialgesetzbuch Erstes Buch (SGB I).

Sozialgesetzbuch Zweites Buch (SGB II).

Sozialgesetzbuch Neuntes Buch (SGB IX).

United Nations—Convention on the Rights of Persons with Disabilities (UN CRPD).

References

1. Deutscher Berufsverband Soziale Arbeit (DBSA). Abgestimmte deutsche Übersetzung des DBSH mit dem Fachbereichstag Sozialer Arbeit. https://www.dbsh.de/profession/definition-der-sozialen-arbeit/deutsche-fassung.html. 2016; Sersheim. Accessed 2 Apr 2024.
2. International Federation of Social Work (IFSW). Globale Definition von Sozialarbeit. https://www.dbsh.de/der-dbsh/internationale-zusammenarbeit/ifsw.html. 2014. Rheinfelden. Accessed 21 Jan 2024.
3. International Association of Schools of Social Work (IASSW). Definition of Social Work. Ifsw.org/wp-content/upload. 2014. Accessed 31 Jan 2025.
4. Dettmers S, Bischkopf J. Handbuch gesundheitsbezogene Soziale Arbeit. München: Reinhardt Verlag; 2021.
5. Deutsche Vereinigung für Soziale Arbeit im Gesundheitswesen e. V. (DVSG). Qualifikationskonzept Gesundheitsbezogene Soziale Arbeit. 2015; Berlin.
6. Thomas A, Schweizer J. Teilhabeorientierung in der Sozialen Arbeit. In: Handbuch gesundheitsbezogene soziale Arbeit. München: reinhardt; 2021. p. 124–9.
7. Thiersch H. Lebensweltorientierte Soziale Arbeit, 9. Auflage. Weinheim: Beltz Juventa; 2014.
8. Rawl J. A theory of justice. Harvard: Harvard University Press; 1971. https://doi.org/10.2307/j.ctvjf9z6v. Accessed 31 Jan 2025.
9. Bartelheimer P, et al. Teilhabe—eine Begriffsbestimmung. Wiesbaden: Springer; 2020. https://doi.org/10.1007/978-3-658-30610-6.
10. Bonfadelli H. In: Gesundheitskommunikation H, von Rossmann C, Hastall M, et al., editors. Wissenskluft-Perspektive und Digital Divide in der Gesundheitskommunikation. Wiesbaden: Springer; 2020.
11. Van Dijk J. Digital divide: impact of access. New York: Wiley; 2017. https://doi.org/10.1002/9781118783764.wbieme0043. Accessed 19 Oct 2023.
12. Deller U, Brake R. Soziale Arbeit. Grundlagen für Theorie und Praxis. Stuttgart: Verlag Barbara Budrich/UTB; 2014.
13. Herriger N. Empowerment in der Sozialen Arbeit. Eine Einführung, 5. Auflage. Stuttgart: Kohlhammer Verlag; 2014.
14. World Health Organization. Ottawa-Charta zur Gesundheitsförderung. 1986. https://iris.who.int/handle/10665/34965. Accessed 31 Jan 2025.
15. Schlichting H, Heusner J. Gesundheit und Gesunderhaltung im Kontext von Pädagogik. In: Maier-Michalitsch N, editor. Gesundheit und Gesunderhaltung bei Menschen mit Komplexer Behinderung. Düsseldorf: Verlag selbstbestimmtes Leben; 2018.
16. World Health Organisation. Ottawa-Charta zur Gesundheitsförderung. Geneva: WHO; 1986. https://iris.who.int/handle/10665/34965. Accessed 19 Oct 2023.
17. Jost A. Gesundheit und Soziale Arbeit. Stuttgart: Kohlhammer; 2013.
18. Spatscheck C, Wolf-Ostermann K. The socio-spatial paradigm in social work—social space analyses as method for practitioners and researchers. In: sozialraum.de (1). 2nd ed. Lund:

Lund University; 2009. https://www.sozialraum.de/the-socio-spatial-paradigm-in-social-work.php. Accessed 31 Jan 2025.
19. Dettmers S. Gesundheitsbezogene Soziale Arbeit. Eine Übersicht. Soziale Arbeit DZI. 2018;67:256–61.
20. Staub-Bernasconi S. Vom beruflichen Doppel- zum professionellen Tripelmandat. Wissenschaft und Menschenrechte als Begründungsbasis der Profession Sozialer Arbeit. In: Zeitschrift für Sozialarbeit in Österreich (SIÖ) 2; 2007. p. 87.
21. Lutz R. Das Mandat der Sozialen Arbeit. Wiesbaden: VS Verlag; 2011.
22. Werwein A. Das politische Mandat Sozialer Arbeit. Eine positionierte Annährung. Esslingen: Hochschule Esslingen; 2008. https://hses.bsz-bw.de/frontdoor/deliver/index/docId/60/file/Das_politische_Mandat_Sozialer_Arbeit.pdf. Accessed 12 Jan 2024.
23. Dahlgren W, Whitehead M. Policies and strategies to promote social equity in health. Strategy paper for Europe. Stockholm: Institute for Future Studies; 1991.
24. Antonovsky A. Salutogenese. Zur Entmystifizierung der Gesundheit. Tübingen: DGVT-Verlag; 1997.
25. Faltermaier T. Salutogenese. In: Bundeszentrale für gesundheitliche Aufklärung (BZgA), editor. Leitbegriffe der Gesundheitsförderung und Prävention. Glossar zu Konzepten, Strategien und Methoden; 2023. https://doi.org/10.17623/BZGA:Q4-i104-3.0.
26. Redlich A. Vorwort—mit dem ganzen Menschen und seinen Ressourcen arbeiten. In: Möbius T, Friedrich S, editors. Ressourcenorientiert arbeiten. Anleitung zu einem gelingenden Praxistransfer im Sozialbereich. Wiesbaden: VS Verlag für Sozialwissenschaften; 2010. p. 7.
27. Plugmann J, Plugmann P. Innovationen in der Gesundheitsversorgung. In: Neue Ansätze und Impulse für Prävention, Gesundheitsförderung und Homecare. Heidelberg: Springer Gabler; 2023.
28. Bartelheimer P, Behrisch B, et al. Teilhabe—Versuch einer Begriffsbestimmung. In: Teilhabeforschung—Konturen eines neuen Forschungsfeldes. Wiesbaden: Springer; 2022. https://doi.org/10.1007/978-3-658-38305-3.
29. Wansing G, Schäfers M, Köbsell S. Teilhabeforschung—Konturen eines neuen Forschungsfeldes. Wiesbaden: Springer SV Verlag; 2022.
30. Schäfers M, Wansing G. Teilhabeforschung—Konturen eines neuen Forschungsfeldes. Heidelberg: Springer VS; 2020.
31. Kastl JM. Einführung in die Soziologie der Behinderung. Wiesbaden: Springer SV; 2017.
32. World Health Organization. Weltbericht Behinderung. Geneva: WHO; 2011. https://iris.who.int/bitstream/handle/10665/199544/9789241509619_eng.pdf;jsessionid=73A6B82B6F4B00DCF4052C03A4935212?sequence=1. Accessed 19 Oct 2023.
33. Kahle U. Inklusion, Teilhabe und Behinderung. In: Herausforderungen und Perspektiven der Transformationsprozesse von Organisationen der Behindertenhilfe aus institutioneller Sicht. Marburg: Lebenshilfeverlag; 2019.
34. Beck I. Partizipation—Aspekte der Begründung und Umsetzung im Feld von Behinderung. Teilhabe. 2013;1:4–11.
35. Deutsches Institut für Menschenrechte. Partizipation—ein Querschnittanliegen der UN-Behindertenrechtskonvention. Positionen Nr. 2010;3:1–4.
36. Behrendt H. Teilhabegerechtigkeit und das Ideal einer inklusiven Gesellschaft. Zeitschrift für Praktische Philosophie, Bd 5 Nr. 2018;1(2018):43–72. https://doi.org/10.22613/zfpp/5.1.2.
37. Fornefeld B. Menschen mit komplexer Behinderung. Selbstverständnis und Aufgaben der Behindertenpädagogik. München: Ernst Reinhardt Verlag; 2009.
38. Hirschberg M. Partizipation—ein Querschnittsanliegen der UN-Behindertenrechtskonvention. In: Deutsches Institut für Menschenrechte, editor. Positionen Nr. 3, Berlin; 2010.
39. Arnstein SR. A ladder of citizen participation. J Am Plan Assoc. 1969;35:216.
40. Bundesverband evangelische Behindertenhilfe. Partizipation sichern und stärken. Berlin: Self-published; 2023.
41. Geyer C. Inklusive Sozialraumpolitik als Aufgabe der Kommune: Herausforderungen und Konzeptbausteine aus einer gemeinwohlökonomischen Perspektive. Sozialer Fortschritt. 2022;71(8):513–30.

42. Fehmel T. Sozialpolitik für die Soziale Arbeit. Nomos Verlag; 2019.
43. Zimmer A, Nährlich S. Zur volkswirtschaftlichen Bedeutung der Sozialwirtschaft. In: Arnold U, Maelicke B, editors. Lehrbuch der Sozialwirtschaft. Baden-Baden: Nomos; 1998. p. 64f.
44. Jüster M. Transformation der Subsidiarität. In: von Grunwald K, Langer A, editors. Handbuch für Wissenschaft und Praxis, hrsg. Bielefeld: Nomos Verlag; 2018. p. 699.
45. Hinte W. von der Gemeinwesenarbeit über die Sozialraumorientierung zur Initiierung bürgerschaftlichen engagements. In: Grundriss soziale Arbeit. Cham: Springer; 2012. p. 663–76.
46. Klafki W. Neue Studien zur Bildungstheorie und Didaktik. 5. Auflage. Weinheim: Beltz Verlag; 1996.
47. Deutsche Gesellschaft für Soziale Arbeit (DGSA). Kerncurriculum Soziale Arbeit, https://www.dgsa.de/ueber-uns/kerncurriculum-soziale-arbeit. 2016; Sersheim. Accessed 21 Jan 2024.
48. Pape P. Digitalization in rehabilitation. In: Glauner P, Plugmann P, Lerzynski G, editors. Digitalization in healthcare. Implementing innovation and artificial intelligence. Heidelberg: Springer; 2023. p. 65–71.
49. Kahle U, Schädler J, Bächle L, Hünefeld L et al. Digitale Teilhabe und Assistive Technologien—vorläufige Eckpunkte einer Forschungsagenda. In: Zeitschrift für Sozialmanagement, Band 21, Nr. 2/2023; 2023. p. 105–12.

The Healthy Longevity Challenge: Closing the Gap Between Lifespan and Healthspan

10

Henri Michael von Blanquet

10.1 Introduction

Traditional medicine focuses on disease: Healthcare as we know it around the globe over the last few decades is a *disease-reactive* healthcare business and *siloed* Health Sciences Industry. Twentieth-Century Medicine has approached health from the perspective of individual diseases in silos: In clinical medicine, biomedical research, drug development, and many more fragmented and subspecialized medical fields. Typically, medicine waits till people are sick with one or more diseases, and then the system optimally tries to cure those diseases, but in reality, what we end up doing is treating the symptoms in organs most of the time. Medicine has been successful in keeping sick people alive, and the healthcare systems have been less successful at keeping people healthy. This is the fundamental challenge: To transform "sickcare" caused by *imprecision medicine* [1, 2]—with its increasing "sickspans" over the last few decades—towards sustainable biology and molecular-based medicine for sustainable health in order to expand the healthspan on an individual and population level (Precision Health). The expansion of the lifespan during the last 150 years opened the gap between lifespan and healthspan dramatically, and our classic disease-reactive healthcare systems will collapse sooner or later by the acceleration of the demographic shift limited by the power of our national economies. *"By 2030, for the first time in recorded history, the old will begin to outnumber the young,"* as the National Academy of Medicine stated as it began the grand global Healthy Longevity Challenge in 2023 [3–6].

H. M. von Blanquet (✉)
The Health Captains Club, Föhr, Germany
e-mail: michael@blanquet.de; President@healthcaptains.institute

P. Plugmann, D. Portius (eds.), *Innovations in Healthcare and Outcome Measurement*, https://doi.org/10.1007/978-3-031-77302-0_10

10.2 Targeting Aging Is Twenty-First-Century Medicine

The biological aging processes are the "mother of all diseases." Closing the gap between lifespan and healthspan for all is the paradigm shift [7]. Aging is the greatest risk factor for disease, e.g.:

- Arthritis.
- Cancer.
- Kidney disease.
- Cardiovascular disease.
- Autoimmune disorders.
- Type II diabetes.
- Immune decline.
- Cognitive decline.

The biology of aging is well described, and the Hallmarks of Aging are summarized by a molecularly and biologically interdependent concept:

10.3 The Hallmarks of Aging

Biological aging processes are characterized by a progressive loss of physiological and molecular integrity, leading to impaired function and increased vulnerability to the full spectrum of diseases and, ultimately, death. Aging research has experienced an unprecedented advance over recent years, particularly with the discovery that the rate of aging is controlled, at least to some extent, by genetic pathways and biochemical processes conserved in evolution. The hallmarks of biological aging are described as:

1. Genomic instability.
2. Telomere attrition.
3. Epigenetic alterations.
4. Loss of proteostasis.
5. Disabled macroautophagy.
6. Deregulated nutrient sensing.
7. Mitochondrial dysfunction.
8. Cellular senescence.
9. Stem cell exhaustion.
10. Altered intercellular communication.
11. Chronic inflammation.
12. Dysbiosis [8, 9].

Aging is driven by these 12 hallmarks, which fulfill the following three premises: (1) their age-associated manifestation, (2) the acceleration of aging by experimentally accentuating them, and (3) the opportunity to decelerate, stop, or reverse

Genomic Instability	Primary Hallmarks of Aging	1
Telomere Attrition	Primary Hallmarks of Aging	2
Epigenetic Alterations	Primary Hallmarks of Aging	3
Loss of Proteostasis	Primary Hallmarks of Aging	4
Disabeled Automarcophagy	Primary Hallmarks of Aging	5
Deregulated Nutrient-sensing	Antagonsitic Hallmarks of Aging	6
Mitochondrial Dysfunction	Antagonsitic Hallmarks of Aging	7
Cellular Senescence	Antagonsitic Hallmarks of Aging	8
Stem Cell Exhausition	Integrative Hallmarks of Aging	9
Altered Intracellular Communication	Integrative Hallmarks of Aging	10
Chronic Inflamation	Integrative Hallmarks of Aging	11
Dysbiosis	Integrative Hallmarks of Aging	12

Fig. 10.1 The Hallmarks of Aging are fulfilling the following three premises: (1) their age-associated manifestation, (2) the acceleration of aging by experimentally accentuating them, and (3) the opportunity to decelerate, stop, or reverse aging by therapeutic interventions on them. Source: 2013 and 2023 in Cell [8, 9]

aging by therapeutic interventions on them. These hallmarks are interconnected with each other, along with the recently proposed hallmarks of health, which include organizational features of spatial compartmentalization, maintenance of homeostasis, and adequate responses to stress [8, 9].

The interdependence of aging hallmarks means that the experimental accentuation or attenuation of one specific hallmark usually affects other hallmarks as well. This underscores the fact that aging is a complex process that has to be conceived as a whole. Accordingly, each of the hallmarks should be considered as a point of entry for future exploration of the aging process, as well as for the development of new anti-aging medicines [6, 8–10] (Fig. 10.1).

10.4 The Five Pillars of Healthy Longevity

Here is an overview of the key pillars for sustainable healthy longevity, all with a positive impact on the expansion of the healthspan to decrease the sickspan:

1. **Healthy exercise.**
2. **Healthy Longevity Medicine.**
3. **Healthy nutrition.**
4. **Healthy sleep.**
5. **Mental, emotional, intellectual and social healthy longevity.**

The fundament for Healthy Longevity seems to be long-term healthy social relationships as the "Harvard Study of Adult Development," which started over 80 years ago, describes loneliness as one of the most powerful killers and "the people who were the most satisfied in their relationships at age 50 were the healthiest at age 80" [11].

Holistic Brain Health should be the basic key towards Healthy Longevity to give the other pillars more substance and effective power to expand the healthspan.

By the definition provided by the Healthy Longevity Medicine Society, "*Healthy Longevity Medicine* is optimizing healthspan by targeting aging processes across the lifespan" [5, 6]. Healthy Longevity at scale, therefore, needs the self-navigation of exercise, nutrition, sleep, and 360° brain health. All of these pillars need more basic science and direct knowledge transfer to medical communities and societies at the same level: "The healthy patient will be the CEO of his own health by navigating his Healthy Longevity with his fingertips on his smartphone to expand his individual healthspan over his lifetime "[1, 2, 12].

10.5 Healthy Longevity Medicine for all Is Based on Scaleable Precision Health

The current "taxonomy of medicine" is a barrier to progress (Source: Keith R. Yamamoto, UCSF, USA):

- **Descriptive**: Disease classification is based predominantly on symptoms and organs.
- **Inflexible**: Creates rigid silos in research, diagnosis & therapy, education, and funding.
- **Narrow**: No natural fit for new fundamental discoveries; no rationale for building a continuum of research and clinical care.
- **Not sustainable: The Hallmarks of Aging—the biology of aging as the greatest risk factor for disease is not part of the current taxonomy—a new symbiosis of an integrated taxonomy of disease and health is the basis for scaleable Precision Health for All.**

Don't forget that "normal" biology is complicated; therefore, the Hallmarks of Aging as a deviation from health and the biology of disease are similarly complex. We need an integrated understanding of the new multiple molecular and traditional levels of medicine, as well as the integration of the Hallmarks of Aging, to deeply understand individual disease and health status on multiple levels in order to bring a tailored Healthy Longevity diagnostic ($n = 1$) and Healthy Longevity therapeutic interventions ($n = 1$) to each individual to expand the Healthspan for All. The traditional "one-size-fits-all" disease-reactive pharma concept delivers value only to a small subgroup of patients. This **imprecision medicine** is absolutely unethical in our modern societies and damages the lives of patients and national economies to the extent of billions of dollars [1, 7, 9]:

Today, medicine is moving through an inflection point from "sickcare" in "silos" towards "lifecare" in scaleable "ecosystems," based on the superconvergence found in the crossover of infotech and biotech. Based technologically and synchronically on the integration and development of a working continuum to create a Precision Health value chain:

- The integration: Aggregate and analyze biological information, incorporating concepts and technologies of physical sciences, engineering, and computer science.

- The working continuum: From fundamental discovery to translation, to clinical research, to clinical practice, to citizens—"from bench to bedside & from bedside to bench, and towards society and industry."
- The Superconvergence: From Imprecision to Precision Medicine [1, 12, 13]—Eric Topol 2013 "The Creative Destruction of Medicine – How the digital revolution will create better healthcare" [14].

10.6 The Precision Health Value-Chain for Healthy Longevity and the Big-Data Challenge

The molecular-digital transformation of medicine towards Healthy Longevity Medicine in the transformation of "sickcare" towards "lifecare" is creating a new multistakeholder value chain for a sustainable Healthy Longevity Industry.

- Precision Health for Healthy Longevity will aggregate, integrate, and analyze biological information, drawing on vast collections of data to produce health advice and predictions and aging and disease diagnoses tailored to the individual.
- Precision Health for Healthy Longevity will be enabled by computational information commons, within which correlations produce a knowledge network, generating new hypotheses, illuminating mechanisms of disease and the Hallmarks of Aging, and establishing links between the Hallmarks of Aging and diseases thought to be unrelated.
- Precision Health for Healthy Longevity will revolutionize the development and deployment of therapies and Healthy Longevity Medicine interventions, as well as principles of clinical practice, by allowing all stakeholders to benefit from and participate in the research data, health data, and health industry data sets.

This multilayer Precision Health Value Chain needs in the long run, to scale for sustainable health, the synchronization of hundreds of academic public hospital providers on a scaleable international platform to share the knowledge network like an information common in a certified democratic, value-based, open-source system to deliver this individualizable medical and health information to every patient needed. By data ethics rules, there should be no limitation of access to medical information in the age of Precision Health [1, 13].

10.7 Precision Health for Healthy Longevity Medicine Will Be Organized in Database-Layers

Today, every patient needs to be digitized, like in Google Maps, for an accurate diagnosis at several molecular levels (genomics, transcriptomics, epigenomics, microbiomes, exposome, and biomarkers of aging) [15]; see (Fig. 10.2). Precision Health for Healthy Longevity takes individual variation into account—in our genes, environment, lifestyle, Hallmarks of Aging, and even in the microscopic organisms

Google Maps: GIS Layers organized by Geographical Positioning	Precision Health Information Commons: Organized arround indivudual Patient Data
GIS Layers:	*Health Data Layers:*
Traffic Layer	Evironment
Land Use Layer	Lifestyle
Forest Use Layer	Individual Wearable Data
Water Use Layer	Electronic Health Record
Weather Layer	Biomarkers
Industry Layer	Radioomics
Census Tracts	Microbiome
Infrastructure Layers	Metabolomics
City Layers	Proteomics
Postal Codes	Transcriptomics
Geographic Raster	Epigenomics
Satelite Raster Imagery	Genomics

Fig. 10.2 "Towards Precision Medicine," Source: National Academy of Sciences (USA) 2011 [15]

that are living inside of us. "The best chance of favorable outcome is getting the initial health intervention to expand the healthspan after molecular individual diagnosis of age-related biomarkers right" (**Precision Health for Healthy Longevity First**; [1, 10]).

Beyond the genome and biomarker measurement of the molecular hallmarks of aging: Understanding how genetic variations contribute to health is just one aspect of Precision Health. While the genome is set for life, the expression of our genes fluctuates over time and in response to the environment. Additional approaches to Precision Health involve measuring levels of proteins, RNA, or metabolic products—biomarkers of aging. Along with genomics—proteomics, epigenomics, and metabolomics can help inform medical choices for individual patients. The field also incorporates what we are learning about the microbes that live in and on our bodies and how they can be manipulated to influence health and disease [1, 8, 9].

10.8 Beyond Targeting Aging in Diagnostics and Therapy, Precision Health Includes Approaches to Diagnostics, Extremely Early Prevention, and Screening of Health

- Methods for identifying those who are at risk before disease strikes.
- Analytical tools for predicting which prevention strategies will work best for which patients.
- Screening methods that can identify early signs of disease before symptoms emerge.
- Diagnostic methods for identifying subtypes of disease that may look the same on the surface but respond very differently to treatment.
- Tests that can identify disease carrier status for prospective parents.
- Devices for managing diseases and for tracking and guiding recovery.

High-performing **Precision Health Ecosystems** will reduce healthcare costs. To achieve this tipping point in the transformational process, the leadership of all stakeholders is needed to save our national health economies, our civilizations, and our ethical belief systems. Continuing on the trajectory of permanently rising healthcare costs caused by imprecise medicine and sickcare will sooner or later lead to the collapse of all our healthcare systems worldwide. The move towards Precision Health for Healthy Longevity Medicine is a fundamental transformation of healthcare politics, national health economics, and the traditional business models of the "old" stakeholders in the healthcare industry that will need to change [1, 7].

The key driving force towards value-based Precision Health for Healthy Longevity for All patients is by democratization of health information at their fingertips via smartphones towards a totally transparent medicine. We have to measure the medical outcomes in a global standardized setting—this is key in Precision Health and starting to implement Precision Health for Healthy Longevity in Academic Medical Center Networks:

10.9 Precision Health Longevity Departments at Public Academic Medical Centers

As Healthy Longevity Medicine powered by Precision Health is a new holistic Medical Specialty field, Longevity Departments for scaleable **Precision Health** should be anchored in public academic medical centers to integrate these four pillars:

1. Academic Medical Center Healthy Longevity **Clinical Center.**
2. Academic Medical Center Healthy Longevity **Research Center.**
3. Academic Medical Center Healthy Longevity **Innovation Hub.**
4. Academic Medical Center Healthy Longevity **Education Hub.**

Since 2023, we have seen the first openings of Healthy Longevity Medical Centers inside academic medical centers towards Healthy Longevity for All. These new Healthy Longevity Departments inside university medical centers act on an international level together to exchange knowledge and to create synchronized standards for a scaleable Healthy Longevity together with Healthy Longevity Research centers like the Buck Institute in California. Prototypes for this new kind of academically anchored Healthy Longevity are the National University of Singapore and the Sheba Medical Center in Tel Aviv, among others.

The Healthy Longevity Department at Sheba Medical Center is based on their **"4A" strategy,** which should be the Healthy Longevity Department fundament at all academic medical centers at scale:

A1: **Accessible**: Healthy Longevity Clinic in public academic medical center.

A2: **Affordable**: Healthy Longevity for All.

A3: **Academic**: 1. Healthy Longevity Clinical Hub 2. Research Hub 3. Innovation Hub.

A4: **Artificial Intelligence**: Big data–driven knowledge networks and information commons.

The political will of the Government in Singapore is to expand the healthspan by plus 3 years in the next 10 years. Though Singapore is just the blueprint for the beginning transformation towards 360° Next Generation Life Care, and because of the beginning and acceleration of the collapse of sickcare, more governments and national economies will follow to close the gap between healthspan and lifespan:

10.10 Closing the Gap Between Healthspan and Lifespan

Research has shown that healthspan is more valuable economically and personally than lifespan [7]. Using a value of statistical life economic model (which places a monetary value on gains from longer life, better health, and changes in the rate of aging), Scott et al. found that compressing the period of morbidity to improve health in older age was more valuable than further increases in life expectancy [7]. *The economic value of gains from an extra year of healthy life expectancy always exceeded those from an extra year of life expectancy.* Targeting biological aging instead of individual diseases offered potentially larger economic gains than the eradication of individual diseases, with an attenuation of aging that increased life expectancy by 1 year worth $38 trillion [7].

Closing the gap between healthspan and lifespan is critical for our national economies and will be one of the main drivers for the transformation from "sickcare" towards "lifecare" to increase the healthspan and decrease the sickspans at the same time.

The Healthy Longevity Industry resonates with the idea of a 360-degree One-Health-Concept (OHC), including Blue Zone Care and One Health Life Care. Instead of expanding the market for sickcare, we must invest in lifecare as a strategic asset from the micro, meso, and macro level to overcome the obstacles and constraints of sick, caring institutions, which brings our national economies towards a collapse instead of creating together a new sustainable multitrillion-dollar Healthy Longevity Industry worldwide.

This transformation will bring the biggest industry of all time to fruition and will have additional effects through the value-based convergence of Healthy Longevity, Blue Zone Community Care, and One Health Life Care:

10.11 Healthy Longevity Medicine, Blue Zone Community Care, and One Health Life Care Are Interdependent and Are a Next-Level Academic Convergence Challenge

In the field of *360° Next Generation Lifecare* in Human Medicine, the professional community is aware that the Hughes parallelity of innovation areas happening at the same time are interdependent and therefore, the industry is creating a "superconvergence" driven by the growing innovations horizon towards new technologies in the transformation of the outdated locally, regionally, and nationally siloed, disease-reactive healthcare systems into sustainable lifecare, by integrating Healthy

Longevity [5], Blue Zone Community Care [16], and One Health Life Care [17] in international medical ecosystems based on scaleable platforms towards a multitrillion-dollar Healthy Longevity Industry [7].

Blue Zone Community Care: A *Blue Zone* is a region in the world where people are claimed to have exceptionally long healthy lives and many centenarians with compressed morbidity due to a lifestyle combining physical activity, low stress, rich social interactions, a local whole-foods diet, and low disease incidence, as found in the Blue Zones in Okinawa (Japan), Sardinia (Italy), Nicoya (Costa Rica), Icaria (Greece), and Lome Linda (California) [16].

Blue Zone Community Care is a new public health concept to create new Blues Zones Communities by combining the knowledge out of the classic Blue Zones, Healthy Longevity for All, and One Health:

One Health is built on a simple understanding—that human health, animal health, and our shared environment are part of a deeply interconnected system. Healthy Longevity Medicine [and Blue Zone Community Care] can be understood as an additional integral part to add towards the "One Health Umbrella" (Fig. 10.3), [17–22].

In One Health Life Care, along with Healthy Longevity Medicine and Blue Zone Community Care, we still lack convergence strategies. These fields are notably different from human healthcare, which has hundreds of university hospitals and thousands of academic research institutions globally acting as *360° Next Generation Healthcare Transformation Hubs.* These hubs facilitate "from bench to bedside and bedside to bench" cycles of established innovation and education, and they support thousands of startups across various fields of innovation. However, we are missing

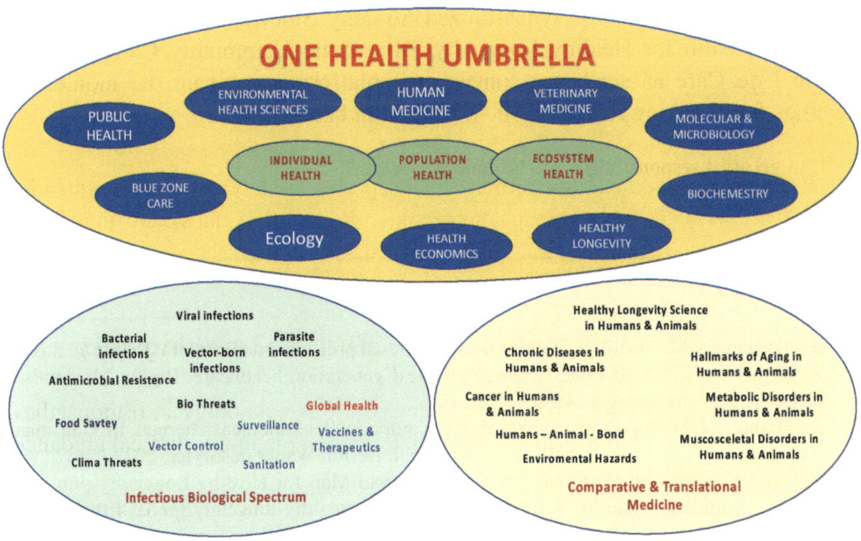

Fig. 10.3 Schematic representation of the One Health Umbrella integrating Blue Zone Care and Healthy Longevity. (Source: One Health Sweden and the One Health Initiative [17])

the establishment of combined *One Health Life Care, Healthy Longevity,* and *Blue Zone Community Care Research Institutions*. Additionally, there is a need to support *One Health Innovation Technology Parks* to create new business models for a genuine One Health Industry.

One Health Life Care, as Healthy Longevity and Blue Zone Community Care, is still not established in the academic institutional training of doctors, veterinarians, and the many environmental, planetary, and blue zone health scientific fields as a whole. The not-yet-existent One Health Education and Research strategies of national and international universities are the missing link towards new One Health Innovations and new One Health Business Platforms. Still, we see the investment in One Health Education as the key factor to opening this transdisciplinary field toward a new sustainable health business beyond the upcoming Healthy Longevity Industry [2, 15–17].

This article should inspire the community to take action, and we are looking forward to making it happen together [12].

Without the breakthrough in the Convergence Challenge of academic institutions, One Health, in combination with Healthy Longevity Medicine and Science and Blue Zone Community Care, as a scientific and strategic approach, remains far too much in the theoretical field. This article is a call to action for the whole community to build a new sustainable health industry at scale for the next generations to come.

University Medical Center, Academic Medical Center, and Health Foundations should bring the leadership together for this convergence to create new health sciences, integrated research, and education, surrounded by new start-up champions, in an effort to create a new international sustainable health industry. The author, therefore, opened The Health Captain's Institute to unite academic medical centers and health foundations for synchronized Strategy Studies, as well as to anchor Precision Health for Healthy Longevity, Blue Zone Community Care, and One Health Life Care as academic convergence platforms to create the momentum together. I am looking forward to it. Welcome on board!

> "Our **greatest responsibility** is to be **good ancestors**."
> –Jonas Salk

References

1. von Blanquet HM. Creating solutions for value-based precision medicine. In: Pieper U, Steidel A, Werner J, editors. XPOMET 360-degree next generation healthcare. Berlin: Medizinisch Wissenschaftliche Verlagsgesellschaft; 2019.
2. von Blanquet HM. Präzisionsmedizin als basis individueller Patientensicherheit. In: Gausmann P, et al., editors. Patientensicherheitsmanagement. Berlin: Walter de Gryter; 2022.
3. National Academy of Medicine—The Global Road Map for Healthy Longevity published 2023. https://nam.edu/initiatives/grand-challenge-healthy-longevity/global-roadmap-for-healthy-longevity.
4. The Grand Global Healthy Longevity Challenge published 2023. https://healthylongevitychallenge.org/about-us/.

5. The Healthy Longevity Medicine Society Healthy Longevity Medicine Definition published 2022. https://hlms.co.
6. Anon. Is ageing a disease? Lancet Healthy Longevity. 2022;3(7):E448. https://doi.org/10.1016/S2666-7568(22)00154-4.
7. Khan M, Al Saud H, Sierra F, et al. Global healthspan summit 2023: closing the gap between healthspan and lifespan. Nat Aging. 2024;4:445–8. https://doi.org/10.1038/s43587-024-00593-4.
8. Lo C, Pez-Otın, Blasco MA, Partridge L, Serrano M, Kroemer G. Hallmarks of aging. Cell. 2013;153(6):1194–217.
9. Lo C, Pez-Otın, Blasco MA, Partridge L, Serrano M, Kroemer G. Hallmarks of aging: an expanding universe. Cell. 2023;186(2):243–87.
10. Zhavoronkov A, Bischof E, Lee KF. Artificial intelligence in longevity medicine. *Nat*. Aging. 2021;1:5–7. https://doi.org/10.1038/s43587-020-00020-4.
11. Harvard Study of Adult Development 1938–2022. https://www.adultdevelopmentstudy.org.
12. von Blanquet HM. Precision medicine und Systemmedizin-Plattformen. In: Matusiewicz D, Martin A, editors. Smarte Medizin. hogrefe Bern; 2023.
13. Eric J. Topol, individualized medcine from Prewomb to tomb. Cell. 2014;157(1):241–53.
14. Topol EJ. The creative destruction of medicine—how the digital revolution will create better healthcare. New York: Basic Books; 2013.
15. National Research Council. Towards precision medicine: building a knowledge network for biomedical research and a new taxonomy of disease. Washington, DC: National Academies Press; 2011. www.nap.edu/catalog/13284/toward-precision-medicine-building-a-knowledge-network-for-biomedical-research.
16. Buettner D, Skemp S. Blue zones: lessons from the World's longest lived. Am J Lifestyle Med. 2016;10(5):318–21. https://doi.org/10.1177/1559827616637066. PMID: 30202288; PMCID: PMC6125071.
17. von Blanquet HM, Friebe M. Navigating towards a future of One Health. In: Friebe M, editor. Novel innovation design for the future of Health: entrepreneurial concepts for patient empowerment and health democratization. Berlin: Springer; 2022.
18. Mackenzie JS, Jeggo M. The One Health Approach-Why Is It So Important? Trop Med Infect Dis. 2019;4(2):88. Published 2019 May 31. https://doi.org/10.3390/tropicalmed4020088.
19. Togami E, Gardy JL, Hansen GR, Poste GH, Rizzo DN, Wilson ME, JAK M. Core competencies in one health education: what are we missing? In: NAM perspectives. Discussion Paper. Washington, DC: National Academy of Medicine; 2018. https://doi.org/10.31478/201806a.
20. Frankson R, Hueston W, Christian K, Olson D, Lee M, Valeri L, Hyatt R, Annelli J, Rubin C. One health core competency domains. Front Public Health. 2016;4:192. Published Sep 13, 2016. https://www.ncbi.nlm.nih.gov/pmc/articles/PMC5020065/.
21. Rabinowitz PM, Natterson-Horowitz BJ, Kahn LH, Kock R, Pappaioanou M. Incorporating one health into medical education. BMC Med Educ. 2017;17:45. https://doi.org/10.1186/s12909-017-0883-6.
22. Binot A, Duboz R, Promburom P, Phimpraphai W, Cappele J, Lajaunie C, Goutard FL, Pinyopommintr T, Fiquie M, Roger FL. A framework to promote collective action within the One Health community of practice: Using participatory modelling to enable interdisciplinary, cross-sectoral and multi-level integration. One Health. 2015;1(2015):44–8. https://www.ncbi.nlm.nih.gov/pubmed/28616464.

Part III

Cutting-Edge Approaches in Medical Treatment

Insights and Innovations in Vascular Medicine

11

Tobias Abt

Dedicated to my dear parents, who have done everything for me.

Abbreviations

AAA	Abdominal aortic aneurysm
ABI	Ankle-brachial index
Aix	Augmentation Index
CAS	Carotid artery stenting
CDT	Complete decongestive therapy
CEA	Carotid endarterectomy
CEUS	Contrast-enhanced ultrasound
CT	Computed tomography
CTA	Computed tomography angiography
CVI	Chronic venous insufficiency
DOAC	Direct oral anticoagulant
DSA	Digital subtraction angiography
DVT	Deep vein thrombosis
EVAR	Endovascular aneurysm repair
EVLA	Endovenous laser ablation
LVA	Lymphaticovenous anastomosis
MR	Magnetic resonance
MRA	Magnetic resonance angiography
MRI	Magnetic resonance imaging
OCT	Optical coherence tomography
PAD	Peripheral arterial disease
PET	Positron emission tomography

T. Abt (✉)
Hamburg, Germany
e-mail: tobiasabt@gmx.net

P. Plugmann, D. Portius (eds.), *Innovations in Healthcare and Outcome Measurement*, https://doi.org/10.1007/978-3-031-77302-0_11

POCUS	Point-of-care ultrasound
PVR	Pulse volume recording
PWV	Pulse wave velocity
RFA	Radiofrequency ablation
TBI	Toe-brachial index
TCAR	Transcarotid artery revascularization
TCD	Transcranial doppler
VLNT	Vascularized lymph node transfer

11.1 Introduction

Vascular diseases, including peripheral artery disease, carotid stenosis, aortic diseases, thrombosis, varicosis, and lipedema/lymphedema pose global health challenges [1]. The field of vascular medicine has recently advanced significantly [2].

Vascular medicine specializes in diagnosing and treating circulatory system disorders, specifically focusing on blood vessels [3]. This field covers various conditions impacting arteries, veins, and lymphatic vessels throughout the body [4]. The circulatory system is vital for supplying blood, oxygen, and nutrients to tissues and organs; disruptions can cause serious health issues [5].

Vascular medicine addresses arterial and venous disorders [6]. Arterial diseases involve conditions that affect the arteries, which carry oxygen-rich blood away from the heart to the rest of the body [7]. Common arterial diseases include those resulting from atherosclerosis, which is the most cause of many arterial conditions, as well as aneurysms [8].

Venous diseases pertain to conditions affecting the veins, responsible for returning deoxygenated blood to the heart [9]. Conditions such as deep vein thrombosis (DVT), chronic venous insufficiency, and varicose veins also fall under the purview of vascular medicine [10].

In addition, there are lymphatic vessels that play a crucial role in circulating lymph, removing waste, and supporting immune function [11].

Diagnosis of vascular conditions often includes functional measurements like ankle and toe brachial index, as well as noninvasive imaging like ultrasound, CT, and MRI, to visualize blood vessels and detect abnormalities [12]. Treatment options depend on the condition and may include lifestyle changes, medications, minimally invasive procedures, and, if necessary, surgery [13].

Vascular medicine specialists collaborate with healthcare professionals like vascular surgeons, interventional radiologists, and cardiologists to provide comprehensive care for patients with vascular disorders [14]. The goal is to manage and improve circulatory health, preventing complications and enhancing overall well-being.

11.2 Diagnostics

11.2.1 Functional Examinations and Imaging Modalities

Vascular medicine has shifted towards noninvasive functional assessments, improving early detection and intervention for conditions such as peripheral arterial disease [15]. Standard tools like ankle-brachial index (ABI) and toe-brachial index (TBI) are now cost-effective means of preventing complications, including amputations [16].

Noninvasive functional assessments evaluate blood vessel function without surgery [17]. Crucial for understanding blood flow and identifying abnormalities, these assessments include the following:

1. **ABI/TBI:** These examinations compare blood pressure measurements at the ankle/toe with those at the arm, indicating the risk of PAD and potential cardiovascular issues [18].
2. **Pulse Volume Recording (PVR):** This noninvasive test measures blood volume changes in limbs during each heartbeat, evaluating arterial disease and peripheral arterial circulation [19].
3. **Pulse Wave Velocity (PWV) and Augmentation Index (AIx):** Assessment of PWV and AIx gauge arterial pulse speed and central arterial pressure waveform augmentation, aiding in risk evaluation and personalized treatment [20].
4. **Segmental Pressure Measurements:** Measuring blood pressure at various limb segments helps identify areas with reduced blood flow, aiding in diagnosing conditions and determining vascular disease severity [21].
5. **Ergometric Procedure for Walking Distance Determination (Treadmill):** This noninvasive procedure evaluates walking distance on a treadmill [22]. It assesses leg blood circulation and performance under stress, aiding in vascular disease diagnosis and severity determination.
6. **Venous Occlusion Plethysmography:** This method allows the noninvasive measurement of volume changes in the veins [23]. It plays a role in assessing venous circulation and supports the diagnosis of venous thrombosis.
7. **Light Reflection Rheography:** Light reflection rheography is a noninvasive method used to measure skin blood flow and assess vascular function [24]. By capturing reflections of infrared light on the skin, changes in blood circulation can be detected, which is helpful in assessing chronic-venous insufficiency.
8. **Duplex Ultrasound:** Combining traditional and Doppler ultrasound, it provides detailed images and information about blood flow, diagnosing conditions like DVT [25, 26].

Noninvasive assessments significantly aid in early detection, diagnosis, and managing vascular conditions, improving patient outcomes and preventing complications [27].

11.2.2 Advanced Imaging Modalities

Advanced imaging modalities, such as contrast-enhanced ultrasound and magnetic resonance angiography, revolutionize vascular medicine, offering precise visualization of lesions for improved preoperative planning and postoperative assessment [28].

Advanced imaging details blood vessel structure and function, aiding in diagnosing and managing various vascular conditions [29]. Notable modalities include:

1. **3D Ultrasound:** Enhanced with three-dimensional capabilities, traditional ultrasound provides more detailed and realistic imaging, valuable for real-time assessment of vascular structures, e.g. in the aorta and carotid artery [30].
2. **Contrast-Enhanced Ultrasound (CEUS):** By enhancing ultrasound imaging with a contrast agent, CEUS improves the detection of vascular abnormalities, especially in aortic, carotid, and peripheral vessels [31].
3. **Digital Subtraction Angiography (DSA):** Although invasive, DSA is highly precise, visualizing blood vessels using X-rays and contrast dye, detecting abnormalities like stenosis or aneurysms [32].
4. **Computed Tomography Angiography (CTA)/Computed Tomography (CT) Venography:** This powerful technique combines X-rays with computer technology, creating detailed cross-sectional images effective in visualizing arterial or venous structures as well as pulmonary embolism [33, 34].
5. **Magnetic Resonance Angiography (MRA)/Magnetic Resonance (MR) Venography:** Utilizing magnetic fields and radio waves, MRA and MR venography generate detailed images without ionizing radiation, valuable for imaging blood vessels, e.g. arteries or DVT/pulmonary embolism [34, 35].
6. **Positron Emission Tomography (PET) Imaging:** Combined with CT (PET/CT), PET imaging detects radioactive tracers to assess blood flow, inflammation, and metabolic status in vascular tissues [36].

These advanced imaging modalities are crucial for accurate diagnosis, treatment planning, and monitoring of vascular conditions [37]. This contributes to more precise patient care and improved outcomes [38].

11.2.3 Ultrasound Technology

Ultrasound technology has advanced significantly, providing detailed imaging of vascular structures for early detection of conditions such as aortic diseases, carotid stenosis, and venous thrombosis [39]. This noninvasive technique utilizes high-frequency sound waves to produce real-time images, aiding healthcare professionals in assessing blood flow, identifying abnormalities, and detecting potential issues at an early stage [40].

Key aspects of ultrasound in early detection are:

1. **Arterial and Venous Imaging:** Ultrasound visualizes arteries and veins, enabling the identification of conditions like atherosclerosis, thrombosis, and aneurysms in their early stages [41].
2. **Early Detection of Atherosclerosis:** Ultrasound detects early signs of atherosclerosis, allowing for timely intervention and lifestyle modifications to prevent further progression [42].
3. **DVT Screening:** Early detection of DVT reduces the risk of complications, such as pulmonary embolism [43].
4. **Monitoring Blood Flow:** Doppler ultrasound assesses blood flow patterns, aiding in the early detection of vascular issues [44].
5. **Screening for Aneurysms:** Ultrasound identifies aneurysms, allowing for monitoring and surgical intervention if necessary [45].
6. **Safe for Repeat Imaging:** Nonionizing ultrasound is safe for repeat imaging, making it suitable for ongoing assessment of chronic vascular diseases [46].

In summary, ultrasound plays a crucial role in the early detection of vascular conditions, providing noninvasive, real-time imaging for timely intervention and improved outcomes [47].

11.2.4 Point-of-Care Ultrasound (POCUS)

Point-of-Care Ultrasound (POCUS) in vascular medicine involves bedside ultrasound for real-time evaluation of vascular conditions [48]. Compact and affordable POCUS devices enhance convenience, speed, and the ability to provide rapid diagnostic information, supporting personalized treatment plans [49].

Key aspects of POCUS in vascular medicine are:

1. **Immediate Bedside Assessment:** POCUS allows healthcare providers to perform ultrasound examinations directly at the bedside, providing valuable information in emergency situations [50].
2. **Quick Diagnostic Information:** POCUS offers fast diagnostic information for assessment of blood flow, detection of abnormalities, and preliminary diagnoses, crucial in time-sensitive scenarios [51].
3. **Vascular Access Guidance:** POCUS guides vascular access procedures, improving accuracy in central line placement and arterial catheterization [52].
4. **Emergency and Critical Care Applications:** POCUS is used in emergency and critical care settings for rapid assessment of conditions like DVT, arterial injuries, and other acute vascular issues [53].

5. **Screening for Abdominal Aortic Aneurysms:** POCUS efficiently screens for aortic aneurysms, enabling early detection and prevention of rupture [54].
6. **Monitoring Fluid Status:** POCUS assesses fluid status, aiding in evaluating factors like inferior vena cava collapsibility for fluid responsiveness and management guidance [55].
7. **Portable and Versatile:** Portable and versatile POCUS devices enhance accessibility in various healthcare settings, including clinics, emergency departments, and intensive care units [56].
8. **Integration into Physical Examination:** POCUS extends the physical examination, allowing real-time visual assessment of vascular structures, enhancing clinician's ability to correlate imaging findings with clinical symptoms [57].
9. **Training and Education:** POCUS serves as a valuable tool in medical education, enabling healthcare professionals to develop and enhance ultrasound skills for interpreting vascular images [58].

In summary, POCUS in vascular medicine provides a quick and accessible method for bedside assessment of vascular conditions [59]. Its versatility and immediate diagnostic capabilities make it valuable in various clinical scenarios, especially in time-sensitive critical situations where quick decisions are crucial for patient outcomes [60].

11.3 Vascular Diseases

The following will present some important vascular diseases. In this context, both established and new innovative procedures are described consecutively (except for what has already been partially mentioned above), as the transition between established and innovative methods is often fluid and not strictly separable. Established procedures are frequently further developed, becoming innovative in the process.

11.3.1 Peripheral Arterial Disease

Peripheral arterial disease (PAD) involves plaque buildup in arteries supplying blood to the extremities, particularly the legs [61]. This leads to reduced blood flow, resulting in symptoms like leg pain and cramping, especially during exercise [62]. Atherosclerosis, characterized by plaque accumulation in arterial walls, often causes PAD, exacerbated by factors such as smoking, diabetes, high blood pressure, and high cholesterol [63]. Untreated PAD poses risks, including nonhealing wounds, infections, and cardiovascular events [64]. Management encompasses lifestyle changes, medications, and, in severe cases, surgical interventions to enhance blood flow [65]. For additional details, refer to Table 11.1 [66].

Recent innovations in PAD diagnosis and treatment aim to elevate patient care, outcomes, and overall disease management [67]. Key innovations include the following:

Table 11.1 Characteristics of peripheral arterial disease regarding definition, epidemiology, etiology, clinical presentation, diagnostics, therapy, and prognosis [66]

	Peripheral arterial disease
Definition	a condition involving the narrowing or blockage of arteries outside the heart, most commonly affecting the limbs
Epidemiology	Common, especially among older individuals, and is associated with risk factors such as smoking, diabetes mellitus type 2, arterial hypertension, dyslipidemia, and obesity. The incidence increases with age
Etiology	Primarily caused by atherosclerosis, leading to plaque buildup in the arteries and reduced blood flow to the extremities
Clinical presentation	Intermittent claudication (pain during physical activity), reduced exercise tolerance, and, in severe cases, rest pain or ulcers due to inadequate blood supply
Diagnostics	Combination of clinical evaluation, ankle-brachial index (ABI) and toe-brachial index (TBI) measurements, and imaging studies (such as ultrasound or angiography)
Treatment	Lifestyle modifications, medications (e.g., antiplatelet drugs, statins), and interventions such as angioplasty or in severe cases bypass surgery to restore blood flow. Smoking cessation and regular exercise are crucial for treatment success
Prognosis	Depending on the severity of the disease and adherence to treatment. Early detection and intervention can improve outcomes, but advanced cases may lead to complications like limb amputation or cardiovascular events. Regular follow-up examinations (e.g. ABI/TBI measurements, ultrasound) are essential for monitoring and managing the condition

1. **Advanced Imaging Technologies:** High-resolution CTA and MRA offer improved visualization of peripheral arteries, aiding clinicians in assessing location and severity of arterial blockages [68].
2. **Walking Exercise:** Structured walking programs play a crucial role in enhancing mobility for PAD patients [69].
3. **Vascular Exercise Groups**: Collaborative exercise programs focusing on vascular health contribute to overall well-being in PAD patients [70].
4. **Drug-Eluting Technologies:** Drug-eluting balloons and stents in endovascular interventions reduce restenosis rates by releasing medications preventing vessel re-narrowing, contributing to more durable and effective results post-vascular interventions [71].
5. **Minimally Invasive Interventions:** Advances in endovascular procedures, like atherectomy and angioplasty, allow less invasive PAD treatments, targeting plaque buildup and improving blood flow, often minimizing the need for open surgical procedures [72].
6. **Intravascular Ultrasound:** Utilizing intravascular ultrasound provides detailed imaging for precise assessment during vascular interventions [73].
7. **Genomic Medicine and Biomarker Research:** Progress in genomics and biomarker research enhances understanding of genetic factors influencing PAD risk, aiding in identifying high-risk individuals and tailoring treatment approaches based on genetic profiles [74, 75].

8. **Gene Therapy for Chronic Limb Threatening Ischemia (CLTI):** Innovative gene therapy approaches show promise in improving outcomes for patients with CLTI [76].
9. **Home-Based Exercise Training/Smartphone:** Utilizing home-based exercise programs facilitated by smartphones enhances accessibility and adherence to exercise routines for PAD patients [77].
10. **Telemedicine and Remote Monitoring:** Integration of telemedicine and remote patient monitoring allows continuous surveillance of PAD patients outside traditional healthcare settings, enabling early issue detection, improving patient adherence, and facilitating timely intervention [78].
11. **Patient-Centered Care and Shared Decision-Making:** A shift toward patient-centered care involves patients in treatment decisions, tailoring therapies to individual preferences and lifestyles [79]. Shared decision-making empowers patients to actively participate in their care, potentially leading to better treatment plan adherence [80].

These innovations collectively contribute to a comprehensive and effective approach to managing PAD [81]. Ongoing advancements in vascular medicine hold the promise of further improving outcomes for individuals affected by PAD [82].

11.3.2 Carotid Stenosis

Carotid stenosis, the narrowing of carotid arteries supplying blood to the brain, is often linked to atherosclerosis, posing the risk of complications like strokes [83]. To access further insights, consult Table 11.2 [66, 84]. Innovations in diagnosis and

Table 11.2 Characteristics of carotid stenosis regarding definition, epidemiology, etiology, clinical presentation, diagnostics, therapy, and prognosis [66, 84]

	Carotid stenosis
Definition	Narrowing of the carotid arteries, the major blood vessels in the neck that supply blood to the brain, typically due to the buildup of atherosclerotic plaques
Epidemiology	Commonly associated with aging and atherosclerosis. It is a significant risk factor for stroke, particularly in older individuals
Etiology	Atherosclerosis, characterized by the accumulation of fatty deposits in the artery walls, is the primary cause of carotid stenosis. Other contributing factors include hypertension, smoking, and dyslipidemia
Clinical presentation	May be asymptomatic, but the condition can lead to transient ischemic attacks (TIAs) or strokes. Symptoms may include sudden weakness, numbness, paresis, or difficulty speaking
Diagnostics	Imaging studies, including carotid ultrasound, CT angiography, or magnetic resonance angiography, to assess the degree of stenosis and stroke risk.
Treatment	Lifestyle changes, medication (e.g., antiplatelet drugs, statins), and in severe cases, surgical/endovascular interventions like carotid endarterectomy or carotid artery stenting to reduce the risk of stroke
Prognosis	Depends on the severity of stenosis and the effectiveness of interventions. Timely diagnosis and appropriate treatment can significantly improve outcomes and reduce the risk of stroke. Regular follow-up and management of cardiovascular risk factors are crucial for long-term prognosis

treatment aim to enhance accuracy, reduce stroke risk, and improve overall management [85].

1. **Transcranial Doppler (TCD) Monitoring:** TCD offers real-time assessment of cerebral blood flow, aiding in monitoring the impact of carotid stenosis and assessing stroke risk by detecting emboli [86]. To ensure a comprehensive evaluation of cerebrovascular health, this procedure should also be applied alongside the widely used Doppler and duplex ultrasound of the extracranial vessels.
2. **Advancements in Carotid Artery Imaging:** High-resolution imaging modalities like duplex ultrasound, CTA, and MRA provide detailed images, aiding precise diagnosis of stenotic lesions [87].
3. **Carotid Artery Stenting (CAS):** As a minimally invasive intervention, CAS involves the placement of a stent to widen narrowed carotid arteries, addressing carotid stenosis and mitigating the risk of complications such as strokes [88].
4. **Embolic Protection Devices:** Used during carotid stenting, these devices capture and remove debris, minimizing embolic stroke risk and enhancing the safety of the procedure [88].
5. **Advancements in Carotid Endarterectomy (CEA):** Traditional CEA sees refinements, including techniques like eversion endarterectomy and regional anesthesia options, contributing to better outcomes and shorter recovery times [89].
6. **Transcarotid Artery Revascularization (TCAR):** TCAR, a minimally invasive procedure, combines aspects of CEA and stenting [90]. It minimizes cerebral emboli risk by temporarily reversing blood flow during stent placement [91].
7. **3D Models for Surgical Planning:** Patient-specific 3D models of carotid arteries aid surgeons in preoperative planning, enabling precise and personalized approaches to interventions [92].
8. **Optical Coherence Tomography (OCT):** OCT utilizes light waves for detailed images of the carotid artery wall, providing high-resolution insights into plaque composition and vulnerability, guiding treatment decisions [93].
9. **Remote Monitoring and Telehealth:** Innovations in telehealth and remote monitoring enable closer monitoring of patients with carotid stenosis, facilitating early detection of changes and timely intervention to prevent adverse events [94].

These innovations collectively advance the diagnosis, treatment, and management of carotid artery stenosis, focusing on improving patient outcomes and reducing stroke risk [95].

11.3.3 Abdominal Aortic Aneurysm

Abdominal aortic aneurysms (AAA) involve the abnormal enlargement of the lower aorta, posing a risk of life-threatening rupture [96]. Often asymptomatic, AAA is influenced by factors like age, gender, smoking, and family history [97]. Early detection through ultrasound is crucial, with treatment options ranging from monitoring to surgical intervention [98]. For more comprehensive information, please consult Table 11.3 [66, 99]. Recent innovations in aortic care aim to enhance outcomes and precision in interventions [100].

1. **Advanced Imaging Techniques:** High-resolution imaging modalities, including CTA and MRA, offer detailed 3D images, aiding accurate diagnosis and treatment planning [101].
2. **Endovascular Aneurysm Repair (EVAR):** EVAR, a minimally invasive procedure for AAA, has evolved with innovations in stent graft design, access and delivery systems, and imaging guidance [102]. These advancements improve safety, speed recovery, and reduce postoperative complications [103].
3. **Fenestrated and Branched Endografts:** Customized devices such as fenestrated and branched endografts address complex aortic aneurysms, providing a tailored approach to interventions [104].
4. **Robot-Assisted Surgery:** Robotics enhance precision and control in aortic surgery, allowing surgeons to perform complex procedures with smaller incisions, potentially reducing complications and improving recovery [105].
5. **Hybrid Operating Rooms:** Combining surgical capabilities with advanced imaging, hybrid operating rooms enable a seamless transition between open surgeries and endovascular interventions, offering a comprehensive approach to aortic care [106].
6. **Genetic and Biomarker Research:** Advances in genetics and biomarkers aid in understanding genetic factors influencing aortic diseases, helping to identify

Table 11.3 Characteristics of abdominal aortic aneurysm regarding definition, epidemiology, etiology, clinical presentation, diagnostics, therapy, and prognosis [66, 99]

	Abdominal aortic aneurysm
Definition	Abnormal dilation or bulging of the aorta, the body's main artery, exceeding ≥3 cm, which can occur in various segments of the vessel
Epidemiology	More common in older individuals, associated with risk factors such as smoking and arterial hypertension. Prevalence increases with age and is higher in men than in women
Etiology	Atherosclerosis and genetic predisposition are common causes of aortic aneurysms. Other contributing factors may include inflammation and infections
Clinical presentation	Often asymptomatic but can lead to symptoms such as abdominal or flank pain, and distal embolism. Rupture is a life-threatening complication
Diagnostics	Imaging studies like ultrasound, CT scans, or MRI to assess the size and location of the aneurysm. Monitoring is crucial to prevent rupture
Treatment	Varies based on the size and location of the aneurysm. Small aneurysms may be monitored, while larger ones (≥5,5 cm) may require surgical intervention, such as open repair or endovascular stent grafting
Prognosis	Depends on the size, growth rate, and timely intervention. Small aneurysms may have a good prognosis with surveillance, while larger or rapidly growing ones pose a higher risk of rupture and require prompt treatment. Regular monitoring and lifestyle modifications are recommended

CT computed tomography, *MRI* magnetic resonance imaging

higher-risk individuals and tailor treatment approaches based on genetic profiles [107].

7. **Aortic Dissection Management:** Hybrid procedures, combining surgical and endovascular techniques, provide individualized treatment strategies for complex cases of aortic dissections [108].
8. **Remote Monitoring and Telehealth:** The integration of remote monitoring and telehealth facilitates continuous observation of patients with aortic diseases, allowing timely adjustments to treatment plans based on early complication signs [109].
9. **Patient-Specific 3D Printing:** Patient-specific 3D printing creates anatomical models for preoperative planning, enhancing understanding and supporting precise interventions in complex cases [110].
10. **Artificial Intelligence (AI) Applications:** Integration of AI in the management of AAA enhances diagnostic accuracy, risk stratification, and treatment planning, contributing to a more tailored and efficient approach in patient care [111].

These innovations collectively advance aortic care, emphasizing minimally invasive approaches, personalized treatments, and multidisciplinary collaboration for improved patient outcomes [112].

11.3.4 Thrombosis

Thrombosis, the formation of blood clots within blood vessels, disrupts normal blood flow and poses serious health risks, including pulmonary embolism and stroke [113]. Factors contributing to thrombosis involve blood vessel damage, changes in blood flow, and genetic predispositions (Virchow's triad) [114]. DVT, commonly occurring in the legs, can lead to severe complications if untreated [115]. Preventive measures include lifestyle changes and, in some cases, anticoagulant medications [116]. Table 11.4 provides additional information for reference [66].

In recent years, innovations in thrombosis care aim to enhance outcomes, reduce complications, and improve healthcare efficiency [117]. Notable advancements include:

1. **Direct Oral Anticoagulants (DOACs):** DOACs represent a breakthrough, offering predictable effects without frequent monitoring, simplifying treatment regimens, and improving patient compliance [118].
2. **Compression Therapy:** Innovative approaches to compression therapy contribute to improved management and prevention of thrombosis-related conditions [119].
3. **Biomarkers and Diagnostic Tools:** Advances in biomarker research and diagnostic imaging, including D-dimer levels, ultrasound, and CT/MR phlebography imaging, enable earlier and more accurate detection, allowing for timely intervention [120]. Thrombophilia is also a crucial aspect of diagnostic advancements [121].

Table 11.4 Characteristics of deep vein thrombosis regarding definition, epidemiology, etiology, clinical presentation, diagnostics, therapy, and prognosis [66]

	Deep vein thrombosis
Definition	Formation of a blood clot (thrombus) within a vein, obstructing the normal blood flow
Epidemiology	Can affect individuals of all ages and is associated with various conditions such as immobility, surgery, or genetic predisposition. It is a common medical condition with diverse risk factors, including adipositas, heart failure, and chronic venous insufficiency
Etiology	Combination of factors in Virchow's triad: Alterations in blood flow, damage to the vessel wall, and changes in blood composition. Risk factors also involve genetics, certain medical conditions, and lifestyle factors
Clinical presentation	Depends on the location of the thrombosis. Common signs include pain, swelling, overheating, and feeling of pressure. In severe cases, thrombosis can lead to complications like pulmonary embolism and stroke
Diagnostics	Clinical evaluation, imaging studies (such as ultrasound, CT or MRI phlebography), and blood tests to detect markers of clotting, e.g. D-dimers
Treatment	Anticoagulant medications to prevent further clotting, and in certain cases, interventions like thrombectomy or the placement of a vena cava filter. Addressing underlying causes and lifestyle modifications are also important
Prognosis	Varies based on the location and extent of thrombosis. Timely diagnosis and appropriate treatment can prevent complications and improve outcomes. However, thrombosis can have serious consequences if not promptly addressed, leading to long-term complications such as a postthrombotic syndrome, or even death

4. **Venous Stents:** Utilizing venous stents provides effective solutions in managing venous disorders [122].
5. **Vena Cava Filters:** The implementation of vena cava filters contributes to preventing complications related to thrombosis and ensuring patient safety [123].
6. **Personalized Medicine:** Tailoring treatment plans based on individual patient characteristics, including genetic factors, allows for more targeted and effective thrombosis management, minimizing adverse effects and optimizing therapeutic outcomes [124]. Diagnostic workups for tumor screening in idiopathic thrombosis (e.g., chest X-ray, abdominal sonography, esophagogastroduodenoscopy, colonoscopy, as well as gynecological consultation [women] or urological consultation [men]) further enhance personalized approaches [125].
7. **Telemedicine and Remote Monitoring:** Telemedicine is vital for managing chronic conditions like thrombosis, because combining telemedicine technology and a virtual examination pathway can help to evaluate remote triage and assessment of patients with suspected thrombosis [126].
8. **Patient Education and Engagement:** Innovations in patient education tools, such as mobile apps and online resources, empower individuals to understand and manage their thrombosis risk [127]. Increased awareness contributes to proactive prevention strategies and early symptom detection [128].
9. **Bioengineering and Clot-Resistant Materials:** Researchers explore bioengineering solutions and clot-resistant materials for medical devices like stents and vascular grafts, aiming to reduce clot formation risks associated with certain interventions [129].

Ongoing research and technological advancements continue driving innovation in thrombosis care, focusing on improving patient care, optimizing treatment strategies, and enhancing the quality of life for individuals at risk of or affected by thrombotic events [130].

11.3.5 Chronic Venous Insufficiency

Chronic venous insufficiency (CVI) results from impaired venous system function, leading to inadequate blood return from the legs to the heart [131]. Common causes include DVT, obesity, prolonged sitting or standing, and leg injuries [132]. Symptoms encompass leg swelling, pain, skin changes, and venous ulcers [133]. Diagnosis involves clinical examination and imaging studies like duplex ultrasound [134]. Management includes lifestyle changes, compression therapy, and surgical interventions [135]. Detailed information can be found in Table 11.5 [66, 136].

Innovations in CVI care aim to enhance outcomes and overall management [137]. Key innovations include:

1. **Advanced Imaging Technologies:** High-resolution imaging modalities, such as duplex ultrasound and venous Doppler studies, provide detailed images of venous anatomy and blood flow, aiding in identifying underlying causes [138].
2. **Compression Therapy Advances:** More comfortable and effective compression garments, intermittent pneumatic compression devices, and inelastic wraps enhance patient adherence and outcomes [139].

Table 11.5 Characteristics of chronic venous insufficiency regarding definition, epidemiology, etiology, clinical presentation, diagnostics, therapy, and prognosis [66, 136]

	Chronic venous insufficiency (CVI)
Definition	a condition, in which the veins, primarily in the legs, fail to efficiently return blood to the heart, leading to blood pooling and associated symptoms
Epidemiology	a common vascular disorder, more prevalent in older individuals. Risk factors include a history of deep vein thrombosis (DVT), obesity, and prolonged standing
Etiology	Primarily involves venous hypertension due to damaged valves in the veins, often resulting from DVT, prolonged standing, or venous obstruction
Clinical presentation	Symptoms range from mild, such as leg swelling and varicose veins, to severe, including skin changes, venous ulcers, and significant discomfort. Edema, pain, and skin discoloration are common
Diagnostics	Clinical evaluation, ultrasound to assess blood flow, and other imaging studies. Light reflection rheography can also be used to assess venous function
Treatment	Includes compression therapy to reduce swelling, lifestyle modifications, and, in some cases, surgical interventions like vein stripping or minimally invasive procedures such as endovenous laser therapy
Prognosis	Varies based on the severity of CVI. Early intervention and adherence to treatment can alleviate symptoms and prevent complications. Advanced cases may lead to chronic leg ulcers and decreased quality of life. Regular monitoring and comprehensive care are essential for managing CVI

3. **Endovenous Ablation Techniques:** Minimally invasive procedures like radiofrequency ablation (RFA) and endovenous laser ablation (EVLA) offer alternatives to surgery, reducing pain and speeding up recovery [140].
4. **Stripping:** Traditional surgical techniques like stripping are still relevant and performed in clinics as an effective option for addressing CVI [141].
5. **Biohybrid Venous Valves:** Innovative biohybrid venous valves contribute to improved venous function, addressing valvular incompetence and promoting better blood flow [142]. This development is still in the research and development phase and may not yet be widely available.
6. **Venous Ulcer Therapies:** Advanced wound care products and therapies accelerate venous ulcer healing, aiming to reduce the risk of recurrence [143].
7. **Telemedicine and Remote Monitoring:** Integration of telemedicine and remote monitoring allows ongoing care for CVI patients, enabling remote consultations and proactive management, which can also be utilized for long-term home care. For instance, a wireless wearable pressure sensing system, which is still in the research phase, enables continuous monitoring of interface pressure in compression garments, providing real-time data that guides therapy and enhances self-management [144].
8. **Patient Education Platforms:** Digital health platforms and patient education tools increase awareness and understanding of CVI, empowering patients to make informed choices and actively participate in their care [145].

These innovations collectively advance the diagnosis and treatment of CVI, emphasizing minimally invasive procedures, personalized care, and improved patient outcomes [146].

11.3.6 Lipedema and Lymphedema

Lipedema and lymphedema are chronic conditions characterized by abnormal fat accumulation and impaired lymphatic drainage [147]. Lipedema results in abnormal fat distribution, mainly in the lower and occasionally in the upper extremities, while lymphedema involves the chronic accumulation of lymphatic fluid due to lymphatic system dysfunction, leading to swelling, typically in the arms or legs [148]. While lipedema primarily affects women, lymphedema can occur in both men and women. For further information, please refer to Table 11.6 [66, 149, 150].

Innovations in the diagnosis and management of these conditions aim to enhance patient outcomes and contribute to a comprehensive approach to these chronic disorders [151]. Key innovations include:

1. **Advanced Imaging Modalities:** High-resolution imaging technologies, such as lymphoscintigraphy and magnetic resonance imaging (MRI), provide detailed insights into lymphatic function, fat distribution, and tissue composition, advancing diagnostic capabilities for both conditions [152].

Table 11.6 Characteristics and comparison of lipedema and lymphedema regarding definition, epidemiology, etiology, clinical presentation, diagnostics, therapy, and prognosis [66, 149, 150]

	Lipedema	Lymphedema
Definition	chronic condition characterized by abnormal fat accumulation, primarily in the legs and sometimes the arms, often causing disproportionate swelling and pain	Condition characterized by the accumulation of excess lymphatic fluid, leading to swelling, typically in the arms or legs
Epidemiology	More common in women, often beginning during puberty or other hormonal changes. Prevalence is higher in individuals with a family history	Can be primary (genetic) or secondary, often associated with cancer treatments like surgery or radiation. It can affect individuals of all ages and genders
Etiology	The exact cause of lipedema is unknown, but genetic and hormonal factors are believed to play, possibly involving disturbed adipogenesis or micro-vascular changes in small blood and lymph vessels	Primary lymphedema is often due to developmental issues in the lymphatic system, while secondary lymphedema results from damage to lymph nodes or vessels, commonly from cancer treatments, surgery, or infection
Clinical presentation	Include bilateral, symmetrical, disproportional fat deposition in the upper and/or lower extremities. Pain, heaviness, and easy bruising are common, and the condition is often resistant to weight loss efforts	Includes persistent swelling, pain, a feeling of heaviness or tightness in the affected limb, and decreased flexibility. Skin changes and recurrent infections can occur in advanced cases
Diagnostics	Primarily clinical, based on physical examination and patient history. Imaging studies such as lymphoscintigraphy or MRI may be used to assess fat distribution and rule out other conditions	Involves clinical evaluation, medical history, and imaging studies like lymphoscintigraphy. Identifying the underlying cause is essential for appropriate management
Treatment	Focuses on symptom relief and may include conservative measures such as compression garments, manual lymphatic drainage, and specialized exercises. Liposuction can be considered for more significant fat reduction	Aims to reduce swelling and manage symptoms. Approaches include manual lymphatic drainage, compression therapy, exercise, and in some cases, surgical interventions
Prognosis	chronic condition without a cure. While symptoms can be managed, the prognosis depends on individual response to treatment. Early intervention and holistic care can improve quality of life, but the condition may progress over time. Regular monitoring and a multidisciplinary approach are often recommended	Depends on the cause and severity of lymphedema. While it is a chronic condition, proper management can significantly improve symptoms and prevent complications. Early intervention and adherence to treatment are crucial for a better long-term prognosis

CT computed tomography, *MRI* magnetic resonance imaging

2. **Lymphatic Microsurgery:** Microsurgical techniques, including lymphaticovenous anastomosis (LVA) and vascularized lymph node transfer (VLNT), offer innovative surgical options for lymphedema [153]. While LVA enhances drainage by connecting lymphatic vessels to veins, VLNT involves transplanting healthy lymph nodes to improve lymphatic function [154].
3. **Compression Garments and Devices:** Innovations in compression garments and devices, such as multilayer bandaging and adjustable compression wraps, improve patient comfort and adherence to compression therapy [155]. These advancements aim to reduce swelling and manage symptoms associated with both conditions, e.g. open wounds.
4. **Complete Decongestive Therapy (CDT) Innovations:** CDT, a standard treatment for lymphedema, has seen innovations with the integration of advanced modalities like pneumatic compression devices and sequential compression pumps, enhancing the efficiency of lymphatic drainage [156, 157].
5. **Liposuction Techniques:** Evolving liposuction procedures tailored for lipedema offer more precise and less invasive methods to remove excess fat deposits [158]. Tumescent liposuction and water-assisted liposuction represent innovations in lipedema management [159].
6. **Lipedema Medications:** Ongoing research explores medications targeting inflammation and fat metabolism as potential treatments for lipedema [160]. While no specific medication has been universally adopted, innovations in pharmaceutical approaches are being investigated [161].
7. **Telehealth and Remote Monitoring:** Integration of telehealth and remote monitoring technologies facilitates ongoing care for patients with both conditions [162]. Telehealth consultations and remote monitoring help healthcare providers assess symptoms, monitor progress, and make necessary adjustments to treatment plans [163].
8. **Nutritional and Lifestyle Interventions:** Innovations in nutritional and lifestyle interventions, including diet counseling and exercise programs, play a role in managing lipedema, aiming to promote overall health, weight management, and improved quality of life, especially in lipedema patients [164, 165].
9. **Educational Resources and Support Groups:** Digital health platforms and online support groups provide valuable resources and a sense of community for individuals with both conditions [166]. These platforms offer educational materials, support, and a space for sharing experiences and coping strategies.

These innovations collectively advance the diagnosis, treatment, and overall management of lipedema and lymphedema, aiming to provide more effective and patient-centered approaches to improve the quality of life for those affected by these conditions [167].

11.4 Conclusions

Recent advancements in vascular medicine mark a transformative era, promising earlier diagnoses, more effective treatments, and personalized care [168]. The integration of noninvasive functional examinations, ultrasound technology, digitalization, sustainability, and personalized medicine reflects the medical community's commitment to enhancing patient well-being [169]. These advancements could notably ease the burden of vascular diseases, improving overall vascular healthcare quality [170].

Vascular medicine has undergone remarkable transformations, driven by technological advances, diagnostic modalities, and treatment strategies [171]. These innovations enhance our grasp of vascular diseases, enabling more precise, personalized, and minimally invasive interventions [172]. Key developments in various aspects of vascular medicine reveal overarching themes [173].

1. **Early Detection and Precision Diagnosis:** Advanced imaging modalities, including ultrasound, CT, and MRI, revolutionize early detection and accurate diagnosis, offering detailed anatomical information for timely and targeted interventions [39, 174].
2. **Minimally Invasive Interventions:** The shift toward minimally invasive procedures reshapes vascular interventions, providing benefits such as reduced recovery times, lower complication rates, and improved overall outcomes [175].
3. **Novel Therapeutics and Targeted Treatments:** The development of novel medications and targeted therapies expands the therapeutic arsenal, addressing the underlying pathophysiology of vascular diseases for more effective and tailored approaches [176].
4. **Patient-Centric Care and Remote Monitoring:** Integration of telehealth, remote monitoring, and digital health platforms ushers in a patient-centric era, enhancing communication, providing real-time data, and empowering patients to actively manage their conditions [177].
5. **Multidisciplinary Collaboration:** The complexity of vascular diseases requires a multidisciplinary approach, with collaborations between specialists contributing to comprehensive care plans [178].
6. **Personalized Medicine and Genetic Insights:** Advances in genetics and personalized medicine shape individualized treatment strategies, offering insights into conditions like aortic diseases and thrombophilia for risk assessment and tailored interventions [179].
7. **Continuous Innovation in Education:** The rapid evolution of vascular medicine necessitates ongoing education and professional development through training programs, conferences, and online resources [180].

In conclusion, ongoing innovations in vascular medicine transform patient care and broaden possibilities in preventing, diagnosing, and treating vascular diseases [181]. Embracing these insights and innovations is crucial to addressing evolving challenges in vascular health and improving the lives of those affected [182]. Collaborative efforts among clinicians, researchers, and industry partners promise greater breakthroughs, propelling vascular medicine into a new era of excellence.

References

1. Roth GA, Mensah GA, Johnson CO, Addolorato G, Ammirati E, Baddour LM, Barengo NC, Beaton AZ, Benjamin EJ, Benziger CP, Bonny A, Brauer M, Brodmann M, Cahill TJ, Carapetis J, Catapano AL, Chugh SS, Cooper LT, Coresh J, Criqui M, DeCleene N, Eagle KA, Emmons-Bell S, Feigin VL, Fernández-Solà J, Fowkes G, Gakidou E, Grundy SM, He FJ, Howard G, Hu F, Inker L, Karthikeyan G, Kassebaum N, Koroshetz W, Lavie C, Lloyd-Jones D, Lu HS, Mirijello A, Temesgen AM, Mokdad A, Moran AE, Muntner P, Narula J, Neal B, Ntsekhe M, Moraes de Oliveira G, Otto C, Owolabi M, Pratt M, Rajagopalan S, Reitsma M, Ribeiro ALP, Rigotti N, Rodgers A, Sable C, Shakil S, Sliwa-Hahnle K, Stark B, Sundström J, Timpel P, Tleyjeh IM, Valgimigli M, Vos T, Whelton PK, Yacoub M, Zuhlke L, Murray C, Fuster V. GBD-NHLBI-JACC Global burden of cardiovascular diseases writing group. Global burden of cardiovascular diseases and risk factors, 1990-2019: update from the GBD 2019 study. J Am Coll Cardiol. 2020;76(25):2982–3021.
2. Behera SS, Pramanik K, Nayak MK. Recent advancement in the treatment of cardiovascular diseases: conventional therapy to nanotechnology. Curr Pharm Des. 2015;21(30):4479–97.
3. Udan RS, Culver JC, Dickinson ME. Understanding vascular development. Wiley Interdiscip Rev Dev Biol. 2013;2(3):327–46.
4. Deng X, Guidoin R. Arteries, veins and lymphatic vessels. In: Black J, Hastings G, editors. Handbook of biomaterial properties. Boston, MA: Springer; 1998.
5. Noordergraaf A. Circulatory system dynamics, vol. 1. Amsterdam: Elsevier; 2012.
6. Boulpaep EL. Arteries and veins. Med Physiol. 2012;2:467–81.
7. Thomas B, Sumam KS. Blood flow in human arterial system-a review. Proc Technol. 2016;24:339–46.
8. O'Rourke M. Mechanical principles in arterial disease. Hypertension. 1995;26(1):2–9.
9. Black CM. Anatomy and physiology of the lower-extremity deep and superficial veins. Tech Vasc Interv Radiol. 2014;17(2):68–73.
10. Chaar C, Ochoa I. Current management of venous diseases. Cham: Springer; 2018.
11. O'Driscoll C. Anatomy and physiology of the lymphatics. In: Lymphatic transport of drugs. London: Routledge; 2019. p. 1–30.
12. Creager M, Loscalzo J, Beckman JA. Vascular medicine E-book: a companion to Braunwald's heart disease. Amsterdam: Elsevier; 2012.
13. Luther B, Kröger K, Katoh M. Kompaktwissen Gefäßmedizin. Berlin: Springer; 2021.
14. Weiss N, Bergert H. Universitäts GefäßCentrum–Wege zur Zertifizierung und daraus resultierende Verbesserungen der Prozesse und der Qualität der Patientenversorgung. In: Handbuch changemanagement im Krankenhaus: 20-Punkte Sofortprogramm für Kliniken. Berlin: Springer; 2017. p. 771–86.
15. Olin JW, et al. Peripheral artery disease: evolving role of exercise, medical therapy, and endovascular options. J Am Coll Cardiol. 2016;67(11):1338–57.
16. Anand V, et al. Comparison of ankle brachial index (ABI), toe brachial index (TBI), and trans-cutaneous partial pressure of oxygen (TcPO2) in prediction of limb outcome among patients with diabetic foot ulcers (DFUs). Indian J Surg. 2023;86:1–5.
17. Sandoo A, Kitas GD. A methodological approach to non-invasive assessments of vascular function and morphology. JoVE. 2015;96:e52339.

18. Hyun S, et al. Ankle-brachial index, toe-brachial index, and cardiovascular mortality in persons with and without diabetes mellitus. J Vasc Surg. 2014;60(2):390–5.
19. Benitez E, Sumpio BE. Pulse volume recording for peripheral vascular disease diagnosis in diabetes patients. J Vasc Diagn. 2015;3:33–9.
20. Husmann M, Jacomella V, Thalhammer C, Amann-Vesti BR. Markers of arterial stiffness in peripheral arterial disease. Vasa. 2015;44(5):341–8.
21. Høyer C, Sandermann J, Paludan JPD, Pavar S, Petersen LJ. Diagnostic accuracy of laser Doppler flowmetry versus strain gauge plethysmography for segmental pressure measurement. J Vasc Surg. 2013;58(6):1563–70.
22. McDermott MM. Medical Management of Functional Impairment in Peripheral artery disease: a review. Prog Cardiovasc Dis. 2018;60(6):586–92.
23. Wilkinson IB, Webb DJ. Venous occlusion plethysmography in cardiovascular research: methodology and clinical applications. Br J Clin Pharmacol. 2001;52:631.
24. Mosti G, Iabichella ML, Picerni P, De Marco G. Quantification of venous reflux by means of some duplex scanner and light reflection rheography parameters and its correlation with chronic venous insufficiency symptoms. Minerva Cardioangiol. 2000;48(11):331–9.
25. Meola M, et al. Basics for performing a high-quality color Doppler sonography of the vascular access. J Vasc Access. 2021;22(1_suppl):18–31.
26. Revzin MV, et al. The radiologist's guide to duplex ultrasound assessment of chronic mesenteric ischemia. Abdom Radiol. 2020;45:2960–79.
27. Hinchliffe RJ, et al. Guidelines on diagnosis, prognosis, and management of peripheral artery disease in patients with foot ulcers and diabetes (IWGDF 2019 update). Diabetes Metab Res Rev. 2020;36:e3276.
28. Settecase F, Rayz VL. Advanced vascular imaging techniques. Handb Clin Neurol. 2021;176:81–105.
29. François CJ. Noninvasive imaging workup of patients with vascular disease. Surg Clin North Am. 2013;93(4):741–60. vii.
30. Golemati S, Cokkinos DD. Recent advances in vascular ultrasound imaging technology and their clinical implications. Ultrasonics. 2022;119:106599.
31. Thakrar DB, Sultan MJ. The role of contrast-enhanced ultrasound in managing vascular pathologies. J Med Imaging Radiat Sci. 2019;50(4):590–5.
32. Krug B, Kugel H, Harnischmacher U, Heindel W, Fischbach R, Altenburg A, Krings F. Diagnostic performance of digital subtraction angiography (DSA) and magnetic resonance angiography (MRA): preliminary results in vascular occlusive disease of the abdominal and lower-extremity arteries. Eur J Radiol. 1995;19(2):77–85.
33. Rajiah P. Updates in vascular computed tomography. Radiol Clin North Am. 2020;58(4):671–91.
34. Karande GY, Hedgire SS, Sanchez Y, Baliyan V, Mishra V, Ganguli S, Prabhakar AM. Advanced imaging in acute and chronic deep vein thrombosis. Cardiovasc Diagn Ther. 2016;6(6):493–507.
35. Roditi G, Wieben O, Prince MR, Hecht EM. MR angiography series: abdominal and pelvic MR angiography. Radiographics. 2022;42(3):E94–5.
36. Sammartino AM, Falco R, Drera A, Dondi F, Bellini P, Bertagna F, Vizzardi E. Vascular inflammation and cardiovascular disease: review about the role of PET imaging. Int J Cardiovasc Imaging. 2023;39(2):433–40.
37. Nishimiya K, Matsumoto Y, Shimokawa H. Recent advances in vascular imaging. Arterioscler Thromb Vasc Biol. 2020;40(12):e313–21.
38. Takx RA, Partovi S, Ghoshhajra BB. Imaging of atherosclerosis. Int J Cardiovasc Imaging. 2016;32(1):5–12.
39. Gettle LM, Revzin MV. Innovations in vascular ultrasound. Radiol Clin North Am. 2020;58(4):653–69.
40. Kim ES, Sharma AM, Scissons R, Dawson D, Eberhardt RT, Gerhard-Herman M, Hughes JP, Knight S, Marie Kupinski A, Mahe G, Neumyer M, Poe P, Shugart R, Wennberg P, Williams DM, Zierler RE. Interpretation of peripheral arterial and venous Doppler waveforms: a

consensus statement from the Society for Vascular Medicine and Society for vascular ultrasound. Vasc Med. 2020;25(5):484–506.
41. Saati AA, Nielsen C, Bishop GJ. Vascular imaging for the primary care provider: venous and arterial disease. Med Clin North Am. 2023;107(5):925–43.
42. Meng H, Ruan J, Yan Z, Chen Y, Liu J, Li X, Meng F. New progress in early diagnosis of atherosclerosis. Int J Mol Sci. 2022;23(16):8939.
43. Kruger PC, Eikelboom JW, Douketis JD, Hankey GJ. Deep vein thrombosis: update on diagnosis and management. Med J Aust. 2019;210(11):516–24.
44. Aziz MU, Eisenbrey JR, Deganello A, Zahid M, Sharbidre K, Sidhu P, Robbin ML. Microvascular flow imaging: a state-of-the-art review of clinical use and promise. Radiology. 2022;305(2):250–64.
45. Benson RA, Meecham L, Fisher O, Loftus IM. Ultrasound screening for abdominal aortic aneurysm: current practice, challenges and controversies. Br J Radiol. 2018;91(1090):20170306.
46. Mehrsheikh AL, Strnad BS, Shetty AS, Itani M. Second-opinion interpretation of outside facility general ultrasound studies: rate of discrepancies and management change. Abdom Radiol (NY). 2023;48(8):2716–23.
47. Liu H, Wang H. Early detection system of vascular disease and its application prospect. Biomed Res Int. 2016;2016:1723485.
48. Arnold MJ, Jonas CE, Carter RE. Point-of-care ultrasonography. Am Fam Physician. 2020;101(5):275–85.
49. Johnson GGRJ, Kirkpatrick AW, Gillman LM. Ultrasound in the surgical ICU: uses, abuses, and pitfalls. Curr Opin Crit Care. 2019;25(6):675–87.
50. Barrosse-Antle ME, Patel KH, Kramer JA, Baston CM. Point-of-care ultrasound for bedside diagnosis of lower extremity DVT. Chest. 2021;160(5):1853–63.
51. Li L, Yong RJ, Kaye AD, Urman RD. Perioperative point of care ultrasound (POCUS) for anesthesiologists: an overview. Curr Pain Headache Rep. 2020;24(5):20.
52. Pouryahya P, McR Meyer AD, Koo MPM. Prevalence and utility of point-of-care ultrasound in the emergency department: a prospective observational study. Aust J Ultrasound Med. 2019;22(4):273–8.
53. Chen L, Malek T. Point-of-care ultrasonography in emergency and critical care medicine. Crit Care Nurs Q. 2018;41(2):94–101.
54. Rhudy AK, Patel S, Houser A, Irfan W, Sheahan M. Point-of-care ultrasound for identification of ruptured infrarenal abdominal aortic aneurysm. Echocardiography. 2022;39(6):841–3.
55. Argaiz ER, Koratala A, Reisinger N. Comprehensive assessment of fluid status by point-of-care ultrasonography. Kidney 360. 2021;2(8):1326–38.
56. Portable Ultrasound Devices in the Pre-Hospital Setting. A review of clinical and cost-effectiveness and guidelines. Ottawa, ON: Canadian Agency for Drugs and Technologies in Health; 2015.
57. Bhagra A, Tierney DM, Sekiguchi H, Soni NJ. Point-of-care ultrasonography for primary care physicians and general internists. Mayo Clin Proc. 2016;91(12):1811–27.
58. Andersen CA, Holden S, Vela J, Rathleff MS, Jensen MB. Point-of-care ultrasound in general practice: a systematic review. Ann Fam Med. 2019;17(1):61–9.
59. Fernando SM, Tran A, Cheng W, Rochwerg B, Strauss SA, Mutter E, McIsaac DI, Kyeremanteng K, Kubelik D, Jetty P, Nagpal SK, Thiruganasambandamoorthy V, Roberts DJ, Perry JJ. Accuracy of presenting symptoms, physical examination, and imaging for diagnosis of ruptured abdominal aortic aneurysm: systematic review and meta-analysis. Acad Emerg Med. 2022;29(4):486–96.
60. Atkinson P, Bowra J, Milne J, Lewis D, Lambert M, Jarman B, Noble VE, Lamprecht H, Harris T, Connolly J, and members of the International Federation of Emergency Medicine Sonography in Hypotension, Cardiac Arrest working group: Romolo Gaspari, Kessler R, Raio C, Sierzenski P, Hoffmann B, Pham C, Woo M, Olszynski P, Henneberry R, Frenkel O, Chenkin J, Hall G, Rang L, Valois M, Wurster C, Tutschka M, Arntfield R, Fischer J, Tessaro M, Bomann JS, Goudie A, Blecher G, Salter A, Rose M, Bystrzycki A, Dass S, Doran O, Large R, Poncia H, Murray A, Sadewasser J, Breitkreutz R, Toh HC, Cevik AA,

Hu AS, Melniker L. International Federation for Emergency Medicine Consensus Statement: Sonography in hypotension and cardiac arrest (SHoC): an international consensus on the use of point of care ultrasound for undifferentiated hypotension and during cardiac arrest. CJEM. 2017;19(6):459–70.
61. Criqui MH, Matsushita K, Aboyans V, Hess CN, Hicks CW, Kwan TW, MM MD, Misra S, Ujueta F, American Heart Association Council on Epidemiology and Prevention, Council on Arteriosclerosis, Thrombosis and Vascular Biology, Council on Cardiovascular Radiology and Intervention, Council on Lifestyle and Cardiometabolic Health, Council on Peripheral Vascular Disease, Stroke Council. Lower extremity peripheral artery disease: contemporary epidemiology, management gaps, and future directions: a scientific statement from the American Heart Association. Circulation. 2021;144(9):e171–91.
62. Firnhaber JM, Powell CS. Lower extremity peripheral artery disease: diagnosis and treatment. Am Fam Physician. 2019;99(6):362–9. Erratum in: Am Fam Physician. 2019 Jul 15;100(2):74.
63. Mandaglio-Collados D, Marín F, Rivera-Caravaca JM. Peripheral artery disease: Update on etiology, pathophysiology, diagnosis and treatment. Med Clin (Barc). 2023;161(8):344–50.
64. Bierowski M, Galanis T, Majeed A, Mofid A. Peripheral artery disease: overview of diagnosis and medical therapy. Med Clin North Am. 2023;107(5):807–22.
65. Campia U, Gerhard-Herman M, Piazza G, Goldhaber SZ. Peripheral artery disease: past, present, and future. Am J Med. 2019;132(10):1133–41.
66. Herold G. Innere medizin 2023. Walter de Gruyter GmbH & Co KG; 2022.
67. Bevan GH, White Solaru KT. Evidence-based medical management of peripheral artery disease. Arterioscler Thromb Vasc Biol. 2020;40(3):541–53.
68. Cina A, Di Stasi C, Semeraro V, Marano R, Savino G, Iezzi R, Bonomo L. Comparison of CT and MR angiography in evaluation of peripheral arterial disease before endovascular intervention. Acta Radiol. 2016;57(5):547–56.
69. Li Y, Rother U, Rosenberg Y, Hinterseher I, Uhl C, Mylonas S, Grambow E, Gombert A, Busch A, Bresler A, Öz T, Görtz H, Pfister K, Dovzhanskiy D, Trenner M, Behrendt CA. A prospective survey study on the education and awareness about walking exercise amongst inpatients with symptomatic peripheral arterial disease in Germany. Vasa. 2023;52(4):218–23.
70. Treat-Jacobson D, Ratchford EV. Vascular disease patient information page: exercise for peripheral artery disease. Vasc Med. 2020;25(1):95–7.
71. Rykowska I, Nowak I, Nowak R. Drug-eluting stents and balloons-materials, structure designs, and coating techniques: a review. Molecules. 2020;25(20):4624.
72. Galyfos G, Liakopoulos D, Sigala F, Filis K. New paradigms in minimally-invasive vascular surgery. Expert Rev Cardiovasc Ther. 2022;20(3):207–14.
73. Loffroy R, Falvo N, Galland C, Fréchier L, Ledan F, Midulla M, Chevallier O. Intravascular ultrasound in the endovascular treatment of patients with peripheral arterial disease: current role and future perspectives. Front Cardiovasc Med. 2020;7:551861.
74. Catalano M, Cortelazzo A, Santi R, Contino L, Demicheli M, Yilmaz Y, Zorzetto M, Campo I, Lanati N, Emanuele E. The Pro12Ala polymorphism of peroxisome proliferator-activated receptor-gamma2 gene is associated with plasma levels of soluble RAGE (receptor for advanced glycation Endproducts) and the presence of peripheral arterial disease. Clin Biochem. 2008;41(12):981–5.
75. Hernández-Aguilera A, Nielsen SH, Bonache C, Fernández-Arroyo S, Martín-Paredero V, Fibla M, Karsdal MA, Genovese F, Menendez JA, Camps J, Joven J. Assessment of extracellular matrix-related biomarkers in patients with lower extremity artery disease. J Vasc Surg. 2018;68(4):1135–1142.e6.
76. Simon F, Duran M, Garabet W, Schelzig H, Jacobs M, Gombert A. Gene therapy of chronic limb-threatening ischemia: vascular medical perspectives. J Clin Med. 2022;11(5):1282.
77. Chan C, Sounderajah V, Normahani P, Acharya A, Markar SR, Darzi A, Bicknell C, Riga C. Wearable activity monitors in home based exercise therapy for patients with intermittent claudication: a systematic review. Eur J Vasc Endovasc Surg. 2021;61(4):676–87.

78. West NEJ, Juneja M, Pinilla N, De Loose KR, Henry TD, Baumgard CS, Kraineva O. Personalized vascular healthcare: insights from a large international survey. Eur Heart J Suppl. 2022;24(Suppl H):H8–H17.
79. Provance JB, Spertus JA, Decker C, Jones PG, Smolderen KG. Assessing patient preferences for shared decision-making in peripheral artery disease. Circ Cardiovasc Qual Outcomes. 2019;12(8):e005730.
80. Smolderen KG, Gosch K, Patel M, Jones WS, Hirsch AT, Beltrame J, Fitridge R, Shishehbor MH, Denollet J, Vriens P, Heyligers J, Stone MEd N, Aronow H, Abbott JD, Labrosciano C, Tutein-Nolthenius R, Spertus JA. PORTRAIT (Patient-centered outcomes related to treatment practices in peripheral arterial disease: investigating trajectories): overview of design and rationale of an international prospective peripheral arterial disease study. Circ Cardiovasc Qual Outcomes. 2018;11(2):e003860.
81. Shamaki GR, Markson F, Soji-Ayoade D, Agwuegbo CC, Bamgbose MO, Tamunoinemi BM. Peripheral artery disease: a comprehensive updated review. Curr Probl Cardiol. 2022;47(11):101082.
82. Chioncel V, Brezeanu R, Sinescu C. New directions in the management of peripheral artery disease. Am J Ther. 2019;26(2):e284–93.
83. Arasu R, Arasu A, Muller J. Carotid artery stenosis: an approach to its diagnosis and management. Aust J Gen Pract. 2021;50(11):821–5.
84. Eckstein HH, Kühnl A, Berkefeld J, Diel R, Dörfler A, Kopp I, Langhoff R, Lawall H, Ringleb P, Sander D, Storck M. S3-Leitlinie zur Diagnostik, Therapie und Nachsorge der extracraniellen Carotisstenose. Gefässchirurgie. 2012;17(6):495–6.
85. Carreira M, Duarte-Gamas L, Rocha-Neves J, Andrade JP, Fernando-Teixeira J. Management of the Carotid Artery Stenosis in asymptomatic patients. Rev Port Cir Cardiotorac Vasc. 2020;27(3):159–66.
86. Bonow RH, Young CC, Bass DI, Moore A, Levitt MR. Transcranial Doppler ultrasonography in neurological surgery and neurocritical care. Neurosurg Focus. 2019;47(6):E2.
87. Saba L, Loewe C, Weikert T, Williams MC, Galea N, Budde RPJ, Vliegenthart R, Velthuis BK, Francone M, Bremerich J, Natale L, Nikolaou K, Dacher JN, Peebles C, Caobelli F, Redheuil A, Dewey M, Kreitner KF, Salgado R. State-of-the-art CT and MR imaging and assessment of atherosclerotic carotid artery disease: the reporting-a consensus document by the European Society of Cardiovascular Radiology (ESCR). Eur Radiol. 2023;33(2):1088–101.
88. Spiliopoulos S, Vasiniotis Kamarinos N, Reppas L, Palialexis K, Brountzos E. Carotid artery stenting: an update. Curr Opin Cardiol. 2019;34(6):616–20.
89. Zhang X, Bai X, Feng Y, Zhang Y, Yang R, Yang Y, Wang T, Xu R, Ma Y, Jiao L. Modified eversion carotid endarterectomy: a novel surgical technique for carotid artery stenosis treatment. Neurol India. 2022;70(5):1787–92.
90. Piper K, Farooq J, Yeung E, Flores-Milan G, Van Loveren H, Lau T. Transcarotid artery revascularization (TCAR) stenting or angioplasty for intracranial carotid artery stenosis: case series and novel application. Interv Neuroradiol. 2023;29(4):351–7.
91. Dakour-Aridi H, Ramakrishnan G, Zarrintan S, Malas MB. Outcomes of transcarotid revascularization with dynamic flow reversal versus carotid endarterectomy in the TCAR surveillance project. Semin Vasc Surg. 2020;33(1–2):24–30.
92. Memon S, Friend E, Samuel SP, Goykhman I, Kalra S, Janzer S, George JC. 3D printing of carotid artery and aortic arch anatomy: implications for preprocedural planning and carotid stenting. J Invasive Cardiol. 2021;33(9):E723–9.
93. İncekalan TK, Taktakoğlu D, Şimdivar GHN, Öztürk İ. Optical cohorence tomography angiography findings in carotid artery stenosis. Int Ophthalmol. 2022;42(8):2501–9.
94. Palombo D, Mugnai D, Mambrini S, Robaldo A, Rousas N, Mazzei R, Bianca P, Spinella G. Role of interactive home telemedicine for early and protected discharge 1 day after carotid endarterectomy. Ann Vasc Surg. 2009;23(1):76–80.
95. Lalla R, Raghavan P, Chaturvedi S. Trends and controversies in carotid artery stenosis treatment. F1000Res. 2020;9:F1000 Faculty Rev-940.

96. Sakalihasan N, Limet R, Defawe OD. Abdominal aortic aneurysm. Lancet. 2005;365(9470):1577–89.
97. Haque K, Bhargava P. Abdominal aortic aneurysm. Am Fam Physician. 2022;106(2):165–72.
98. De Freitas S, D'Ambrosio N, Fatima J. Infrarenal abdominal aortic aneurysm. Surg Clin North Am. 2023;103(4):595–614.
99. Eckstein HH. Abdominelles Aortenaneurysma. In: Akutes abdomen: diagnose–differenzial-diagnose–erstversorgung–therapie. Cham: Springer; 2016. p. 441–8.
100. Golledge J, Thanigaimani S, Powell JT, Tsao PS. Pathogenesis and management of abdominal aortic aneurysm. Eur Heart J. 2023;44(29):2682–97.
101. Duquette AA, Jodoin PM, Bouchot O, Lalande A. 3D segmentation of abdominal aorta from CT-scan and MR images. Comput Med Imaging Graph. 2012;36(4):294–303.
102. Sharma A, Sethi P, Gupta K. Endovascular abdominal aortic aneurysm repair. Interv Cardiol Clin. 2020;9(2):153–68.
103. Debono S, Nash J, Tambyraja AL, Newby DE, Forsythe RO. Endovascular repair for abdominal aortic aneurysms. Heart. 2021;107(22):1783–9.
104. Atkins AD, Atkins MD. Branched and fenestrated aortic endovascular grafts. Methodist Debakey Cardiovasc J. 2023;19(2):15–23.
105. Rusch R, Hoffmann G, Rusch M, Cremer J, Berndt R. Robotic-assisted abdominal aortic surgery: evidence and techniques. J Robot Surg. 2022;16(6):1265–71.
106. Di Marco L, Murana G, Lovato L, Gliozzi G, Buia F, Attinà D, Pacini D. Endovascular solutions for aortic arch diseases: total and hybrid. Surg Technol Int. 2021;38:331–8.
107. Groeneveld ME, Meekel JP, Rubinstein SM, Merkestein LR, Tangelder GJ, Wisselink W, Truijers M, Yeung KK. Systematic review of circulating, biomechanical, and genetic markers for the prediction of abdominal aortic aneurysm growth and rupture. J Am Heart Assoc. 2018;7(13):e007791.
108. Nienaber CA, Clough RE. Management of acute aortic dissection. Lancet. 2015;385(9970):800–11.
109. Kaspersen JH, Aasland J, Leira HO, Odegård A, Nagelhus B, Størset G, Lundbom J, Rosenlund TT, Tjora A, Myhre HO. Three-dimensional teleradiology for surveillance following endovascular aortic aneurysm repair: a feasibility study. J Endovasc Ther. 2005;12(2):196–9. https://doi.org/10.1583/04-1422.1.
110. Bortman J, Mahmood F, Schermerhorn M, Lo R, Swerdlow N, Mahmood F, Matyal R. Use of 3-dimensional printing to create patient-specific abdominal aortic aneurysm models for preoperative planning. J Cardiothorac Vasc Anesth. 2019;33(5):1442–6.
111. Raffort J, Adam C, Carrier M, Ballaith A, Coscas R, Jean-Baptiste E, Hassen-Khodja R, Chakfé N, Lareyre F. Artificial intelligence in abdominal aortic aneurysm. J Vasc Surg. 2020;72(1):321–333.e1.
112. Golledge J. Abdominal aortic aneurysm: update on pathogenesis and medical treatments. Nat Rev Cardiol. 2019;16(4):225–42.
113. Di Nisio M, van Es N, Büller HR. Deep vein thrombosis and pulmonary embolism. Lancet. 2016;388(10063):3060–73.
114. Kushner A, West WP, Khan Suheb MZ, Pillarisetty LS. Virchow triad. In: StatPearls. Treasure Island (FL): StatPearls Publishing; 2022.
115. Khan F, Tritschler T, Kahn SR, Rodger MA. Venous thromboembolism. Lancet. 2021;398(10294):64–77.
116. Lutsey PL, Zakai NA. Epidemiology and prevention of venous thromboembolism. Nat Rev Cardiol. 2023;20(4):248–62.
117. Monteleone PP, Rosenfield K, Rosovsky RP. Multidisciplinary pulmonary embolism response teams and systems. Cardiovasc Diagn Ther. 2016;6(6):662–7.
118. Long B, Gottlieb M. Direct oral anticoagulants versus conventional anticoagulants for deep vein thrombosis. Acad Emerg Med. 2023;30(9):974–6.
119. Amin EE, Joore MA, Ten Cate H, Meijer K, Tick LW, Middeldorp S, Mostard GJM, ten Wolde M, van den Heiligenberg SM, van Wissen S, van de Poel MHW, Villalta S, Serne EH, Otten H-M, Klappe EH, Prandoni P, ten Cate-Hoek AJ. Clinical and economic

impact of compression in the acute phase of deep vein thrombosis. J Thromb Haemost. 2018;16(8):1555–63.
120. Xu L, Ji C, Miao X, Ge J, Li F, Xu C. Combination of circulating miR-125a-5p, miR-223-3p and D-dimer as a novel biomarker for deep vein thrombosis. Am J Med Sci. 2022;364(5):601–11.
121. Colucci G, Tsakiris DA. Thrombophilia screening revisited: an issue of personalized medicine. J Thromb Thrombolysis. 2020;49:618–29.
122. Williams ZF, Dillavou ED. A systematic review of venous stents for iliac and venacaval occlusive disease. J Vasc Surg Venous Lymphat Disord. 2020;8(1):145–53.
123. Young T, Sriram KB. Vena caval filters for the prevention of pulmonary embolism. Cochrane Database Syst Rev. 2020;10(10):CD006212.
124. Nagalla S, Bray PF. Personalized medicine in thrombosis: back to the future. Blood. 2016;127(22):2665–71.
125. Khorana AA, Mackman N, Falanga A, Pabinger I, Noble S, Ageno W, Moik F, Lee AYY. Cancer-associated venous thromboembolism. Nat Rev Dis Primers. 2022;8(1):11.
126. Iyengar KP, Jain VK, Soni M, Hakim Z. Virtual risk assessment pathway for deep venous thrombosis: a preliminary model. Postgrad Med J. 2022;98(1155):24–8.
127. Ranganathan P, Aggarwal R, Pramesh CS. Virtual clinical trials. Perspect Clin Res. 2023;14(4):203–6.
128. Cheng C-W, Wu H, Thompson PJ, Taylor JR, Zehnbauer BA, Wilson KK, Wang MD. Anticoagulation manager: development of a clinical decision support mobile application for management of anticoagulants. Annu Int Conf IEEE Eng Med Biol Soc. 2016;2016:2582–5.
129. Al Meslmani B, Mahmoud G, Strehlow B, Mohr E, Leichtweiß T, Bakowsky U. Development of thrombus-resistant and cell compatible crimped polyethylene terephthalate cardiovascular grafts using surface co-immobilized heparin and collagen. Mater Sci Eng C Mater Biol Appl. 2014;43:538–46.
130. Yamashita Y, Morimoto T, Kimura T. Venous thromboembolism: recent advancement and future perspective. J Cardiol. 2022;79(1):79–89.
131. Youn YJ, Lee J. Chronic venous insufficiency and varicose veins of the lower extremities. Korean J Intern Med. 2019;34(2):269–83.
132. Raffetto JD. Pathophysiology of chronic venous disease and venous ulcers. Surg Clin North Am. 2018;98(2):337–47.
133. White JV, Ryjewski C. Chronic venous insufficiency. Perspect Vasc Surg Endovasc Ther. 2005;17(4):319–27.
134. Santler B, Goerge T. Chronic venous insufficiency—a review of pathophysiology, diagnosis, and treatment. J Dtsch Dermatol Ges. 2017;15(5):538–56.
135. Azar J, Rao A, Oropallo A. Chronic venous insufficiency: a comprehensive review of management. J Wound Care. 2022;31(6):510–9.
136. Engelberger RP, Kern P, Ney B, Dabiri A, Merminod T, Mazzolai L. Chronisch-venöse insuffizienz. Swiss Med Forum. 2016;16(15):337–43.
137. Attaran RR. Latest innovations in the treatment of venous disease. J Clin Med. 2018;7(4):77.
138. García Carriazo M, Gómez de Las Heras C, Mármol Vázquez P, Ramos Solís MF. Doppler ultrasound study and venous mapping in chronic venous insufficiency. Radiologia. 2016;58(1):7–15. English, Spanish.
139. Källman U, Fallenius M, Bååth C. A new compression stocking with well-defined pressure-a randomized controlled pilot study. Phlebology. 2023;38(10):683–94.
140. El Kilic H, Bektas N, Bitargil M, Balkaya IA, Demir T, Koramaz I. Long-term outcomes of endovenous laser ablation, n-butyl cyanoacrylate, and radiofrequency ablation for treatment of chronic venous insufficiency. J Vasc Surg Venous Lymphat Disord. 2022;10(4):865–71.
141. Pittaluga P, Chastanet S, Guex JJ. Great saphenous vein stripping with preservation of sapheno-femoral confluence: hemodynamic and clinical results. J Vasc Surg. 2008;47(6):1300–4.
142. González-Pérez F, Acosta S, Rütten S, Emonts C, Kopp A, Henke HW, Bruners P, Gries T, Rodríguez-Cabello JC, Jockenhoevel S, Fernández-Colino A. Biohybrid elastin-like venous valve with potential for *in situ* tissue engineering. Front Bioeng Biotechnol. 2022;10:988533.

143. Bieniek E, Skołucka-Szary K, Brzeziński J, Piaskowski S, Lewiński A. Innovative biodegradable dibutyrylchitin dressing for the treatment of ulcers occurring during chronic venous insufficiency in patients with type 2 diabetes. Int J Occup Med Environ Health. 2021;34(4):565–73.
144. Li R, Nie B, Zhai C, Cao J, Pan J, Chi YW, Pan T. Telemedical wearable sensing platform for management of chronic venous disorder. Ann Biomed Eng. 2016;44(7):2282–91. https://doi.org/10.1007/s10439-015-1498-x. Epub 2015 Nov 3. PMID: 26530542.
145. Carpentier PH, Satger B, Sandrin B. Patient education in Spa resorts: experience from a French National Program for patients with chronic venous insufficiency. Int J Environ Res Public Health. 2022;19(3):1176.
146. Davies AH. The seriousness of chronic venous disease: a review of real-world evidence. Adv Ther. 2019;36(Suppl 1):5–12.
147. Wagner S. Lymphedema and lipedema—an overview of conservative treatment. Vasa. 2011;40(4):271–9.
148. Duhon BH, Phan TT, Taylor SL, Crescenzi RL, Rutkowski JM. Current mechanistic understandings of lymphedema and lipedema: Tales of fluid, fat, and fibrosis. Int J Mol Sci. 2022;23(12):6621.
149. Kruppa P, Ghods M. Lipödem. In: Klinische angiologie. Berlin: Springer; 2022. p. 1–8.
150. Ludwig M, Ludwig M. Lymphödem. In: Facharztwissen Angiologie: zur Vorbereitung auf die Facharztprüfung. Cham: Springer; 2020. p. 233–40.
151. Blome C, Augustin M, Heyer K, Knöfel J, Cornelsen H, Purwins S, Herberger K. Evaluation of patient-relevant outcomes of lymphedema and lipedema treatment: development and validation of a new benefit tool. Eur J Vasc Endovasc Surg. 2014;47(1):100–7.
152. Nowak S, Henkel A, Theis M, Luetkens J, Geiger S, Sprinkart AM, Pieper CC, Attenberger UI. Deep learning for standardized, MRI-based quantification of subcutaneous and subfascial tissue volume for patients with lipedema and lymphedema. Eur Radiol. 2023;33(2):884–92.
153. Yang JC, Wu SC, Hayashi A, Lin WC, Huang GK, Tsai PY, Chien PC, Hsieh CH. Lower limb lymphedema patients can still benefit from Supermicrosurgical Lymphaticovenous anastomosis (LVA) after vascularized lymph node flap transfer (VLNT) as delayed lymphatic reconstruction-a retrospective cohort study. J Clin Med. 2021;10(14):3121.
154. Ramachandran S, Chew KY, Tan BK, Kuo YR. Current operative management and therapeutic algorithm of lymphedema in the lower extremities. Asian J Surg. 2021;44(1):46–53.
155. Macdonald JM, Sims N, Mayrovitz HN. Lymphedema, lipedema, and the open wound: the role of compression therapy. Surg Clin North Am. 2003;83(3):639–58.
156. Atan T, Bahar-Özdemir Y. The effects of complete decongestive therapy or intermittent pneumatic compression therapy or exercise only in the treatment of severe lipedema: a randomized controlled trial. Lymphat Res Biol. 2021;19(1):86–95.
157. Vignes S. Les lymphœdèmes : du diagnostic au traitement [Lymphedema: from diagnosis to treatment]. Rev Med Interne. 2017;38(2):97–105. French.
158. Bellini E, Grieco MP, Raposio E. A journey through liposuction and liposculture: review. Ann Med Surg (Lond). 2017;24:53–60.
159. Dadras M, Mallinger PJ, Corterier CC, Theodosiadi S, Ghods M. Liposuction in the treatment of lipedema: a longitudinal study. Arch Plast Surg. 2017;44(4):324–31.
160. Ernst AM, Bauer H, Bauer HC, Steiner M, Malfertheiner A, Lipp AT. Lipedema research-quo Vadis? J Pers Med. 2022;13(1):98.
161. Torre YS, Wadeea R, Rosas V, Herbst KL. Lipedema: friend and foe. Horm Mol Biol Clin Investig. 2018;33(1):/j/hmbci.2018.33.issue-1/hmbci-2017-0076/hmbci-2017-0076.xml.
162. Mangion A, Ivasic B, Piller N. The utilization of e-health in lymphedema care: a narrative review. Telemed J E Health. 2023;30:331.
163. Gall A, Bradford N, Finnane A. Using telehealth to support self-management of lymphoedema: clinicians' and patients' perspectives. J Lymphoedema. 2020;15(1):29–35.
164. Forner-Cordero I, Forner-Cordero A, Szolnoky G. Update in the management of lipedema. Int Angiol. 2021;40(4):345–57.

165. Keith L, Seo CA, Rowsemitt C, Pfeffer M, Wahi M, Staggs M, Dudek J, Gower B, Carmody M. Ketogenic diet as a potential intervention for lipedema. Med Hypotheses. 2021;146:110435.
166. Gabe-Walters M, Thomas M. Development of the Lymphoedema patient reported outcome measure (LYMPROM). Br J Nurs. 2021;30(10):592–8.
167. Shavit E, Wollina U, Alavi A. Lipoedema is not lymphoedema: a review of current literature. Int Wound J. 2018;15(6):921–8.
168. Kinlay S, Michel T, Leopold JA. The future of vascular biology and medicine. Circulation. 2016;133(25):2603–9.
169. Wongvibulsin S, Martin SS, Steinhubl SR, Muse ED. Connected health technology for cardiovascular disease prevention and management. Curr Treat Options Cardiovasc Med. 2019;21:1–15.
170. Kim ESH, Beckman JA. Introduction to the vascular medicine issue of Progress in cardiovascular diseases. Prog Cardiovasc Dis. 2018;60(6):565–6.
171. Shi R, Babu S. Modern approaches and innovations in the diagnosis and treatment of peripheral vascular diseases. Front Biosci Schol. 2021;13(2):173–80.
172. Gunduz S, Albadawi H, Oklu R. Robotic devices for minimally invasive endovascular interventions: a new dawn for interventional radiology. Adv Intell Syst. 2021;3(2):2000181.
173. Tinajero MG, Gotlieb AI. Recent developments in vascular adventitial pathobiology: the dynamic adventitia as a complex regulator of vascular disease. Am J Pathol. 2020;190(3):520–34.
174. Murphy DJ, Aghayev A, Steigner ML. Vascular CT and MRI: a practical guide to imaging protocols. Insights Imaging. 2018;9(2):215–36.
175. Bacharach JM, Slovut DP. Endovascular therapies for vascular disease. Am Heart Hosp J. 2003;1(1):69–76.
176. Passacquale G, Sharma P, Perera D, Ferro A. Antiplatelet therapy in cardiovascular disease: current status and future directions. Br J Clin Pharmacol. 2022;88(6):2686–99.
177. Lareyre F, Chaptoukaev H, Kiang SC, Chaudhuri A, Behrendt CA, Zuluaga MA, Raffort J. Telemedicine and digital health applications in vascular surgery. J Clin Med. 2022;11(20):6047.
178. Lareyre F, Behrendt CA, Chaudhuri A, Ayache N, Delingette H, Raffort J. Big data and artificial intelligence in vascular surgery: time for multidisciplinary cross-border collaboration. Angiology. 2022;73(8):697–700.
179. Leopold JA, Maron BA, Loscalzo J. The application of big data to cardiovascular disease: paths to precision medicine. J Clin Invest. 2020;130(1):29–38.
180. Eberhardt RT, Bonaca MP, Abu Daya H, Garcia LA, Gupta K, Mena-Hurtado C, Rogers RK, Sethi SS, Young MN, Piazza G. Call for formalized pathways in vascular medicine training: JACC review topic of the week. J Am Coll Cardiol. 2022;79(21):2129–39.
181. Moureau NL. Vessel health and preservation: the right approach for vascular access. Cham: Springer; 2019. p. 303.
182. Alexander Y, Osto E, Schmidt-Trucksäss A, Shechter M, Trifunovic D, Duncker DJ, Aboyans V, Bäck M, Badimon L, Cosentino F, De Carlo M, Dorobantu M, Harrison DG, Guzik TJ, Hoefer I, Morris PD, Norata GD, Suades R, Taddei S, Vilahur G, Waltenberger J, Weber C, Wilkinson F, Bochaton-Piallat ML, Evans PC. Endothelial function in cardiovascular medicine: a consensus paper of the European Society of Cardiology Working Groups on atherosclerosis and vascular biology, aorta and Peripheral vascular diseases, coronary pathophysiology and microcirculation, and thrombosis. Cardiovasc Res. 2021;117(1):29–42.

Tobias Abt MD, MHBA, EU-MSc., completed his studies in medicine at the Universities of Erlangen-Nuremberg, Sydney, the West Indies, and Cape Town, in epidemiology at the Universities of Mainz, Utrecht, Porto, and Turin, as well as in health economics at the University of Erlangen-Nuremberg. After extensive clinical experience at renowned university hospitals in Göttingen, Mainz, and Dresden, as well as at the Asklepios Klinik St. Georg in Hamburg, he is currently practicing as a specialist in internal medicine and angiology in a medical practice in Hamburg.

Furthermore, Dr. Abt is a certified nutritionist, emergency and sports medicine specialist, as well as an investigator for clinical studies and a hygiene officer. In addition to his publication and lecture activities, he serves as a reviewer for a medical journal and is involved with the German Society of Angiology (DGA) as the primary contact for the Hamburg Medical Association, holds membership in the "Guidelines and Quality Assurance" commission, and contributes to the creation/revision of several guidelines. He is a multiple winner of vascular medicine ScienceSlams ("AngioSlams").

Development of Sustainable Aftercare Strategies Following Bariatric Procedures (ABARO-Study)

12

Melanie Klein, Oliver Riedel, Wiebke Zachariassen, and Mark Dankhoff

Melanie Klein and Oliver Riedel share the first authorship.

12.1 Introduction

The prevalence of obesity, which is defined as having a body mass index (BMI) of 30 or more, has substantially increased during the past decades, especially in industrialized countries. It affects approximately 13% of the world population [1] and is associated with a large number of comorbidities, including respiratory, cardiovascular, and metabolic diseases, skin diseases, allergies, orthopedic diseases, psychological suffering as well as a decreased life expectancy [2, 3].

The genesis of overweight and obesity is usually multifactorial and is determined, among others, by psychological, biological, genetic, and early childhood factors as well as by lifestyle, food options, socialization, and socioeconomic status. Therefore, the effective treatment of obesity and its comorbidities should involve a combination of various curative therapeutic measures.

There are also invasive or surgical procedures, which modify the gastrointestinal tract in a reversible or irreversible way in order to support lower food or nutrient absorption. Due to these changes, after most surgical procedures in bariatric surgery, additional electrolytes, vitamins, minerals, and trace elements must be supplied throughout life. However, this so-called bariatric surgery is one of the most efficient weight loss treatments for people with obesity [4, 5].

But the multitude of possible intra—and postoperative complications as well as postoperative impairments of the metabolism, hormonal control mechanisms, and the psyche must also be taken into account. It is known, among other things, that

M. Klein · W. Zachariassen
Health Services Research, DAK-Gesundheit, Hamburg, Germany

O. Riedel
Department of Clinical Epidemiology, Leibniz Institute for Prevention Research and Epidemiology—BIPS, Bremen, Germany

M. Dankhoff (✉)
Hamburg, Germany

P. Plugmann, D. Portius (eds.), *Innovations in Healthcare and Outcome Measurement*, https://doi.org/10.1007/978-3-031-77302-0_12

inadequate food intake often represents a compensation for psychological impairments and it can therefore be assumed that bariatric surgery cannot eliminate the causes of obesity on a psychological level. Whether this results in a shift in impairment, for example in an increase in depression or other conditions, has not yet been investigated.

It should also be noted that long-term success depends upon adequate aftercare through ongoing conservative care of the patient after the procedure. In the first year after surgery, the aim of follow-up care is mainly to avoid postoperative complications; plastic-aesthetic correction operations are often necessary. In addition, following bariatric surgery, nutritional therapy, psychological support, and motivation for sustained exercise are required to optimize weight loss and stabilize it in the long term. New eating rhythms must also be practiced in order to avoid malnutrition. It is important to advise patients regarding pain, nausea, reflux, temporary alopecia, etc. The therapy of concomitant illnesses must also be strictly controlled, as diseases such as diabetes and hypertension can improve quickly, leading to the risk of hypotension and hypoglycemia. However, the number of specialist centers is currently not sufficient to ensure adequate aftercare and primary care practices have not yet been sufficiently trained in this regard to ensure demand.

Therefore, it can be assumed that patients do not receive the necessary follow-up care after bariatric surgery and thus long-term success, the reduction of obesity-related comorbidities and secondary diseases and the improvement of the patients' quality of life, is not achieved.

In Germany, the Innovation Fund, funded by the Federal Joint Committee (G-BA), is a health policy instrument to promote integrated care, innovative cross-sectoral forms of care, and health care research in Germany. The basis is the law to strengthen care in statutory health insurance (GKV Supply Strengthening Act) passed in 2015. Approximately 300 million euros are available every year to generate sustainable projects in the areas of *new forms of care* and *health services research.*

New forms of care (Neue Versorgungsformen) go beyond the current standard care provided by statutory health insurance (SHI). Funding is primarily given to projects that aim to overcome sectoral separation or optimize intra-sector interfaces with the help of innovative processes and structures.

In the area of *health services research* (Versorgungsforschung), the aim is to create a scientific basis for solving relevant care problems in statutory health insurance.

The ABARO-study (**A**uswirkungen nach **BAR**iatrischen **O**perationen; effects after bariatric operations) was accepted by the G-BA for funding in 2019 and was funded from April 1, 2020 to September 30, 2023. As part of our ABARO-study, we examined the aftercare, quality of life, and weight development of the patients several years after the invasive or surgical procedures. The aim of the study was to uncover deficits in the care of bariatric surgery patients in order to develop treatment recommendations and suitable strategies for adequate aftercare in a further step.

The results of this study were used to describe and determine the course of treatment several years after the operation (OP). In order to achieve this goal, billing data from DAK-Gesundheit (with around 5.5 million insured people one of the largest

German statutory health insurance provider) and data from a survey of a total of 2151 insured persons were combined and analyzed. The results made it possible to illustrate deficits in aftercare, risks and secondary diseases as well as the needs of patients that had not yet been examined. The results were used to formulate recommendations for better care and to develop new care concepts.

Therefore, the aim of this study was to describe so-called care deficits in the required (lifelong) aftercare as well as the necessary recommendations for action derived from the findings for sustainable and successful further treatment.

12.2 Methods

12.2.1 Study Design

The present analyses were based on a linked data set comprising longitudinal health claims data and cross-sectional data from a patient survey. The design of the underlying study has been described previously in more detail [6]. In brief, a two-step approach was chosen to combine health claims data from a large German statutory health insurance (secondary data) provider with data collected through a survey (primary data) as follows:

First, the German Pharmacoepidemiological Research Database (GePaRD) [7] was used to identify patients who have undergone bariatric surgery anytime between 2004 and 2018, who were known to be still alive in the last data year available at the time of the study conduction in 2022. GePaRD is based on claims data from four SHI providers in Germany and currently includes information on approximately 25 million persons who have been insured with one of the participating providers since 2004 or later. Since one of the SHIs also initiated the project, only data from this SHI were used in this case, comprising approximately 5, five million insured individuals. In addition to demographic data, GePaRD contains information on drug dispensations as well as outpatient (i.e. from general practitioners and specialists) and inpatient procedures and diagnoses. Next, all identified patients meeting the inclusion criteria were invited to participate in a survey on their bariatric surgery and related information, e.g. sociodemographics, dietary behavior, utilization of medical services since the operation, subjective assessment of the success of therapy, and an assessment of postsurgical quality of life (BQL). In addition, each patient was screened for mental health outcomes with the Mini-Symptom-Checklist (MINI-SCL). The Mini-SCL consists of three scales, each of which comprising six items from the Symptom Checklist (SCL-90). The MINI-SCL measures the presence of depression, anxiety, and somatization, based on the 7 days prior to filling the survey. Each scale assesses specific symptoms (e.g. for depression: loss of interest, feelings of loneliness, worthlessness or hopelessness). A global severity of impairment score can be calculated by summing all scores from all three scales. This score can vary between 35 and 75, with lower scores denoting higher psychological stress [8]. The quality of life was assessed with the bariatric quaility of life (BQL) index [9].

As an indicator for eating disorders, the Eating Disorder Examination-Questionnaire 8 (EDE-8) was used. The EDE-8 scale consists of eight Items, and a global score can vary between 0 and 8, with lower scores denoting higher possibilities of disordered eating behaviors [10].

Moreover, in the survey we asked for body height and for body weight prior to intervention (T0), soon after intervention (T1) and at the time of survey (T2). These Data were used to calculate the Body Mass Index (BMI): the reported body weight (in kilograms) divided by the square of height in meters. The excess weight loss (EWL, in %) in relation to the normal weight was calculated by dividing the number of kilograms lost by the number of kilograms in the patients' excess weight (related to a BMI of 25). The EWL was calculated for T1 and T2.

Overall, 6913 potential candidates for the survey were identified. Hereof, 1691 patients could not be contacted for various reasons (e.g. being no longer insured with this SHI or having objected to receiving mail, for more details on reasons for exclusion please see [6]). Thus, 5222 patients were invited to fill out the survey, 2151 of whom responded and could be considered for the analyses. As for all identified patients, health claims data were available, regardless of their participation in the survey, survey responders and nonresponders could be compared with regard to their sociodemographics and clinical information. They did not differ in terms of sex, years since surgery, or comorbidity profiles. However, responders were about 3 years older than nonresponders (54.6 years vs. 51.5 years).

12.2.2 Statistical Analyses

Summary statistics consisted of counts, percentages, means and standard deviations (SD), medians, and quartiles (Q1, Q3), where appropriate. All statistical analyses were conducted using R version 4.3.1 [11].

12.2.3 Ethics

The study was approved by the Hamburg Medical Chamber Ethics Committee (October 11, 2021, No. 2021–10,543-BO-ff) and has been performed according to ethical standards laid down in the 1964 Declaration of Helsinki. Written informed consent was obtained from all participating patients.

In Germany, the utilization of health insurance data for scientific research is regulated by the Code of Social Law. All involved health insurance providers as well as the German Federal Office for Social Security and the Senator for Health, Women and Consumer Protection in Bremen as their responsible authorities approved the use of GePaRD data for this study. Informed consent for studies based on claims data is required by law unless obtaining consent appears unacceptable and would bias results, which was the case in this study. According to the Ethics Committee of the University of Bremen, studies based on GePaRD are exempt from institutional review board review.

12.3 Results

12.3.1 Sample Characteristics

The study sample is described in Table 12.1. The majority of study participants were female (80.7%). The mean age was 47.9 (SD: 10.9) years at bariatric surgery and 54.5 (SD: 10.8) years at the conduction of the survey. The mean years since bariatric intervention were 6.5 (SD: 3.1). Most of the participants had a gastric bypass (50.0%) or a gastric sleeve (43.0%). The proportion of reversible interventions was less than 6% (gastric band or gastric balloon). The mean BMI before surgery (at T0) was 51.9 (SD: 8.7). At the conduction of the survey, the mean BMI decreased to 34.8 (SD: 7.5) and the proportion of patients who still (or again) had a BMI > 40 after the intervention (at T2) was 22.3%. Following bariatric intervention, the mean BMI was 31.1 (SD: 6.4) and 12.5% reported to never have achieved a BMI < 40. The mean EWL in % in T1 was 79.0% (SD: 29.8%) and decreased to 64.6% (SD: 30.9) in T2 (at survey).

12.3.2 Complaints After Surgery

In Fig. 12.1, the complaints immediately after OP and those still frequently experienced at the time of the survey as stated by the study participants are displayed. The

Table 12.1 Characteristics and clinical parameters of the sample (N = 2.151)

	Total
Sociodemographics	
Males, N (%)	416 (19.3%)
Females, N (%)	1.735 (80.7%)
Age	
Age at conduct of the survey, mean (SD)	54.5 (10.9)
Age at surgery, mean (SD)	47.9 (10.8)
Clinical parameters	
Years since surgery, mean (SD)	6.5 (3.1)
Type of surgery in %	
Gastric bypass	50.0%
Gastric sleeve	43.0%
Gastric band	5.5%
Gastric balloon	0.3%
Other	1.1%
Body-mass-index before surgery (T0)	
Mean (SD)	51.9 (8.7)
Body-mass-index lowest, after surgery (T1)	
Mean (SD)	31.1 (6.4)
Body-mass-index at survey (T2)	
Mean (SD)	34.8 (7.5)
>40 (in %)	22.3%
Excess weight loss in %	
Mean (SD)	
T1 (lowest after surgery)	79.0 (29.8)
T2 (at survey)	64.6 (30.9)

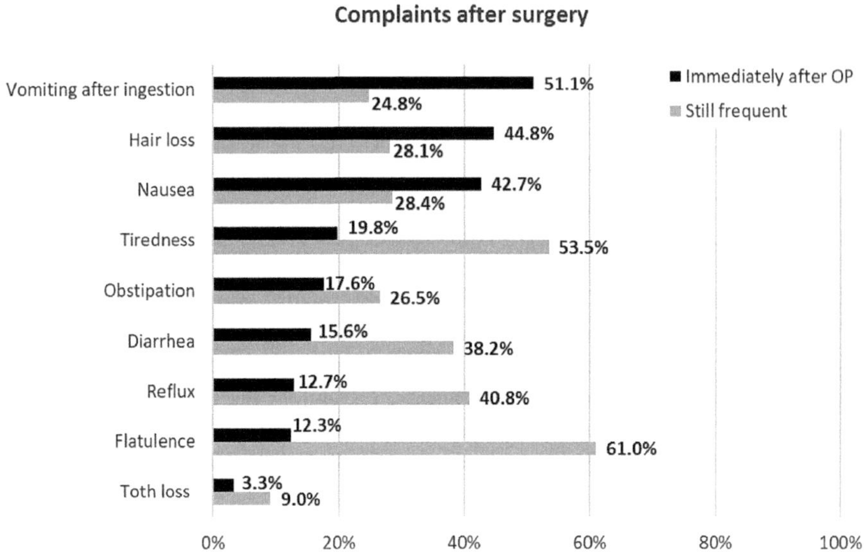

Fig. 12.1 Complaints after surgery reported by the study participants immediately after OP and still frequent at time of the survey

frequency of the complaints changed over time, whereas even several years after surgery some of the stated complaints occurred more frequently than immediately after OP, i.e., fatigue, obstipation, diarrhea, reflux, flatulence, and tooth loss. Moreover, fatigue (53.5%), diarrhea (38.2%), reflux (40.8%), and flatulence (61.0%) were very often rated as still frequently occurring. Diarrhea, nausea, hair loss, obstipation, and vomiting after ingestion were also stated by more than 20% as still frequent and tooth loss by 9%.

In addition, a dumping syndrome was reported by 28.9% of all study participants immediately after the surgery and 33.8% rated it as still frequent later on. Female participants reported more often that they were suffering from dumping syndrome immediately after OP (30.7%) and/or still frequently suffering from it later (36.2%). Male study participants reported this only in 28.9% respectively 33.8% (Fig. 12.2).

12.3.3 Reported Data of Aftercare

Most of the study participants reported that they had at least one postsurgical appointment in the first year after intervention, 57.6% reported that they had three or more (Table 12.2). With regard to the question of how long they had been in medical aftercare, 5.2% reported that they had none, 22.2% reported they had aftercare only in the first year, 18.2% had aftercare for 2 years, 12.5% for 3 years, and more than 40% for 4 years or more. We also asked to rate the quality of the aftercare and 17.1% reported the aftercare as inadequate, 18.4% as adequate, 33.7% rated the quality as good, and 30.8% rated it as very good.

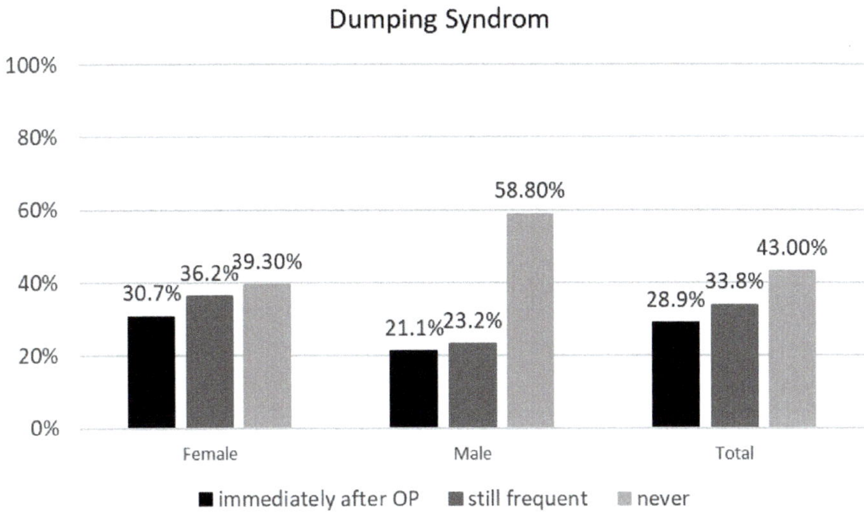

Fig. 12.2 Dumping Syndrome reported by the study participants immediately after OP and still frequent (multiple replies possible)

Table 12.2 Data of postsurgical and aftercare of the sample

	Total
Number of postsurgical appointments in the first year after intervention	
None	3.7%
1 appointment	11.0%
2 appointments	27.7%
3 or more	57.6%
How long have you been in medical aftercare?	
I had no medical aftercare	5.2%
Only in the first year	22.2%
2 years	18.2%
3 years	12.5%
4 years or more	41.9%
How do you rate the quality of your aftercare?	
Inadequate	17.1%
Adequate	18.4%
Good	33.7%
Very good	30.8%

12.3.4 Quality of Aftercare in Relation to Other Variables

In the following section, the results regarding the quality of aftercare in relation to other variables is described.

As shown in Fig. 12.3, the EWL in T1 and especially in T2 decreased with the quality of aftercare. It is also shown, that the quality of aftercare had an effect on weight gain after surgery to the timepoint of the survey: In patients who rated the

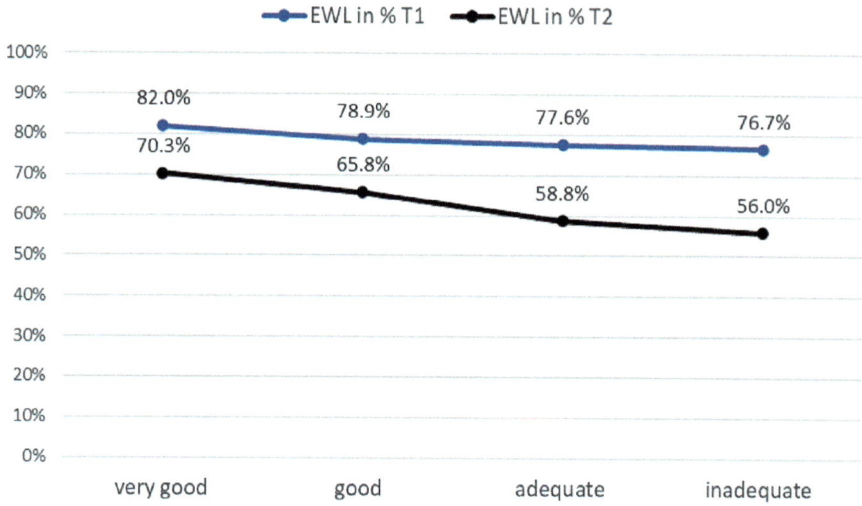

Fig. 12.3 EWL in % in T1 and in T2 in relation to the quality of aftercare rated by the study participants

quality of aftercare as "very good" the mean EWL decreased more or less 12% points over time from T1 to T2, whereas the mean EWL in patients who rated the quality of aftercare as "inadequate" it decreased by 20% points (T1: 76.7, T2: 56.0).

Moreover, with the quality of aftercare the number of study participants, who were satisfied with the progression of their body weight, increased. Only 46.6% of those, who rated the quality of aftercare as inadequate were satisfied with their body weight, whereas this proportion was 82.8% among those, who rated the quality as very good (Fig. 12.4).

About 20% of the patients, who rated the quality as inadequate reported complications or an emergency attendance at a doctor/hospital after the intervention. In the group of patients who rated the quality as very good, this happened only in 11% of cases (Fig. 12.5).

In Fig. 12.6 the association of the quality of aftercare in relation to the BQL, in relation to the Mini-SCL, and in relation to the EDE-8 is displayed. Regarding the BQL a more highly rated quality of aftercare was associated with higher scores on the BQL at the time of survey conduction. Furthermore, regarding the Mini-SCL and the EDE-8 it was shown, that the total score decreased in relation to the quality of aftercare.

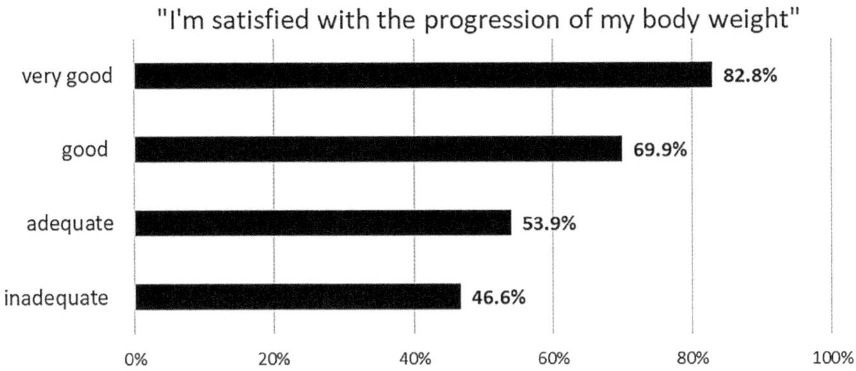

Fig. 12.4 Study participants, who stated that they are satisfied with the progression of their body weight after surgery in relation to the quality of aftercare (in %)

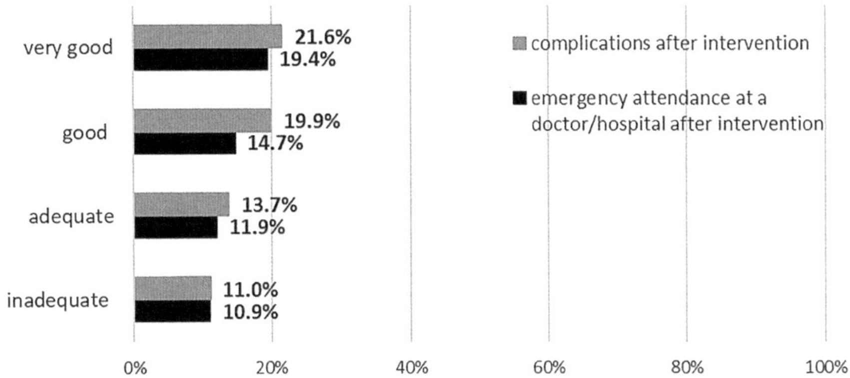

Fig. 12.5 Study participants, who stated that they had complications after intervention and/or that they had an emergency attendance at a doctor/hospital after intervention in relation to the quality of aftercare (in %)

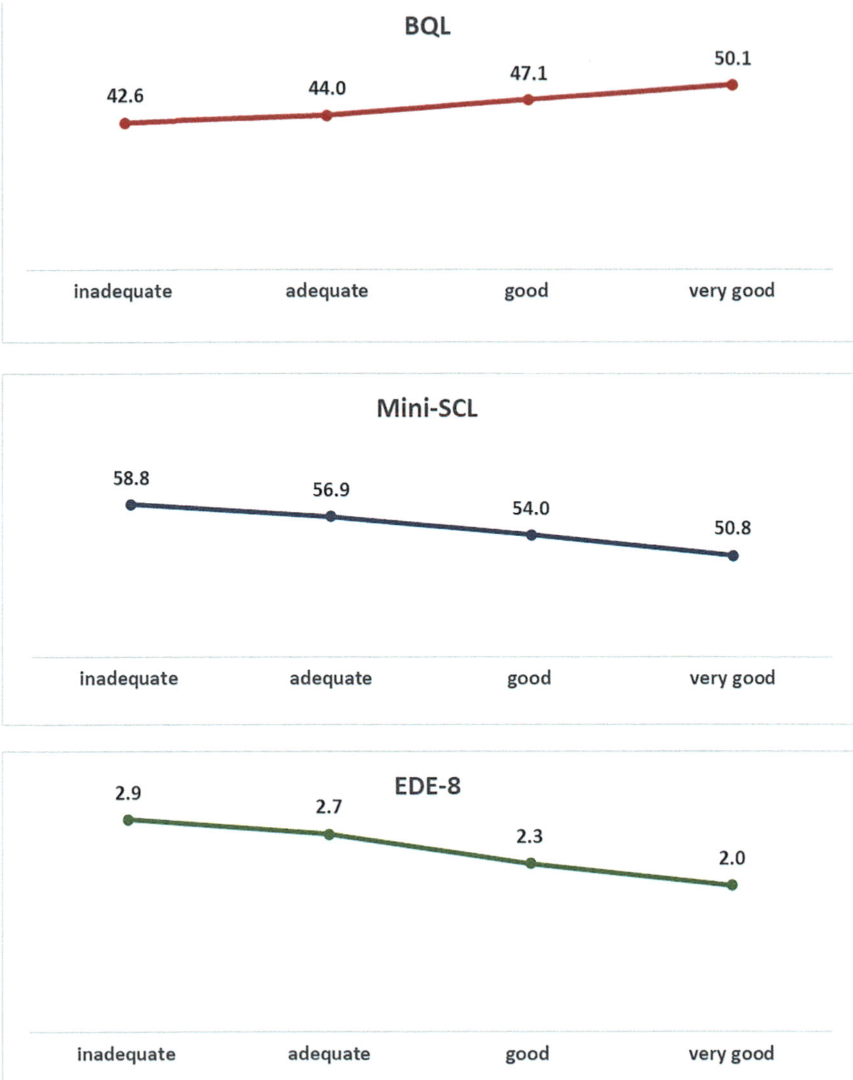

Fig. 12.6 Quality of aftercare in relation to the BQL Score, in relation to the Mini-SCL and in relation to the EDE-8 (indicator for eating disorders)

12.4 Discussion

The aim of our ABARO-Study was to investigate the situation in patients after bariatric surgery, the aftercare as well as the quality of aftercare in relation to the weight development and the quality of life of the patients several years after bariatric surgery in order to uncover deficits in care and to develop treatment recommendations and suitable strategies for adequate aftercare in a further step.

We discovered that even several years after surgery—the mean years since bariatric intervention were 6.5 in our sample—complaints such as fatigue, reflux, and flatulence were very often reported by the study participants. In this regard, it should be mentioned, that the frequency of complaints several years after surgery even increased compared to the frequency of complaints immediately after OP. Moreover, a dumping syndrome was reported by 33.8% as still frequent at the time of the survey. In the literature [12–14], an early dumping syndrome (occurring within 10–30 min after a meal) is present on average in 15.7% of patients and a late dumping syndrome (occurring 1–3 h after a high-carbohydrate meal) can reach up to 25% in a period of 1–5 years after surgery. At this point, it should be mentioned that we only asked if a dumping syndrome was present, we did not distinguish between early or late dumping syndromes. This might explain why we found higher rates. However, the high proportion of patients with complaints and/or a dumping syndrome even several years after surgery underlines the need for action. For example, to avoid a dumping syndrome, appropriate nutrition behavior should be learned and practiced (i.e. several small meals throughout the day, balanced nutrition with low glycemic carbohydrate foods), therefore dietary advice is one important measure in aftercare to ensure long-term treatment success [15].

In Germany, following the S3 guidelines for surgery of obesity and metabolic diseases [16–18], patients after bariatric surgery have lifelong access to structured, inter-professional aftercare. In our study, only 42% of the study participants reported that they had aftercare for 4 years or more. Regarding the aftercare, we also asked the patients to rate the quality and 17.1% reported the aftercare as inadequate. In a further step, we assessed the quality of aftercare in relation to other variables.

First, it was shown that the extent of EWL—both soon after surgery and several years later at the time of study conduction—was correlated with the quality of aftercare, i.e. patients with higher EWL also reported a higher quality of aftercare. Moreover, after bariatric surgery weight regain is a well-known and common factor and challenging for the patients and the healthcare system [19–21]. In this regard, it is particularly interesting that in our study the quality of aftercare had an effect on weight regain after surgery. It was shown, that in patients with inadequate quality of aftercare, the mean EWL decreased more over time from T1 (after surgery) to T2 (at survey) than in patients who rated the quality as very good.

Second, we discovered that in patients who had rated the quality as good or very good, the number of study participants, who were satisfied with the progression of their body weight, increased. Moreover, if the quality of aftercare was rated as good or very good, the postsurgical quality of life (BQL) was also more highly rated. Similar associations were shown regarding psychological stress (Mini-SCL) and the EDE-8 as an indicator for eating disorders—the total score decreased in relation to the quality of aftercare. These findings suggest that the aftercare is an important factor to ensure long-term success of the treatment after bariatric surgery. In this regard, it should be noted that our study design was based on a retrospective identification of patients, and these were invited to fill out the survey. Therefore, we were not able to determine the quality of aftercare and/or the progression of the body weight or other variables over time, which would have enabled us to conduct a pre–post-comparison.

The same limitation is found in a cross-sectional study conducted by [22]. In this study, the quality of care transitions during discharge from the hospital in patients with bariatric surgery up to 24 months after the OP was investigated. Nevertheless, they also found that patients who reported high quality of care transitions had significantly lower weight regain 24 months after surgery compared to patients who reported low quality of care transition in the discharge process.

The overall strength of our study is that it is the first to combine health insurance data with a questionnaire survey while taking into account such a long observation period of up to 12 years after surgery and including a large sample of bariatric patients. Thanks to the survey's high response rate of almost 50% (2151 patients), we were able to gain unique insight into the situation, the long-term consequences of the operation and aftercare. Therefore, this study provides a comprehensive overview of the middle-term and long-term impact of bariatric interventions. In summary, even several years after surgery a dumping syndrome and other complaints such as fatigue, reflux and flatulence are still frequent. Moreover, our findings suggest that the aftercare is an important factor to ensure long-term success of the treatment after bariatric surgery, because we found associations between the quality of aftercare and the weight development (EWL) as well as the quality of life (BQL) and psychological stress (Mini-SCL/EDE-8).

12.5 Recommendations for Action

In terms of postoperative complaints, certain results point to noticeable deficits, i.e. there is a need for sustained action in order to effectively close these current deficits.

In summary, immediately after surgery and in particular even several years after the OP, the study participants stated that they were suffering from a lot of complaints such as fatigue, reflux, and flatulence. The same picture emerges in terms of a dumping syndrome; more than 30% were suffering from it even several years after intervention. Moreover, our findings suggest that the aftercare is an important factor to ensure long-term success of the treatment after bariatric surgery, because we found associations between the quality of aftercare and the weight development (EWL) as well as with the quality of life (BQL) and psychological stress (Mini-SCL/EDE-8).

With regard to these findings, optimization of follow-up and aftercare is absolutely necessary from a medical and therapeutic perspective.

However, the term aftercare does not only refer to the postoperative consultations in the bariatric surgery centers, but also to the long-term and holistic aftercare provided by general practitioners, gastroenterologists, nutritionists, psychologists—and also dermatologists and orthopedists.

This requires various mechanisms, which ultimately only work in combination to sustainably alleviate or eliminate postoperative symptoms, and which must therefore be embedded in a comprehensive and binding (certified) aftercare program.

These offers would be primarily special follow-up appointments, psychological support, nutritional advice, gastroenterological, and dental check-ups as well as dermatological and orthopedic consultations.

Since experience has shown that bariatric surgery requires lifelong follow-up care, appropriate time intervals must be defined for the above-mentioned mechanisms and adhered to by the affected patients.

One possible way to support the aftercare for these patients in Germany would be to develop a new form of care (Neue Versorgungsform), which would go beyond the current standard care and overcome sectoral separation. Such a program is the 18-month ACHT follow-up program, which is a digitally supported, structured, and cross-sectoral program to improve success after bariatric-metabolic surgery [23]. Currently, the program is being evaluated, and the results are not published yet.

However, finally, to optimize the aftercare for all patients, and not only for those taking part in a special program and only for 18 months, it would be necessary to incorporate our findings in the German "S3 guidelines for surgery of obesity and metabolic diseases" (currently being revised, as it was only valid until December 31, 2022).

12.6 Abstract/Summary

12.6.1 Purpose

Obesity has increased enormously in the past decades and is associated with a lot of comorbidities and a decreased life expectancy. One of the most efficient weight loss treatments for people with obesity is bariatric surgery. But it is also known, due to the irreversible changes to the gastrointestinal tract, that long-term success can only be ensured through adequate aftercare. Therefore, the aim of our ABARO-study was to examine the aftercare, complaints, the weight development, and the quality of life of patients even several years after bariatric surgery in order to develop recommendations for adequate aftercare in a further step.

12.6.2 Materials and Methods

The present analyses were based on a linked data set comprising longitudinal health claims data and cross-sectional data from a patient survey. Patients with a bariatric intervention between 2004 and 2018 were identified in the health claims database and invited to fill in the survey, comprising sociodemographic and medical data, information about the complaints, about the aftercare, lifestyle information, and psychometric scales. The BMI and the excess weight loss (EWL) were calculated for the time immediately after bariatric surgery (T1) and when filling out the survey (T2).

12.6.3 Results

The majority of study participants were female (80.7%). The mean ages were 47.9 (SD: 10.9) years at bariatric surgery and 54.5 (SD: 10.8) years at the conduction of the survey. The mean years since bariatric intervention was 6.5 (SD: 3.1). The mean

EWL in % in T1 (immediately after OP) was 79.0% (SD: 29.8%) and decreased to 64.6% (SD: 30.9) in T2 (at survey). A lot of the study participants stated that they suffered from fatigue (53.5%), diarrhea (38.2%), reflux (40.8%), and flatulence (61.0%) even several years after surgery, and more than 30% reported suffering from a dumping syndrome. Moreover, we found strong associations between the quality of aftercare and the weight development (EWL) as well as with the quality of life (BQL) and psychological stress (Mini-SCL/EDE-8).

12.6.4 Discussion

Our findings suggest that the aftercare is an important factor to ensure long-term success of the treatment after bariatric surgery. With regard to these findings, optimization of aftercare is absolutely necessary, which does not only refer to the postoperative consultations in the bariatric surgery centers but also to the long-term and holistic aftercare provided by general practitioners, gastroenterologists, nutritionists, psychologists—and also dermatologists and orthopedists.

Declaration of Competing Interests All authors declare no competing interests.

Acknowledgements The authors would like to thank the statutory health insurance provider "DAK-Gesundheit," which provided data for this study. Moreover, the authors thank Heike Gerds (BIPS) for proofreading the manuscript. Our further thanks go to Willempje Hummel-Bartenschlager (BIPS) and Birgit Wolter (BIPS) for supporting the data entry as well as Philipp Alexander Volkmar (BIPS) and Anja Gabbert (BIPS) for the statistical programming of the data sets.

References

1. Stival C, Lugo A, Odone A, van den Brandt PA, Fernandez E, Tigova O, et al. Prevalence and correlates of overweight and obesity in 12 European countries in 2017-2018. Obes Facts. 2022;24:655.
2. Sarma S, Sockalingam S, Dash S. Obesity as a multisystem disease: trends in obesity rates and obesity-related complications. Diabetes Obes Metab. 2021;23:3–16.
3. Whitlock G, Lewington S, Sherliker P, Clarke R, Emberson J, Halsey J, et al. Body-mass index and cause-specific mortality in 900 000 adults: collaborative analyses of 57 prospective studies. Lancet. 2009;373:1083–96.
4. Velapati SR, Shah M, Kuchkuntla AR, Abu-dayyeh B, Grothe K, Hurt RT, et al. Weight regain after bariatric surgery: prevalence, etiology, and treatment. Curr Nutr Rep. 2018;7:329–34.
5. Voorwinde V, Hoekstra T, Monpellier VM, Steenhuis IHM, Janssen IMC, van Stralen MM. Five-year weight loss, physical activity, and eating style trajectories after ariatric surgery. Surg Obes Relat Dis. 2022;18:911–8.
6. Riedel O, Braitmaier M, Dankhoff M, Hornschuch M, Klein M, Zachariassen W, Hoyer J. Quality of life in bariatric patients up to twelve years after surgery—results from a nationwide retrospective cohort study. Obes Res Clin Pract. 2023;17(4):353–60. https://doi.org/10.1016/j.orcp.2023.08.001. Epub 2023 Aug 15.
7. Haug U, Schink T. German Pharmacoepidemiological research database (GePaRD). In: Sturkenboom M, Schink T, editors. Databases for Pharmacoepidemiological research. Cham: Springer; 2021.

8. Franke GH. Mini-symptom-checklist. Göttingen: Hogrefe; 2017.
9. Weiner S, Sauerland S, Fein M, Blanco R, Pomhoff I, Weiner RA. The bariatric quality of life (BQL) index: A measure of Well-being in obesity surgery patients. Obes Surg. 2005;15:538–45.
10. Kliem S, Mößle T, Zenger M, Strauß B, Brähler E, Hilbert A. The eating disorder examination-questionnaire 8: A brief measure of eating disorder psychopathology (EDE-Q8). Int J Eat Disord. 2016 Jun;49(6):613–6.
11. R Core Team. R: A language and environment for statistical computing. Vienna: R Foundation for Statistical Computing; 2022.
12. D'hoedt A, Vanuytsel T. Dumping syndrome after bariatric surgery: prevalence, pathophysiology and role in weight reduction—a systematic review. Acta Gastro-Enterol Belg. 2023;86:417–27.
13. Van Beek AP, Emous M, Laville M, Tack J. Dumping syndrome after esophageal, gastric or bariatric surgery: pathophysiology, diagnosis, and management. Obes Rev. 2017;18:68–85.
14. Vecht J, Masclee AA, Lamers CB. The dumping syndrome. Current insights into pathophysiology, diagnosis and treatment. Scand J Gastroenterol Suppl. 1997;223:21.
15. Schiller M. Postprandiale Hypoglykämie: Unangenehm und gefährlich. Österreichische Ärztezeitung. 2024:3.
16. Deutsche Gesellschaft für Allgemein-und Viszeralchirurgie. S3-Leitlinie Chirurgie der Adipositas und metabolischer Erkrankungen [Internet]. [cited 2022 Dec 29]. https://register.awmf.org/assets/guidelines/088-001l_ S3_ Chirurgie-Adipositas-metabolische-Erkrankungen_2018-02. PDF.
17. Dietrich A, Aberle J, Wirth A, Muller-Stich B, Schutz T, Tigges H. Obesity surgery and the treatment of metabolic diseases. Dtsch Arztebl Int. 2018;115:705–11.
18. Runkel N, Colombo-Benkmann M, Huttl TP, Tigges H, Mann O, Flade-Kuthe R, et al. Evidence-based German guidelines for surgery for obesity. Int J Color Dis. 2011;26:397–404.
19. Demeglio C, Becouarn G, Topart P, Bodin R, Buisson JC, Ritz P. Weight loss trajectories after bariatric surgery for obesity: mathematical model and proof-of-concept study. JMIR Med Inform. 2020;8:e13672.
20. Istfan NW, Lipartia M, Anderson WA, Hess DT, Apovian CM. Approach to the patient: management of the post–bariatric surgery patient with weight regain. J Clin Endocrinol Metab. 2021;106:251–63.
21. Magro DO, Geloneze B, Delfini R, Pareja BC, Callejas F, Pareja JC. Long-term weight regain after gastric bypass: a 5-year prospective study. Obes Surg. 2008;18:648–51.
22. Marsall M, Bäuerle A, Hasenberg T, Schräpler L, Robitzsch A, Niedergethmann M, Teufel M, Weigl M. Quality of care transition during hospital discharge, patient safety, and weight regain after bariatric surgery: a cross-sectional study. Obes Surg. 2023;33:1143–53. https://doi.org/10.1007/s11695-023-06486-6.
23. Stark R, Renz A, Hanselmann M, Haas C, Neumann A, Martini O, Seyfried F, Laxy M, Stier C, Zippel-Schultz B, Fassnacht M, Koschker A-C. Adipositas care and health therapy (ACHT) after bariatric-metabolic surgery: A prospective non-randomized intervention study. Obes Facts. 2024;17:311. https://doi.org/10.1159/000538264.

Melanie Klein Studies of Health Sciences (Focus on Epidemiology, Surveillance and Prevention) at Hamburg University of Applied Sciences (2001–2007), Scientist at the Department of Occupations Health Research, Institution for Statutory Accident Insurance and Prevention in the Health and Welfare Services (2006–2010). Doctorate at Faculty for Human and Health Sciences, University of Bremen (2013). Postdoctoral Scientist at Competence Centre for Epidemiology and Health Services Research for Healthcare Professionals (Cvcare), University Medical Center Hamburg-Eppendorf (UKE) (2010–2015). Since 2015 working at DAK-Gesundheit (statutory health insurance) in health services research as a specialist for research projects.

Oliver Riedel Studied psychology (specializing in clinical psychology) at the TU Dresden, followed by a doctorate and habilitation at the TU Dresden. He worked as a research assistant at the

Chair of Clinical Psychology and Psychotherapy from 2005 to 2014. Since 2014, he has been a Senior Scientist at the Leibniz Institute for Prevention Research and Epidemiology in Bremen. He has many years of expertise in the design, implementation and evaluation of clinical-epidemiological surveys in field studies and with routine data from statutory health insurance.

Wiebke Zachariassen Studies of human medicine at Universität Hamburg 2001–2007, doctoral thesis in 2007. 2007–2014 internship in general and visceral surgery in Allgemeines Krankenhaus Altona in Hamburg, specialist in general surgery 2014. 2014–2016 honorary doctor in rescue services, 2016–2021 emergency doctor at Sana Klinikum Ostholstein in Oldenburg in Holstein. Since 2021 at DAK-Gesundheit working in health services research as a specialist for research projects among other things for projects funded by the Innovationsfonds.

Mark Dankhoff Study of medicine, license to practice medicine and doctorate at the Georg-August University in Göttingen, Germany. Specialist in general medicine, nutritional medicine, basic diabetological care, hypertensiology DHL, obesiology DAG/DDG and certified obesity trainer AGA. Worked for DAK-Gesundheit, one of the largest German statutory health insurance companies, from 1994 to 2021, including as head physician at the DAK-Gesundheit specialist clinic for children and adolescents on Sylt from 2005 to 2015, then as a consulting physician in the board of health services research department of the DAK-Gesundheit in Hamburg, among other things, responsible for the annual children and adolescent report. Since 2021 working freelance as a medical advisor. Reserve medical officer, currently Lieutenant Colonel Medical Corps at the Bundeswehr Hospital in Hamburg. Founding member of "Im Puls. Think Tank Herz-Kreislauf e.V.". 1993 PRO CORDE KHK sponsorship award. 2013 Prevention Prize of the German Obesity Society (DAG e. V). and the Working Group on Obesity in Children and Adolescents (AGA). E-Mail: dr.dankhoff@t-online.de

Navigating the Future of Dysphagia Management: From Advanced Innovations to Personalized Therapies

13

Stefanie Duchac

13.1 Introduction

Maintaining a healthy lifestyle is paramount for overall well-being, encompassing various aspects such as nutrition, social interactions, physical activity, and mental health [1]. However, individuals with swallowing difficulties or the conditions leading to swallowing difficulties face unique challenges that can significantly disrupt their pursuit of a healthy lifestyle.

13.1.1 The Difficulty of Swallowing

Swallowing is not just a necessity for nutrient and fluid intake but also basis for any social interaction including eating and drinking [2]. In daily life, often performed unconsciously, we swallow hundreds of times a day, ingesting saliva, liquids, and solid foods, fascinatingly enough since the act of swallowing, or deglutition, is a complex and dynamic senso-motor process involving the coordination of numerous muscles and cranial nerves. It encompasses three main domains: the oral, pharyngeal, and esophageal domain [3]. Simply put, during the oral stage, food is manipulated and formed into a cohesive bolus by the tongue and oral muscles, preparing it for propulsion towards the pharynx. Subsequently, in the pharyngeal stage, the soft palate elevates to close off the nasopharynx, while the larynx moves upwards and the epiglottis folds over the laryngeal inlet to prevent food or liquid from entering the airway. When the pharyngoesophageal segment is open, the bolus is pushed into the esophagus by pressure through a pharyngeal stripping wave.

S. Duchac (✉)
SRH University, School of Health, Education and Social Siences, Heidelberg, Germany
e-mail: stefanie.duchac@srh.de

P. Plugmann, D. Portius (eds.), *Innovations in Healthcare and Outcome Measurement*, https://doi.org/10.1007/978-3-031-77302-0_13

Swallowing involves rapid and sequential movements orchestrated by cortical and subcortical structures as well as the brainstem and mediated by the cranial nerves, particularly the trigeminal, facial, glossopharyngeal, vagus, and hypoglossal nerves [4]. Any disruption in this intricate coordination, whether due to neurological impairment, muscular dysfunction, or structural abnormalities, can lead to swallowing difficulties (dysphagia), characterized by symptoms such as difficulty initiating swallowing, material entering the airway resulting in penetration and/or aspiration (Fig. 13.1), coughing or choking during meals, regurgitation, and inefficient swallowing leading to oral and/or pharyngeal residues [5].

Dysphagia encompasses a range of disorders affecting the oral, pharyngeal, and esophageal domains of swallowing, posing significant health risks to individuals. Many diseases, including neurological disorders like stroke, Parkinson's, and Alzheimer's, and also other diseases such as oncologic, endocrine, psychiatric, immunologic causes, infectious disease, surgical complications, injuries, and congenital causes can lead to swallowing difficulties [6]. The prevalence of dysphagia is substantial, with 590 millions of people affected worldwide [7].

13.1.2 Complications Associated with Dysphagia

The complications of dysphagia are diverse and can have significant impacts on the health and quality of life of those affected [5]. Among the most common complications are malnutrition and dehydration, which can arise from difficulties in effective

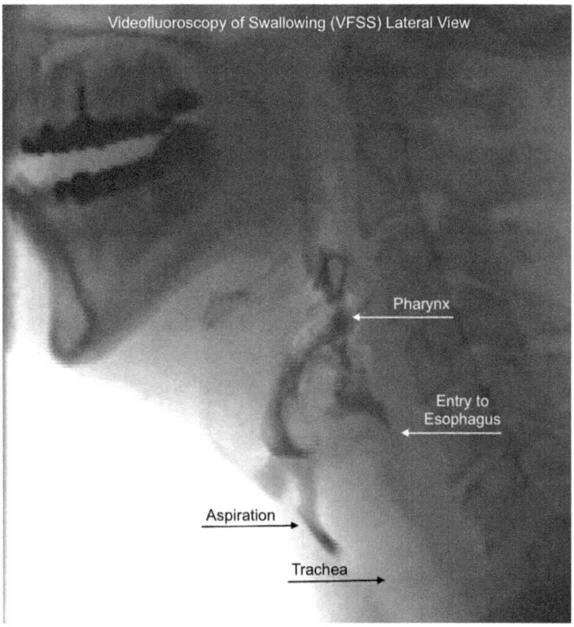

Fig. 13.1 Aspiration (material entering the trachea) visualized by Videofluoroscopy of Swallowing

swallowing and limited oral intake. The lack of adequate nutrient intake and fluid intake can lead to significant weight loss, muscle weakness, and fatigue.

If the safety of the swallow is affected, and material enters the airway, this aspiration of food or liquid particles poses the risk of aspiration pneumonia, a serious lung infection that can lead to life-threatening complications.

In addition to the physical effects, dysphagia also significantly impairs the quality of life of affected individuals. The associated limitations in eating and drinking can cause social isolation, emotional distress, and psychological impairments that greatly affect daily life [8].

As chronic illnesses often associated with dysphagia, this exacerbates challenges and hinder individuals' ability to engage in regular physical activity or maintain a consistent exercise routine [9]. Therefore, comprehensive dysphagia management, which addresses not only swallowing function but also nutrition, fluid intake, and quality of life, is crucial for effective care.

13.2 Diagnostic Advances in Dysphagia

13.2.1 Emerging Technologies in Dysphagia Diagnosis

The clinical diagnosis of dysphagia presents challenges, particularly in capturing the dynamic nature of the swallow and identifying not just symptoms like penetration/aspiration and residue but also the underlying cause of the symptoms. The precise diagnosis of dysphagia poses challenges due to the complexity of swallowing, productivity demands, and the inherent variability of the swallow, aspects that cannot be observed clinically [10]. Overcoming these challenges is essential for accurate diagnosis.

Traditional diagnostic methods do not offer a direct visual of these aspects, emphasizing the need for objective assessment tools in both early screening and comprehensive clinical swallow evaluations. In early detection screenings and clinical swallow function assessments, there is a requirement for procedures that can objectively evaluate swallow function [10].

The challenges are developing methods that provide insights into the mechanisms of swallowing. Even in established imaging techniques like flexible Endoscopic Evaluation of Swallowing (FEES) and Videofluoroscopic Swallow Studies (VFSS), decisions must be made regarding the balance between capturing information about symptoms and biomechanical insights.

Recent advances in diagnostic technologies, such as high-resolution manometry, have improved our ability to assess different aspects of swallowing function. These developments and further innovations in assessment tools, and digitalization will improve diagnostic accuracy and provide clinicians with unprecedented insights into the biomechanics of swallowing, enabling early detection of abnormalities [11].

Emerging technologies offer promising solutions to the challenges associated with swallowing assessment. For example, artificial Intelligence (AI) is becoming integral for data analysis and pattern recognition in dysphagia diagnostics [12–14].

These advanced technologies have the potential to enhance the precision and objectivity of assessments by deciphering complex patterns in swallowing dynamics.

As we delve into the era of advanced technologies, considerations must extend beyond the mere acquisition of data. The focus should be on leveraging these technologies to gain meaningful clinical relevant insights into symptomatic manifestations, biomechanical aspects, but also underlying pathomechanisms of swallowing. By harnessing the power of AI for interpretation and pattern recognition, we might unlock new dimensions in dysphagia diagnosis, ultimately leading to more effective and personalized therapeutic interventions.

13.2.2 Impact on Early Detection and Intervention

The integration of advanced diagnostic tools facilitates early detection. Timely identification of swallowing disorders empowers healthcare professionals to implement personalized treatment strategies, mitigating the risk of complications [15].

Early intervention is crucial, not only for reducing complications but also for addressing the principles of neuroplasticity and complex functionality depending on the cause of the swallowing disorder [16]. The early stages of dysphagia often present opportunities to harness the brain's ability to adapt and reorganize itself [17]. This is particularly relevant in cases where dysphagia is linked to neurological conditions. Early interventions can leverage neuroplasticity, allowing patients to develop compensatory strategies or, in some cases, even restore functions [15].

Furthermore, the complexity of swallowing requires a thoughtful approach to intervention. Understanding the root cause of dysphagia dysphagia, e.g. using Brain Imaging Techniques, allows to implement targeted therapies that go beyond compensatory techniques. Early intervention enables the incorporation of strategies, aiming not only to manage symptoms but also to enhance the overall function of the swallowing mechanism.

> The relevance of early intervention extends beyond the reduction of complications associated with dysphagia. It aligns with the principles of adaptability and complexity, addressing the dynamic nature of swallowing disorders and paving the way for more effective and holistic treatment strategies.

13.2.3 Rehabilitation of Dysphagia

Next to medical or surgical approaches the historical focus in functional dysphagia rehabilitation is on strengthening swallowing muscles. This approach assumes that e.g. conscious effortful swallowing can enhance the pressure development of the swallowing muscles, supporting oropharyngeal bolus transport. However, the traditional emphasis on strength may not always be the most effective approach, especially considering the dynamic and highly coordinative nature of swallowing. Moreover, weakness is not likely the cause of impaired swallowing function [18].

In contrast to the conventional focus on peripheral biomechanical processes, a shift towards central therapy approaches emerges. Research has explored neuromodulatory methods such as pharyngeal electrical stimulation, transcranial direct current stimulation, and repetitive transcranial magnetic stimulation. These approaches aim to achieve enhanced central neuromotor responses through targeted stimulation, demonstrating increasing evidence of their functional effectiveness [19].

In light of the complexity of oropharyngeal swallow function, a crucial question arises: Is there a therapy approach that, through a specific modulation of the swallow process, can affect central sensorimotor control systems, leading to neurophysiological changes with sustained and reliably improved functions? This initiated a shift in rehabilitation thinking towards skill-based approaches in dysphagia therapy [18].

Skill training focuses on improving movement initiation, deviation, and coordination of multiple movement components into a complex functional movement. Such competency- and skill-based approaches induce cortical reorganization of motor networks and have been shown to be more effective than purely strength-focused exercises in various contexts [19, 20].

The exploration of neurogenic dysphagia rehabilitation has increased in recent years yet leaving many questions to be explored. Competency- and skill-based swallow training can be a promising rehabilitative approach for patients with corresponding pathomechanisms, ultimately leading to improved patient care. The integration of biofeedback supports this evolution but is only as effective as the method or maneuver it visualizes. Dysphagia therapists should critically evaluate their actions, considering various factors in their clinical reasoning, including treatment approach, guidance, patient-specific factors, and desires.

13.3 Clinical Decision-Making in Dysphagia Management

In the realm of dysphagia management, the significance of evidence-based clinical decision-making cannot be overstated. As healthcare professionals navigate the complexities of assessing and treating swallowing disorders, the integration of evidence and best practices leads to optimal patient outcomes.

Evidence-based practice (EBP) serves as a guiding framework for clinical decision-making in dysphagia management, leading to interventions with the best available evidence (external evidence) while incorporating clinical expertise (internal evidence) and patient preferences (social evidence).

13.3.1 External Evidence: Incorporating Research Findings

According to Sackett et al. the best available external evidence encompasses clinically relevant research, including medical basic science and patient-oriented investigations into diagnostic accuracy, prognostic factors, and the efficacy and safety of therapeutic, rehabilitative, and preventive measures [21].

Traditionally, the level of evidence has been seen as a fundamental criterion for assessing the quality of research. However, it is important to recognize that the hierarchical view of evidence may not always be appropriate or applicable to every research question or clinical scenario. In recent years, there has been a notable paradigm shift in rehabilitation research, emphasizing the importance of aligning study designs with specific research questions [22]. This shift from a hierarchical understanding of evidence towards a more flexible, circular evidence model acknowledges the diverse and nuanced nature of clinical practice. Especially essential to support translation from knowledge into clinical practice [23].

Furthermore, studies with a very controlled study design may lead to the exclusion of specific patient populations, such as those with advanced age or significant comorbidities, from participating in research studies. This exclusionary practice can result in limiting the applicability of evidence-based interventions in real-world clinical settings [24]. Recognizing the importance of inclusivity and diversity in research, efforts should be made to design studies that reflect the heterogeneity of the patient population encountered in clinical practice.

In the context of dysphagia management, this shift prompts a reconsideration of how external evidence is integrated into the clinical decision-making process. Healthcare practitioners are encouraged to critically evaluate the relevance and applicability of research findings to specific clinical contexts. (e.g. implementation of systematic screening or other diagnostic tools, identification of objective outcome measures based on normative data, selection of effective treatment approaches).

Integrating the best available external evidence into dysphagia therapy involves several crucial aspects:

1. **Literature Review: Identifying Relevant Studies** Conducting a thorough literature review is the initial step in evidence integration. This involves searching for studies that reflect the current evidence base in dysphagia research.
2. **Quality Assessment: Evaluating Studies** Rigorous evaluation of literature is imperative, considering various quality markers. Assessing factors such as study design, sample size, methodology, and statistical analyses ensures the reliability and validity of the evidence.
3. **Knowledge Transfer: Applying Findings to Clinical Decision-Making** Translating research findings into the clinical context requires understanding of the study's implications.

13.3.2 Internal Evidence: Therapeutic Decision-Making Within Multidisciplinary Teams

Internal evidence, often referred to as "clinical experience," plays a crucial role in clinical decision-making, especially when the findings of external evidence and patients' preferences diverge. Therefore, healthcare professionals, as integral team members, contribute their expertise to refine dysphagia management pathways including collective experience of multidisciplinary teams. It is essential to recognize that the number of years of experience alone does not necessarily lead to more thoughtful decision-making. Instead, the ability to think critically and engage in clinical reasoning is paramount. This includes the ability to constantly develop and, if necessary, break away from established routines.

Furthermore, it should be considered that the clinical decision-making process can be influenced by various aspects, such as cognitive biases, cognitive heuristics, and patterns of thinking and behavior. These biases can inadvertently skew the interpretation of clinical information and lead to suboptimal decision-making outcomes. Awareness of these biases and their potential impact on clinical judgment is crucial for therapists, as it enables them to recognize and mitigate their effects through deliberate reflection and decision-making strategies. Additionally, fostering a culture of interdisciplinary collaboration and knowledge-sharing facilitates the exchange of insights and perspectives, enriching therapists' repertoire of clinical reasoning tools and ultimately improving patient care.

> By cultivating a deeper understanding of cognitive biases and actively challenging ingrained patterns of thinking, therapists can enhance the accuracy and effectiveness of their clinical decision making processes.

Internal evidence is therefore much more than just clinical experience, even if it is highly relevant. Spencer et al. use the term "professional judgement" [25]. Professional judgment encompasses a range of factors, including clinical expertise, knowledge of evidence-based practices, and the ability to adapt interventions to suit the unique circumstances of each patient [25]. By embracing professional judgment and remaining open to ongoing learning and growth, therapists can optimize dysphagia care and improve outcomes for their patients.

13.3.3 Social Evidence: Understanding Patient Wishes and Needs

Recognizing the social dimension of dysphagia care involves understanding the unique wishes and needs of patients. Patient-centered care requires a holistic approach that considers not only the physiological aspects of dysphagia but also the psychological and social aspects influencing the patient's experience. Social evidence, in the context of dysphagia management, emphasizes the importance of shifting focus from solely analyzing the functional swallow to considering the patient as a whole. This entails recognizing the social and cultural factors that impact an individual's ability to manage their dysphagia effectively. Factors such as social support networks, living arrangements, access to resources, and cultural beliefs surrounding food and eating habits all play a significant role in shaping the patient's experience of dysphagia and their ability to adhere to treatment recommendations. By incorporating social evidence into dysphagia management, healthcare professionals can suggest interventions to better meet the needs and preferences of patients, ultimately enhancing their quality of life and overall well-being [8].

13.3.4 Integration of Evidence Into Clinical Practice

By integrating empirical research findings, systematic reviews, and clinical practice guidelines, healthcare professionals can discern the most effective and appropriate interventions fitting to each patient's unique needs. Moreover, evidence-based practice empowers clinicians to critically evaluate the validity and applicability of research findings to real-world clinical scenarios, fostering a culture of continuous learning and improvement in dysphagia care.

Rousseau & Gunia identified three critical factors contributing to the successful implementation of evidence-based practice across diverse fields: practitioner ability, motivation, and opportunity to practice [26]. This refers as well to the fact that contextual factors, such as environmental and personal factors, have an impact on an individual's level of functioning. Therefore, Gutenbrunner & Nugraha, (2020) propose that components of the health system (e.g., health insurance coverage, availability of services, treatments, and assistive devices) and the service organization (e.g., spectrum and training level of health professionals, availability of diagnostic and treatment devices) also significantly impact decision-making in individual cases and should be included as a fourth factor in the model of evidence-based decision-making.

> Incorporating external, internal, and social evidence into clinical practice is essential for optimizing patient outcomes and improving the quality of care for individuals with swallowing difficulties.

13.4 Balancing Act: Customizing Dysphagia Management

While advancements in diagnostic techniques provide an increasing amount of information, the challenge still is personalizing interventions to meet the diverse needs of individual patients. A one-size-fits-all approach is inadequate! Healthcare professionals bear a significant responsibility in navigating this complexity, especially amidst the influx of information. It is imperative for therapists not to neglect aspects of clinical decision-making, even with the increasing availability of data. This entails acknowledging and mitigating potential influences of their own personality traits and behavioral patterns on their decision-making processes. Additionally, therapists must prioritize understanding and accommodating the unique needs and preferences of each patient. By encouraging a patient-centered approach and integrating patient perspectives into the decision-making process, therapists can ensure that interventions addressing the specific challenges and goals of individuals with dysphagia, especially in patients at risk.

13.4.1 Integrating Risk Assessment Into Dysphagia Management

Balancing the risks associated with dysphagia requires a comprehensive understanding of the potential complications, such as aspiration pneumonia or malnutrition.

Prevention of aspiration pneumonia by increasing the swallowing safety is one of the major goals in dysphagia management. However, it is important to dispel the myth that every instance of aspiration leads to pneumonia, and that some interventions, such as thickening liquids, are not in principle effective for every patient. While aspiration increases the risk of pneumonia, the development of pneumonia depends on various factors. The three pillars contributing to aspiration pneumonia include the overall health status, oral health (presence of pathogenic microorganisms) as well as impaired defense mechanisms (e.g. cough function). Several factors increase the risk of developing aspiration pneumonia, including advanced age, decreased level of consciousness, compromised immune function, and underlying pulmonary or neurological conditions and the inability of patients to eat by themselves and conduct oral care by themselves [27].

Additionally, oral health emerges as a critical factor in dysphagia management. Poor oral hygiene and dental conditions can exacerbate swallowing difficulties and increase the risk of aspiration pneumonia [28]. By addressing oral health concerns alongside swallowing function, both, the underlying pathology and contributing factors are addressed. Therefore, integrating oral health assessments and preventive measures into dysphagia management protocols is imperative for promoting safe swallowing and overall well-being.

13.4.2 Prioritizing Quality of Life in Dysphagia Care

Quality of life considerations should be at the forefront of dysphagia management. Striking a balance between therapeutic interventions and preserving the patient's overall well-being is important for achieving meaningful outcomes. In this context, participative decision-making emerges as a crucial component of patient-centered care. Empowering patients, if possible, to actively engage in the decision-making process not only fosters a sense of autonomy and agency but also enhances treatment adherence and satisfaction. For instance, if therapeutic techniques share similar mechanisms of action, involving patients in the decision-making process allows them to choose interventions that align with their preferences and experiences. This collaborative approach not only promotes patient autonomy but also increases a therapeutic alliance between patients and healthcare professionals, facilitating better communication, trust, and ultimately, improved treatment outcomes.

> By prioritizing quality of life considerations and integrating participative decision-making into dysphagia management, healthcare providers can enhance the overall patient experience and promote overall well-being

13.4.3 Nutritional Considerations

Nutritional health is an important element of dysphagia care [29]. Beyond addressing the act of swallowing, attention must be given to ensuring patients receive adequate nutrition, emphasizing the interdisciplinary approach of dysphagia management with broader health goals. The nutritional status of patients, particularly those undergoing dietary modifications, holds significant relevance in dysphagia management. Adjustments to food texture or consistency may impact the overall nutritional intake and dietary variety, potentially leading to deficiencies in essential nutrients [30]. Therefore, incorporating nutritional screening as a standardized practice is paramount to identify at-risk individuals and facilitate timely interventions. Collaboration among speech-language pathologists, dietitians, physicians, and other healthcare professionals enables the assessment of patients' nutritional needs and facilitates the best outcome for swallowing function and nutritional health [31].

13.5 Future Directions in Dysphagia Management

13.5.1 Technological Innovations

Continued technological advancements hold the promise of further refining our understanding of dysphagia and enhancing diagnostic and therapeutic approaches. From artificial intelligence applications capable of analyzing imaging studies and predicting patient outcomes to innovative medical devices designed to optimize swallowing function, the future of dysphagia management is indeed filled with possibilities. However, amidst these technological strides, the importance of critical thinking and empathy remains paramount. While technology can provide invaluable insights and tools, it is the critical thinking skills of healthcare providers that enable them to interpret data, evaluate treatment options, and make informed clinical decisions. Empathy plays a crucial role in patient care, fostering trust, rapport, and effective communication between healthcare providers and patients.

> As we continue to embrace technological innovations in dysphagia management, the integration of critical thinking and empathy into clinical practice will be indispensable, ensuring that advancements in technology are harnessed to their fullest potential for the benefit of individuals with swallowing difficulties.

13.5.2 Anticipating Evolving Patient Needs

As healthcare evolves, so do the needs and expectations of patients. Anticipating these changes and adapting dysphagia management strategies accordingly will be essential for providing patient-centered care in the future. With advancements in technology and a growing emphasis on patient empowerment and shared decision-making, healthcare providers must continuously reassess their approach to dysphagia management to meet evolving patient needs. This includes embracing innovative communication tools and platforms that facilitate remote consultations and patient education, as well as incorporating patient-reported outcomes measures to assess treatment efficacy and patient satisfaction. Moreover, recognizing the diverse cultural, linguistic, and socioeconomic backgrounds of patients is crucial in developing interventions to be inclusive and equitable.

13.5.3 Collaboration and Knowledge Sharing in the Field

Cultivating collaboration between healthcare professionals, researchers, and patients is pivotal for advancing dysphagia care, especially in the future. Knowledge sharing and interdisciplinary teamwork contribute to a comprehensive and evolving approach to dysphagia management.

By bringing together experts from various fields such as speech-language pathology, otolaryngology, gastroenterology, nutrition, dentists, and neurology, healthcare teams can leverage diverse perspectives and expertise to address the multifaceted nature of dysphagia effectively. Furthermore, collaboration with researchers from different fields facilitates the translation of scientific discoveries into clinical practice, driving innovation and improving patient outcomes.

Equally important is the active involvement of patients in the care process. By incorporating patient perspectives, preferences, and experiences, healthcare providers can gain valuable insights into the lived experience of dysphagia and tailor interventions to better meet individual needs. Patient engagement also fosters a sense of ownership and empowerment, leading to greater treatment adherence and satisfaction.

Fostering collaboration among healthcare professionals, researchers, and patients is essential for advancing dysphagia care, driving innovation, and improving the quality of life for individuals affected by swallowing difficulties.

13.6 Food for Thought

Navigating the future of dysphagia management requires a synthesis of advanced innovations and personalized therapies. The intricate interplay between diagnostic technologies, evidence-based practice, and patient-centered care forms the foundation for successful dysphagia management.

As we stand at the intersection of technological progress and patient-centered care, a collective call to action is extended to healthcare professionals and researchers. Embracing the challenges and opportunities in dysphagia management will pave the way for a healthier future, one where each patient's unique needs are met with precision and empathy leading to positively impacting the healthy lifestyle of individuals with swallowing difficulties.

References

1. Yokutkhon S. Healthy lifestyle. Int J Soc Sci Interdiscip Res. 2022;11(12):254–9.
2. Leslie P, Broll J. Eating, drinking, and swallowing difficulties: the impacts on, and of, religious beliefs. Geriatrics (Switzerland). 2022;7(2):1–8.
3. Martin-Harris B, Brodsky MB, Michel Y, Castell DO, Schleicher M, Sandidge J, et al. MBS measurement tool for swallow impairment-MBSimp: establishing a standard. Dysphagia. 2008;23(4):392–405.
4. Matsuo K, Palmer JB. Anatomy and physiology of feeding and swallowing: normal and abnormal. Phys Med Rehabil Clin N Am. 2008;19(4):691–707.
5. Daniels SK, Huckabee ML, Gozdzikowska K. Dysphagia following stroke. San Diego, CA: Plural Publishing; 2019.
6. Roden DF, Altman KW. Causes of dysphagia among different age groups: a systematic review of the literature. Otolaryngol Clin N Am. 2013;46(6):965–87.
7. Cichero JAY, Lam P, Steele CM, Hanson B, Chen J, Dantas RO, et al. Development of international terminology and definitions for texture-modified foods and thickened fluids used in dysphagia management: the IDDSI framework. Dysphagia. 2017;32(2):293–314.
8. Smith R, Bryant L, Hemsley B. The true cost of dysphagia on quality of life: the views of adults with swallowing disability. Int J Lang Commun Disord. 2023;58(2):451–66.
9. Maehara T, Nishimura R, Yoshitake A, Tsukamoto M, Kadomatsu Y, Kubo Y, et al. Association of daily physical activity and leisure-time exercise with dysphagia risk in community-dwelling older adults: a cross-sectional study. Sci Rep. 2023;13(1):1–10. https://doi.org/10.1038/s41598-023-37605-z.
10. Doeltgen SH, McAllister S, Murray J, Ward EC, Pretz JE. Reasoning and decision making in clinical swallowing examination. Curr Phys Med Rehabil Rep. 2018;6(3):171–7. https://doi.org/10.1007/s40141-018-0191-z.
11. Labeit B, Michou E, Hamdy S, Trapl-Grundschober M, Suntrup-Krueger S, Muhle P, et al. The assessment of dysphagia after stroke: state of the art and future directions. Lancet Neurol. 2023;22(9):858–70. https://doi.org/10.1016/S1474-4422(23)00153-9.
12. Lai DKH, Cheng ESW, Lim HJ, So BPH, Lam WK, Cheung DSK, et al. Computer-aided screening of aspiration risks in dysphagia with wearable technology: a systematic review and meta-analysis on test accuracy. Front Bioeng Biotechnol. 2023;11(June):1–16.
13. Matsuda Y, Ito E, Kuroda M, Araki K, Nakada W, Hayakawa Y. A basic study for predicting dysphagia in panoramic X-ray images using artificial intelligence (AI) part 2: analysis of the position of the hyoid bone on panoramic radiographs. Eng. 2023;4(4):2542–52.
14. Zifan A, Lin J, Peng Z, Bo Y, Mittal RK. Unraveling functional dysphagia: a game-changing automated machine-learning diagnostic approach. Appl Sci. 2023;13(18):10116.
15. Cheng I, Hamdy S. Metaplasticity in the human swallowing system: clinical implications for dysphagia rehabilitation. Neurol Sci. 2022;43(1):199–209. https://doi.org/10.1007/s10072-021-05654-9.
16. Kamal LH, Abdou RM, Hamouda NH, Said SM. The effect of early intervention of swallowing therapy on recovery from oropharyngeal dysphagia in stroke patients : a cross sectional study. Educ Sci Tech. 2021;8(3):1367–82.
17. Robbins J, Butler SG, Daniels SK, Lazarus CL, Mccabe D. Swallowing and dysphagia rehabilitation: translating principles of neural plasticity into clinically oriented evidence. J Speech Lang Hear Res. 2008;51(February):276–301.

18. Huckabee ML, Flynn R, Mills M. Expanding rehabilitation options for dysphagia: skill-based swallowing training. Dysphagia. 2023;38(3):756–67. https://doi.org/10.1007/s00455-022-10516-3.
19. Cheng I, Sasegbon A, Hamdy S. Evaluating the therapeutic application of neuromodulation in the human swallowing system. Dysphagia. 2023;38(4):1005–24. https://doi.org/10.1007/s00455-022-10528-z.
20. Huckabee ML, Burnip E. Still rethinking rehab: motor learning treatment approaches for dysphagia. Perspect ASHA Spec Interest Groups. 2018;3(13):146–56.
21. Sackett DL, Rosenberg WM, Gray JAM, Haynes RB, Richardson WS. Evidence based medicine: what it is and what it isn't It's. BMJ. 1996;312:3–19.
22. Walach H, Falkenberg T, Fønnebø V, Lewith G, Jonas WB. Circular instead of hierarchical: methodological principles for the evaluation of complex interventions. BMC Med Res Methodol. 2006;6:1–9.
23. Negrini S, Gimigliano F, Arienti C, Kiekens C. Knowledge Translation: the bridging function of Cochrane rehabilitation. Arch Phys Med Rehabil. 2018;99(6):1242–5. https://doi.org/10.1016/j.apmr.2017.11.002.
24. Hirschwald J, Finnegan L, Hofacker J, Walshe M. Underserved groups in dysphagia intervention trials in Parkinson's disease: a scoping review. Ageing Res Rev. 2024;93(2023):102150. https://doi.org/10.1016/j.arr.2023.102150.
25. Spencer TD, Detrich R, Slocum TA. Evidence-based practice: a framework for making effective decisions. Educ Treat Children. 2012;35(2):127–51.
26. Rousseau DM, Gunia BC. Evidence-based practice: the psychology of EBP implementation. Annu Rev Psychol. 2016;67:667–92.
27. Langmore SE, Terpenning MS, Schork A, Chen Y, Murray JT, Lopatin D, et al. Predictors of aspiration pneumonia: how important is dysphagia? Dysphagia. 1998;13(2):69–81.
28. Lee DS, Kim HE, Choi JS. Oral health-related factors associated with dysphagia risk among older, healthy, community-dwelling Korean adults: a pilot study. Healthcare (Switzerland). 2024;12(2):267.
29. Lieber AC, Hong E, Putrino D, Nistal DA, Pan JS, Kellner CP. Nutrition, energy expenditure, dysphagia, and self-efficacy in stroke rehabilitation: a review of the literature. Brain Sci. 2018;8(12):218.
30. Rodd BG, Tas AA, Taylor KDA. Dysphagia, texture modification, the elderly and micronutrient deficiency: a review. Crit Rev Food Sci Nutr. 2022;62(26):7354–69. https://doi.org/10.1080/10408398.2021.1913571.
31. Takeuchi K, Aida J, Ito K, Furuta M, Yamashita Y, Osaka K. Nutritional status and dysphagia risk among community-dwelling frail older adults. J Nutr Health Aging. 2014;18(4):352–7.

Personalized Solutions in Orthopaedic Surgery: The Era of 3D Technology and Future

14

Vikas Jain

14.1 Current Landscape of 3D Technology in Healthcare

Orthopaedic surgery has evolved greatly in recent times, with technology enabling more accurate and successful surgical operations. Personalized orthopaedic surgery is changing the way orthopaedic surgeons approach patient care. Personalized orthopaedic surgery is a proactive approach to orthopaedic patients that focuses on customization.

Rather than using a one-size-fits-all method, it considers each patient's unique anatomy, medical history, and other factors to create a tailored treatment plan. This approach focuses on the planning efforts made before the surgery itself to ensure maximum efficiency and effectiveness in the outcomes of the patient.

By utilizing digital technology, such as virtual twins, 3D printed implants, and preoperative planning software, orthopaedic surgeons can create custom treatment plans and provide proactive patient surgical management orthopaedics and improve patient outcomes.

3D technology has revolutionized the medical device industry and orthopaedic surgeries. In instances, an orthopaedic surgeon must provide out-of-the-box customized solutions in the form of implants and guiding jigs, to optimize the anatomy and function.

Osteointegration and ***intra-articular*** solutions for complex orthopaedic surgeries where the surgeon has no option of off-the-shelf implant, Patient-specific Implant provides the best solutions. Osteointegration has been a challenge for medical device companies and orthopaedic surgeons. However, this technology provides easy and sure shot solution. Similarly, Intra-articular lesions require absolute congruency, again only possible by this technology.

V. Jain (✉)
3D Technology Trailblazer & Orthopaedic Surgeon, Vapi, Gujarat, India

P. Plugmann, D. Portius (eds.), *Innovations in Healthcare and Outcome Measurement*, https://doi.org/10.1007/978-3-031-77302-0_14

Complex defects in the bony structure in once-orthopaedics, trauma and arthroplasty cases where optimized solutions can only be obtained by patient-specific implants.

In cases of ***complex deformities***, in paediatric or adult orthopaedic patients, preoperative planning and guiding jigs and instruments play a very important role in achieving perfect and precise correction, thus not only reducing the surgical time and blood loss but also achieving optimized results in patients.

3D Technology in healthcare refers to the imaging, scanning, modelling, visualization, and printing of objects, the human body, and its parts in three dimensions in a scaled model or implant. This technology has a wide range of applications across healthcare, predominantly in orthopaedics.

14.2 Key Aspects and Applications of 3D Technology

(a) **Medical Imaging**: Techniques like MRI, CT scans, and ultrasound use 3D technology to create detailed images of the inside of the human body, aiding not only in diagnosis and treatment but also in planning, modelling, visualization, and printing (Fig. 14.1).
(b) **3D Scanning** and **Modelling:** Capturing the physical dimensions and shape of any human body part to create a digital 3D model. Bone models of any diseased bone can be created for the study of the surgeon. Even any surgery can be performed on the software or bone model, giving an idea of the steps, dimensions, trajectory of screws, size, and type of implants required (Fig. 14.2).
(c) **3D Visualization** is the display of 3D data through immersive environments like virtual reality (VR) or augmented reality (AR). It is used for simulations, training, and surgeries.

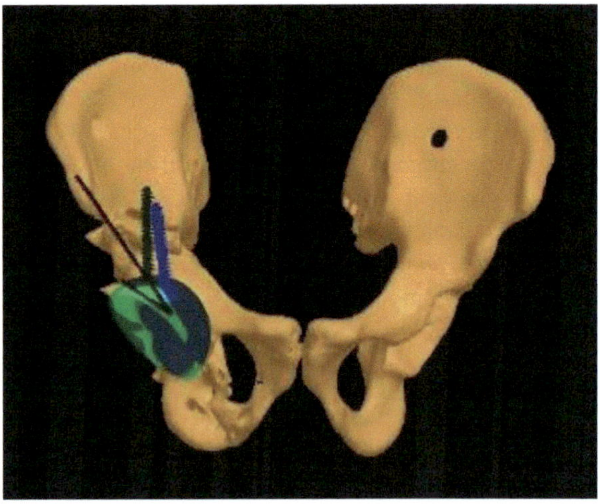

Fig. 14.1 3D modelling

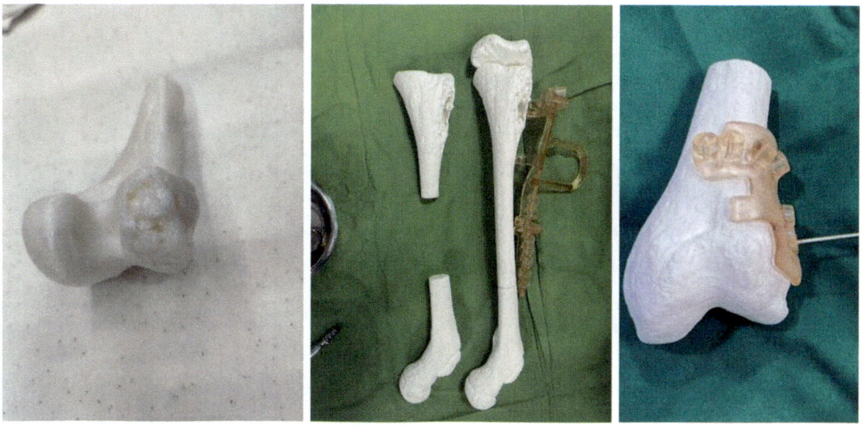

Fig. 14.2 Bone models 3D printed 1:1 scale brings the disease out of the body

- **Virtual Reality (VR)**: A fully immersive digital experience where users can interact with a 3D environment using VR headsets and controllers. VR is used in gaming, orthopaedic training simulations, education, and surgery.
- **Augmented Reality (AR)**: Overlaying digital information (3D models, graphics) onto the real world, viewed through devices like smartphones, tablets, or AR glasses. The virtual model is overlapped over the real bone during surgery to navigate the pre-planned surgery. (HOLOLENS) AR is used in applications for orthopaedic surgery for non-robotic navigation of surgery (Fig. 14.3).

(d) 3D **Printing**: Also known as additive manufacturing, 3D printing involves creating physical objects from digital models by layering materials. Polymers are used to make bone models of diseased bone and jigs are made to correct deformity. Metals like titanium, cobalt, and chromium are used for PSI implants.

- **Patient-Specific Instruments (PSI):** 3D-printed surgical guides and jigs are designed based on the patient's anatomy, allowing for more accurate and efficient surgical procedures. These jigs help in precise cutting, drilling, and alignment, reducing the margin for error. They are mainly printed in Polymers.
- **PSI Implants and Prosthetics**

  These are designed to fill the defect and to fit the patient's unique anatomical features, ensuring better compatibility and reconstructing the patient's anatomy. Advanced materials used in 3D printing, such as biocompatible metals and polymers (PEKK, PEEK), enhance the durability and functionality of implants. The aim is a perpetual prosthetic implant! (Fig. 14.4).

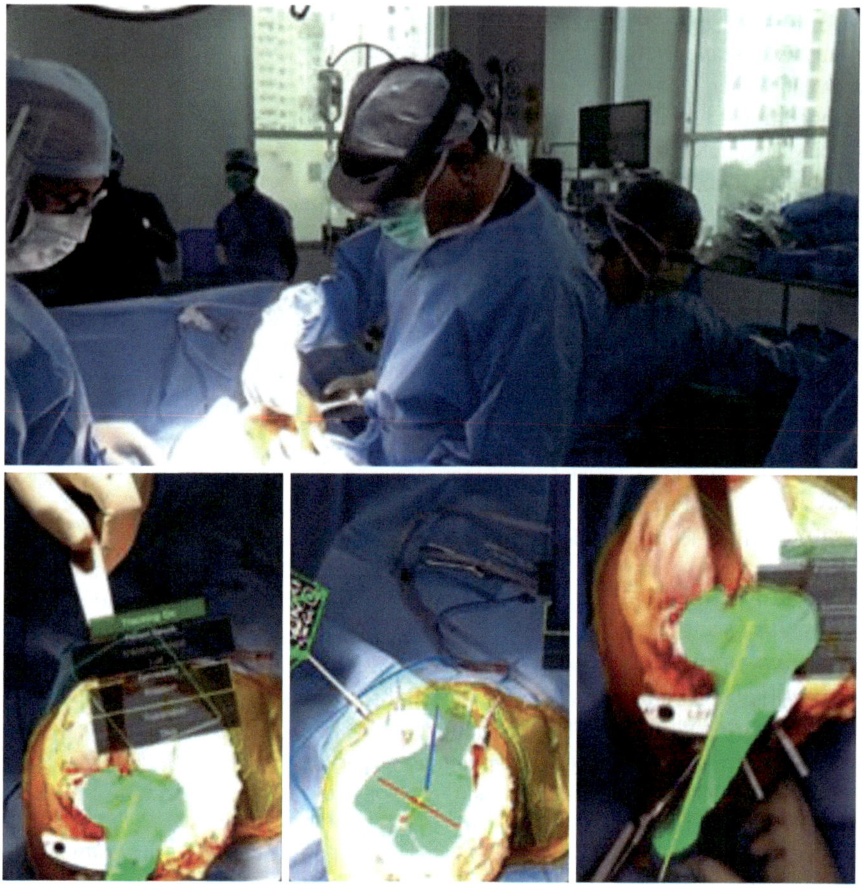

Fig. 14.3 Augmented reality-based total knee arthroplasty using HoloLens

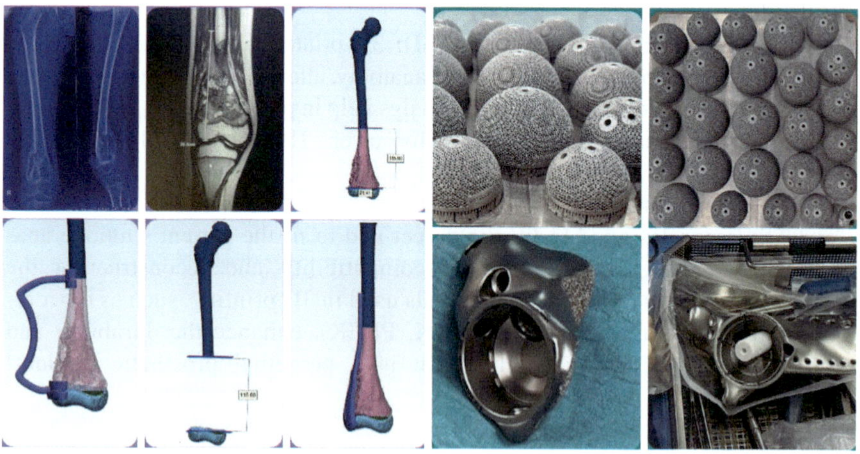

Fig. 14.4 3D printed Jig in case of tumour resection, 3D printed acetabular cups in titanium

14.3 Benefits and Challenges of 3D Technology in Orthopaedic Surgery

14.3.1 Benefits

- **Precision:** Enhanced accuracy in surgical planning and execution.
- **Customization:** Tailored solutions that fit individual patients' bone and joint anatomy.
- **Efficiency:** Reduced surgery time and improved recovery rates, better patient outcomes, reduced surgical stress.
- **Safety:** Lower risk of complications and infections, reduce blood loss.
- **Education:** Better training tools for orthopaedic surgeons and bone models help the patient and relatives to understand the disease better.

14.3.2 Challenges

- **Cost:** High initial investment in 3D technology and equipment.
- **Regulation:** Ensuring regulatory compliance and standardization of 3D-printed medical devices.
- **Integration:** Seamless integration of 3D technology into existing surgical workflows. Time constraints, as the planning and services take time to execute.
- **Research:** Ongoing research and development to enhance the capabilities and applications of 3D technology in orthopaedics. The technology is at a very nascent stage.
- **Poor Adaptation:** The technology adaptation by orthopaedic surgeons is a slow process. It requires efforts to educate, unlearn, and relearn the technological advantages.

Continuous collaboration between medical and biomedical researchers, orthopaedic surgeons, and industry stakeholders will likely be crucial in shaping the future of 3D technology in orthopaedic care.

14.4 Indications of Patient -Specific Solutions in Orthopaedics

PSIs and jigs offer advantages in specific cases, and their use should be carefully considered based on individual patient factors and the surgeon's expertise. Additionally, ongoing research and technological advancements continue to expand the applications of these personalized orthopaedic solutions.

- **Oncological Reconstructions:**
- Patients undergoing tumour resections in the musculoskeletal system often require reconstructive surgery. PSIs can be used to create implants that fit precisely into the defect left by the tumour resection, promoting better functional outcomes. This technique is widely used in many countries (Fig. 14.4).

- **Complex Joint Reconstructions:**
- PSIs are commonly used in joint replacement surgeries, such as complex primary or revision, total knee arthroplasty (TKA) and total hip arthroplasty (THA), especially in cases with complex anatomical variations, defects.
- Patients with severe bone and joint deformities/bone defects may benefit from customized implants that are specifically tailored to their unique anatomy.
- **Revision Surgeries:**
- In cases of revision hip, knee, or any other joint surgery where there may be altered anatomy or bony defects due to previous implants, trauma, or bone loss, PSIs can help address the challenges posed by these complex situations.
- Presently, augments are used to address defect challenges. They are used at the acetabular or glenoid end of either arthroplasty. There are a lot of adjustments that are required to be made with augments. These augments are again trabecular metal, which enables osteointegration. Larger acetabular cups are also used by various surgeons, which alter the centre of the hip many times.
- Having augments pre-planned and 3D printed will give perfection and better patient outcomes.
- **Deformity Corrections:**
- Patients with congenital deformities or acquired deformities due to trauma or diseases require proper preoperative study on 3D software, and if required, customized implants and jigs are designed and manufactured.
- Jigs help correct deformities by aligning osteotomized bones/joints according to the patient's unique anatomy in all three axes. The anatomy that was deformed can now be corrected in all three planes and near normal anatomy can be restored.
- **Trauma Cases:**
- Complex fractures and trauma cases may involve complex situations and geometry that are challenging to address with standard implants. PSIs and jigs can be used to create customized solutions for fracture fixation, ensuring accurate alignment during surgery. In cases of malunion, non-union, or traumatic bone loss, deformity corrections and defect-filling solutions can be achieved using this technology.
- **Minimally Invasive Surgery (MIS):**
- PSIs are increasingly used in minimally invasive orthopaedic procedures. Customized guides aid in accurate implant placement and alignment, reducing the invasiveness of the surgery and promoting faster recovery. A small incision with a corrective jig will enable perfect wire, screw placement, or osteotomy.
- **Patient-Specific Instruments for Precise Bone Cuts:**
- Customized cutting guides can be designed to facilitate precise bone cuts during surgery. This is particularly relevant in joint replacement surgeries, where accurate cuts are crucial for proper implant alignment and function. The same is used for deformity correction as described above (Figs. 14.2, 14.4).
- **Anatomically Challenging Cases:**
- Cases with unusual or complex anatomies, where standard implants may not fit optimally, can benefit from PSIs. The customization allows for a better fit and can contribute to improved stability and longevity of the implant.

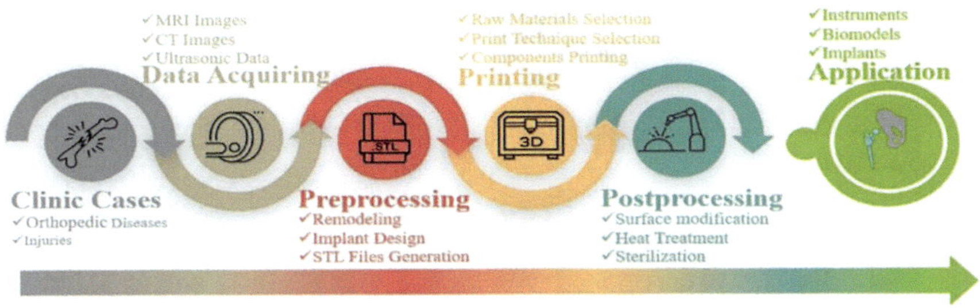

Fig. 14.5 Process of data acquisition, segmentation, designing, printing to product, post-process to application

- **Alignment Corrections:**
- Patients with malalignments in joints may require corrective osteotomies. Patient-specific instruments can assist in precisely planning and executing these corrective procedures.
- **Enhanced Surgical Planning:**
- PSIs n3D Technology Trailblazerot only aid in implant design but also in the preoperative planning process. Surgeons can use virtual models and simulations to plan the surgery more accurately, ensuring a smoother and more predictable procedure. This reduces the surgical time and blood loss (Fig. 14.5).

14.5 Patient-Specific Orthopaedic Implants

14.5.1 Customized Implants

Advantages: It is tailored to the patient's specific anatomy, giving proper anatomical reconstruction and filling the defect where required. Using the trabeculae interface potentially reduces complications such as implant loosening and giving excellent osteointegration.

Process: Typically involves advanced imaging techniques (e.g., CT scans), 3D metal printing, and computer-aided design (CAD) to create implants that match the patient's anatomy precisely.

14.6 Osteointegration Principle: Metal/Other Materials

Metal osteointegration refers to the process by which metal implants integrate or bond with the surrounding bone tissue. This integration is crucial for the stability and long-term success of various ***Prosthetic orthopaedic implants***, such as joint replacements, spinal implants, and orthopaedic fixation devices.

- Achieving a strong and durable integration between metal implants and bone is essential for the functionality and longevity of these devices.

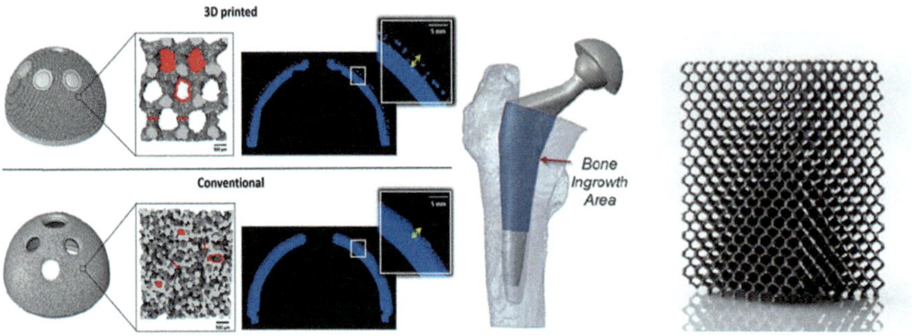

Fig. 14.6 Interface trabecular|lattice for osteointegration

- 3D printing enables the creation of lattice\trabeculae that mimic the bone trabeculae, and the integration is almost certain proven by various studies.
- Metal osteointegration involves a combination of biocompatible materials, surface treatments, implant design, and postoperative care to promote a strong and enduring integration between the metal implant and the surrounding bone tissue. Commonly used metal is Biomedical grade Titanium.
- The matrix formation in trabecular metal prosthetic implants is a dynamic process involving the infiltration of bone cells into the porous structure, leading to the deposition of a bone-like matrix.
- This process is crucial for achieving stable osseointegration, ensuring the long-term success and functionality of orthopaedic implants in clinical applications (Fig. 14.6).

14.7 Intra-Articular Prosthetic Implants

Intra-articular implants using 3D technology represent a cutting-edge approach in orthopaedics, specifically in the development of implants designed to fit within the joint space. These implants are customized for individual patients, leveraging 3D printing to give exact congruency to the native bone and cartilage.

- The **coefficient of friction** and **congruency** are important factors in the design of intra-articular implants, especially in focal or partial intra-articular surgeries.
- These factors influence the performance, wear resistance, and overall functionality of the implants within the joint space.
- A balance between the coefficient of friction and congruency is crucial in the design of intra-articular implants.
- Optimizing these factors helps reduce wear, enhance stability, and improve the long-term performance of joint replacements.
- Advances in materials, fusion imaging, and manufacturing techniques continue to shape the design and customization of intra-articular implants for better patient outcomes.
- Ongoing research and advancements in materials and design are likely to further enhance the efficacy of these implants (Fig. 14.7).

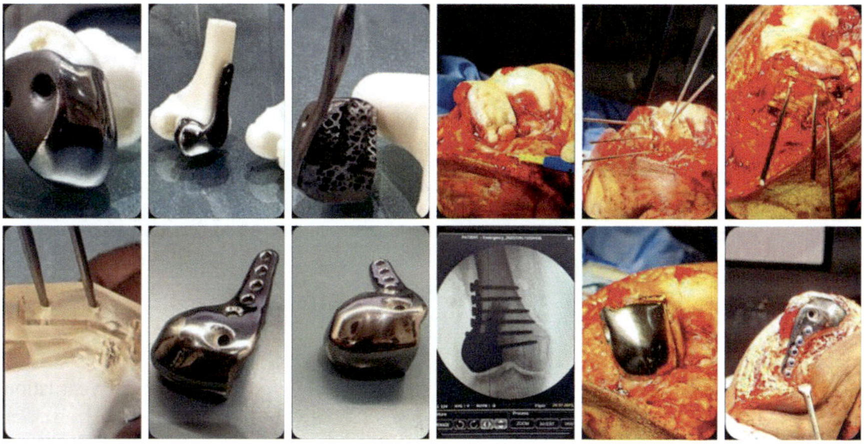

Fig. 14.7 3D Printed titanium, lateral femoral condyle with absolute congruency

Most important point to be considered is the interface of metal and cartilage should not be point loaded and should always have equal surface loading between the congruent surfaces in the entire range of movement under loading.

14.8 Surgical Approach, Steps of Fixation, and Stability of Fixation

- An orthopaedic surgeon gives their insights into the **surgical approach** and **steps** of fixation of the customized implant.
- The designer and surgeon plan the surgical steps of fixation precisely based on the design and application of a customized implant.
- The **stability of fixation** in customized implants is a critical factor in determining the success of orthopaedic surgeries. Achieving **stable fixation** is essential for promoting proper healing, reducing the risk of complications, and ensuring the long-term functionality of the implant.

14.9 Regulatory Considerations

- **Regulatory Approval:** The use of 3D-printed medical devices and implants often requires regulatory approval. Materials chosen should comply with regulatory standards.
- **Biocompatibility Testing:** Before clinical use, materials should undergo rigorous biocompatibility testing to ensure they do not elicit harmful responses in the human body. A Finite Element Analysis of any 3D-printed implant is a must to understand its strength of implant under loading of around one million cycles (Fig. 14.8).

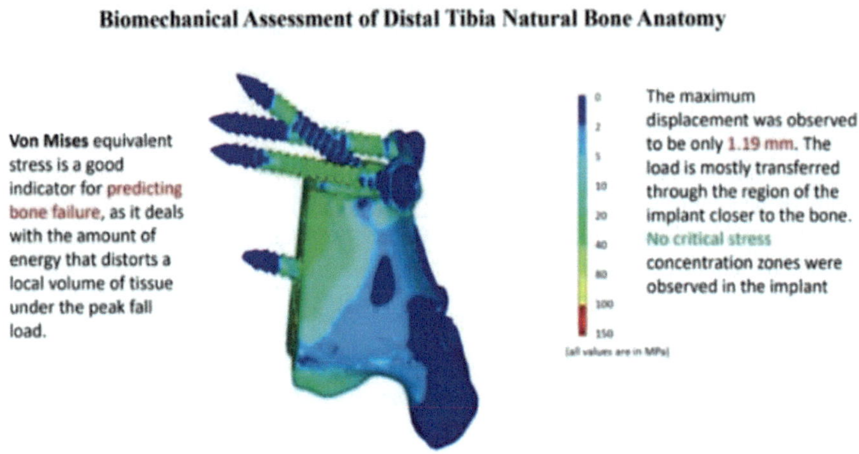

Fig. 14.8 Finite element analysis of any 3D printed implant

- **Application-Specific Requirements:** The specific requirements of the intended application, such as mechanical properties, degradation rates, and interaction with biological tissues, should guide material selection.

14.10 Artificial Intelligence (AI) and Machine Learning (ML)

AI and ML are increasingly being integrated into 3D technology in orthopaedics, offering innovative solutions for diagnostics, treatment planning, surgical guidance, and personalized patient care.

There are many ways in which AI and ML are influencing 3D technology in orthopaedics:

- **Image Analysis and Segmentation** can be automated using AI, process images, isolate anatomical structures, and reduce time for surgeons.
- **Disease Detection and Diagnosis** are possible using AI; ML can identify disease patterns and abnormalities in orthopaedic CT or MRI images.
- **Surgical Planning and Simulation** using AI algorithms can be automated. Implant placement, osteotomy, and jig design for corrective osteotomy can also be automated. Simulation models for surgical practice will reduce surgical time and stress and give the best patient outcomes.
- **Predictive Analytics for Patient Outcomes** by analysing the patient data and predicting potential complications, success rates, and effectiveness of different surgical implants and interventions.
- **Implant Design and Customization** by ML algorithms is the future. An AI model will consider biomechanics, material properties, anatomy, fit, and functionality of medical implants.
- **Rehabilitation and Postoperative Monitoring** using AI can assist in developing personalized rehabilitation plans, recovery trajectory, post-operative

outcomes, as well as in identifying complications and any deviation from the recovery path.

- **Decision Support Systems** can assist surgeons in making informed decisions based on patient data.
- **Natural Language Processing (NLP)** can extract valuable information from unstructured clinical notes, enhancing the richness of datasets used for training ML models in orthopaedic applications.
- **Remote Consultations** and **Virtual Collaboration** are possible using AI-powered tools that can support virtual collaboration between healthcare professionals. The tools allow for remote consultations and the sharing of 3D models and data for collaborative decision-making.
- **Quality Control in 3D Printing** is possible by selecting optimized material, desired properties, and patient-specific factors. AI can monitor quality, identify defects, and ensure industry compliance.
- The integration of AI and ML into 3D technology in orthopaedics holds great potential for enhancing patient care, improving surgical outcomes, and advancing the field of orthopaedic medicine through data-driven insights and personalized approaches.
- It is crucial to address challenges such as data privacy, ethical considerations, and the need for robust validation of AI algorithms in clinical practice.

14.10.1 Future of Orthopaedics Using 3D Technology

In the coming years, the number of cases with bone defects and deformities will increase and become more complex. Preoperative planning using information from CT/MRI, auto-segmentation, and AI-enabled solutions will become the future of orthopaedic surgeries.

The software will suggest the use of corrective jigs, or design customized implants. There will be automated defect or deformity analysis, and solutions will be suggested by computers. The surgeries will be twinned, first on prototype models and then on the patients.

Not only skeletal solutions but also soft tissue solutions in the form of cartilage, meniscus, muscle, nerve, or collagen tissue bioprinting will revolutionize orthopaedic surgery. Biodegradable, advanced polymers with memory will create a new class of implants. The learning of orthopaedics will switch to virtual oculus lenses, and HoloLens will assist surgeons per operative.

Robots will replace surgical hands, and surgeons will operate from remote locations. AI will enable post-operative rehabilitation and monitoring of patients' gait, movements, and recovery.

While these predictions offer a glimpse into potential future developments, it is important to note that the field of 3D technology in orthopaedics is dynamic, and unexpected breakthroughs or changes in the healthcare landscape could influence its trajectory. Advancements in 3D printing technology and material science continue to expand the range of biocompatible materials available for medical applications. Researchers are actively exploring new materials and refining existing ones to meet the diverse needs of medical 3D printing.

14.10.2 Case Study

This is an actual case study of a 3D-technology application for a patient with a Giant Cell Tumour (GCT).

Surgeon: Dr. Lalit Maini, Professor & Head of Dept, Maulana Azad Medical College, New Delhi, INDIA.

Concept & Design: Dr. Vikas Jain.

14.11 Defect Due to GCT Lower End Left Tibia in Young Female

A case of a 32-year-old female with a recurrence of GCT of the right Distal Tibia. She was initially treated with curettage and cementing as primary treatment and had recurrence after 4 years when she presented to us.

- History of right ankle pain, swelling, and stiffness of 4 years' duration.
- On clinical examination and subsequent investigation (X-ray, CT-scan, and MRI), she was diagnosed as a case of recurrence of GCT of the lower end of the right tibia. The patient underwent a biopsy for a definitive diagnosis and imaging of the extent of the tumour.
- Surgical options of ***arthrodesis*** with bone graft were contemplated.
- Another option is to replace that part of the ***ankle plafond with a 3D-printed trabecular prosthetic implant***, which has its articular surface metal on cartilage. The surgeon opted for this option.

14.12 Planning and Design Consideration

- Our team designed and conceptualized an en-bloc resection using 3D software. The resection gap/defect was calculated using opposite limb data mirroring. The model was thus created, meshed, and modified to create an intra-medullary canal, a fixation mechanism for bone and soft tissues.
- The trabecular concept with osteointegration was contemplated.
- The titanium prosthetic implant was 3D printed by additive layering on a DMP FLEX 350 printer. The post-printing processing involved a hydroxyapatite coating on the bone interface and the articular surface was given an excellent mirror finish.
- The articular surface was precisely and perfectly congruent with the superior surface of the talus as metal was contemplated on cartilage bearing.
- The FDA approved, and FEA analysis of the implant was done and was supplied sterile for surgery.

14.13 Intraoperative

- The surgery was successfully executed as per the preoperative plan under regional anaesthesia.
- A jig was used to remove the exact GCT tumour part of the bone with an intra-articular segment as per the preoperative planning on a bone model.
- The implant was perfectly aligned and fixed; the fibular graft was used intra-medullary to give secure secondary fixation; screws were fixed as per plan; on the table, the implant was sturdy, and the ankle range of movements was full. Soft tissues were reconstructed with the holes provided for anchoring (Fig. 14.9).

Info Box—Giant Cell Tumour (GCT)

Giant cell tumours of bone presenting in the distal tibia are rare; however, when they occur, they can present a reconstructive challenge. They are associated with a high local re-occurrence rate with intra-lesional treatment. Therefore, approaches to reconstruct the ankle after en bloc resection warrant study. Not only that, but the defect may not be treated by any off-the-shelf implant available currently in the medical device industry. Ankle arthrodesis with bone grafting would have not enabled joint preservation.

Clinical Outcome

- The patient has been followed up regularly and the expected results were achieved.
- After 9 months of follow-up, there is no recurrence of the tumour, patient has the full weight-bearing capability, and there are pain-free full range of movements at the ankle joint.
- Radiologically the implant has integrated with the bone with excellent joint preservation.
- Excellent osteointegration of the implant is seen on x-rays, and good ankle movements with metal on cartilage is observed. However, long-term follow-up is a must to prove any hypothesis.

Discussion

- 3D technology has enabled anatomical solutions for the described patient thus improving its mobility and quality of life.
- 3D technology enabled not only a detailed study of the tumour but also a proper preoperative plan for the patient—a young active women.
- A unique prosthetic implant has been designed, developed, and made out of titanium to exactly fit into the defect of resection.
- The aim of joint preservation and osteointegration has been achieved. New possibilities of metal on cartilage exist and they work well.

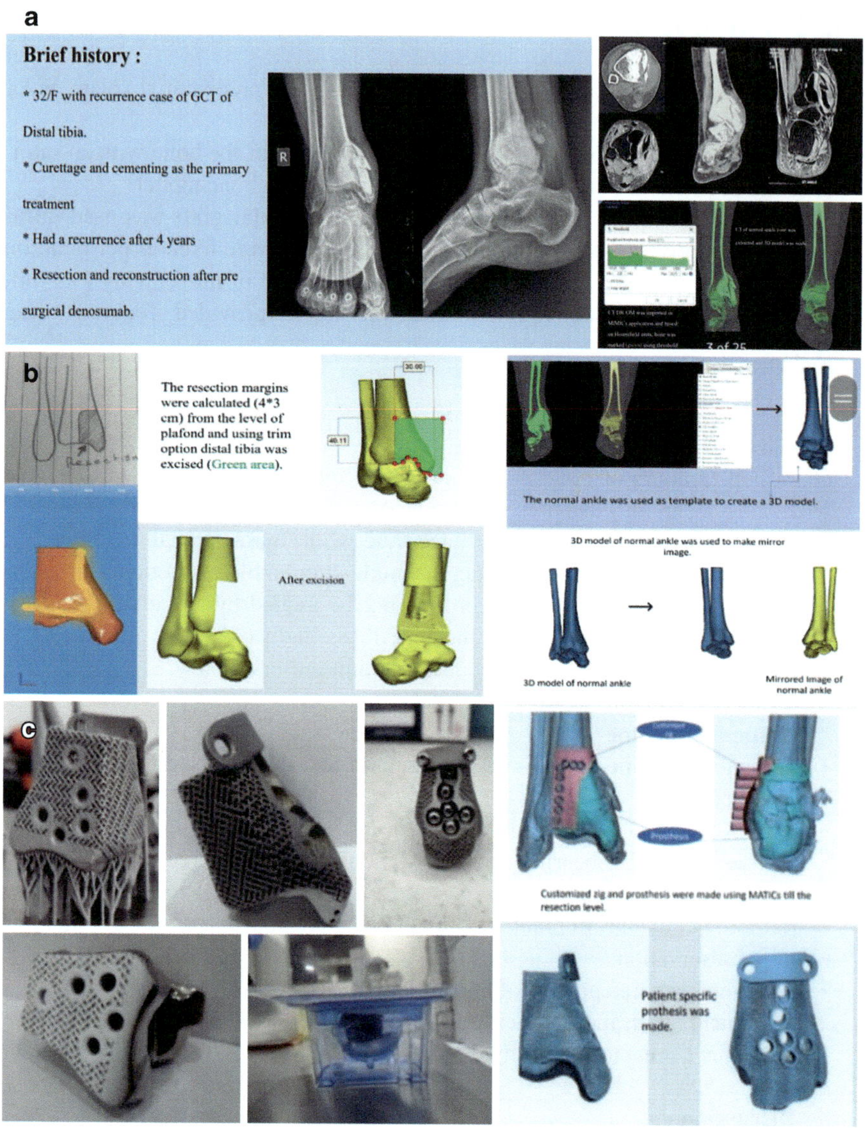

Fig. 14.9 (**a**) X-rays and MRI data of recurrence of GCT distal TIBIA. (**b**) Pencil drawing, CT segmentation, osteotomy cut, intra-articular planning. (**C**). 3D Printed plafond, unfinished, after finishing and sterile packaging. (**d**) Intraoperative, radiological, and fluoroscopic images. (**e**) Post-operative X-ray and ankle image in full flexion and full extension. (**f**) FEA of this implant, forces, and various studies citing ankle partial replacement

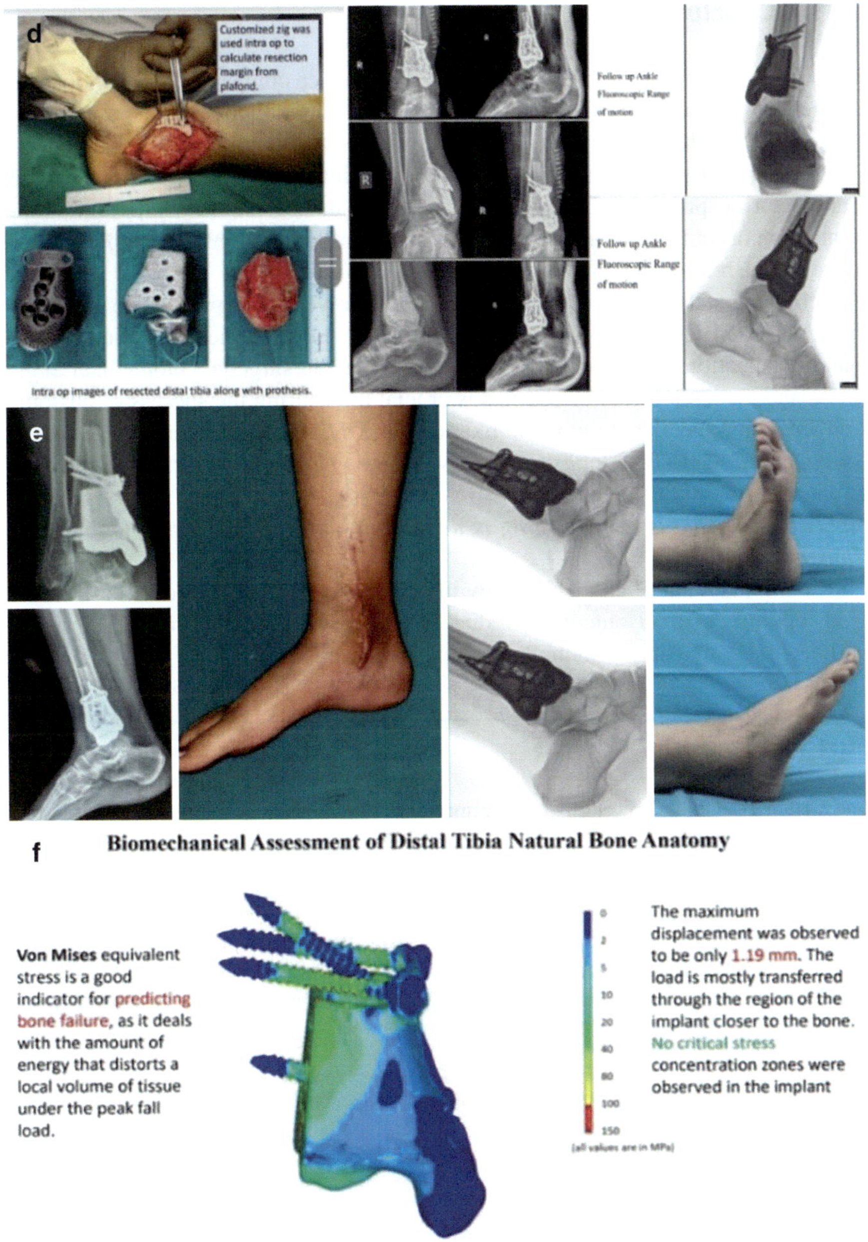

Fig. 14.9 (continued)

14.14 Conclusion

3D technology has opened new doors to medical device companies and orthopaedic surgeons. This technology is also evolving, has slow adoption, and poses many challenges, which in turn enable newer innovations.

3D printing (additive manufacturing) has revolutionized the design theory and manufacturing processes in orthopaedic medical device industry, providing substantial opportunities for easy prototyping, small production runs with opportunities for real-time refinement, and customizability.

Achieving stability in customized implants involves a comprehensive approach that considers patient-specific anatomy, biomechanics, surgical techniques, and material selection. Collaboration between orthopaedic surgeons, biomedical engineers, and medical device companies is crucial to ensuring the success of customized implants and the stability of fixation in orthopaedic surgeries. A complete ecosystem needs to be established in this technology. Research should be the core of optimization of this technology.

*"**The thing that is transforming is not technology, it is the technology that is transforming us!** "*

The ultimate aim of any technology in orthopaedics should be to better humankind, optimize patient outcomes, reduce any form of surgical stress, and enable optimized learning and wisdom through planning and surgery.

Further Reading

Gao CH, Wang CY, Jin H, et al. Additive manufacturing technique-designed metallic porous implants for clinical application in orthopedics. RSC Adv. 2018;8(44):25210–27. https://doi.org/10.1039/c8ra04815k.

Hollister SJ. Scaffold design and manufacturing: from concept to clinic. Adv Mater. 2009;21(32–33):3330–42. https://doi.org/10.1002/adma.200802977.

Javaid M, Haleem A. Current status and challenges of additive manufacturing in orthopaedics: an overview. J Clin Orthop Trauma. 2019;10(2):380–6. https://doi.org/10.1016/j.jcot.2018.05.008.

Li ZH, Wang CY, Li C, et al. What we have achieved in the design of 3D printed metal implants for application in orthopedics? Personal experience and review. Rapid Prototyp J. 2018;24(8):1365–79.

Morrison RJ, Kashlan KN, Flanangan CL, et al. Regulatory considerations in the design and manufacturing of implantable 3D-printed medical devices. Clin Transl Sci. 2015;8(5):594–600. https://doi.org/10.1111/cts.12315.

Osman RB, van der Veen AJ, Huiberts D, et al. 3D-printing zirconia implants; a dream or a reality? An in-vitro study evaluating the dimensional accuracy, surface topography and mechanical properties of printed zirconia implant and discs. J Mech Behav Biomed Mater. 2017;75:521–8. https://doi.org/10.1016/j.jmbbm.2017.08.018.

Rengier F, Mehndiratta A, von Tengg-Kobligk H, et al. 3D printing based on imaging data: review of medical applications. Int J Comput Assist Radiol Surg. 2010;5(4):335–41. https://doi.org/10.1007/s11548-010-0476-x.

Roohani-Esfahani SI, Newman P, Zreiqat H. Design and fabrication of 3D printed scaffolds with a mechanical strength comparable to cortical bone to repair large bone defects. Sci Rep. 2016;6:19468. https://doi.org/10.1038/srep19468.

Taniguchi N, Fujibayashi S, Takemoto M, et al. Effect of pore size on bone ingrowth into porous titanium implants fabricated by additive manufacturing: an in vivo experiment. Mat Sci Eng C-Mater. 2016;59:690–701. https://doi.org/10.1016/j.msec.2015.10.069.

Van der Stok J, Van der Jagt OP, Yavari SA, et al. Selective laser melting-produced porous titanium scaffolds regenerate bone in critical size cortical bone defects. J Orthop Res. 2013;31(5):792–9. https://doi.org/10.1002/jor.22293.

Wang XJ, Xu SQ, Zhou SW, et al. Topological design and additive manufacturing of porous metals for bone scaffolds and orthopaedic implants: a review. Biomaterials. 2016;83:127–41. https://doi.org/10.1016/j.biomaterials.2016.01.012.

Wang H, Su KX, Su LZ, et al. The effect of 3D-printed Ti6Al4V scaffolds with various macropore structures on osteointegration and osteogenesis: a biomechanical evaluation. J Mech Behav Biomed Mater. 2018;88:488–96. https://doi.org/10.1016/j.jmbbm.2018.08.049.

Wu H, Fahy WP, Kim S, et al. Recent developments in polymers/polymer nanocomposites for additive manufacturing. Prog Mater Sci. 2020;111:10638.

Wu Y, Liu J, Kang L, Tian J, Zhang X, Hu J, Huang Y, Liu F, Wang H, Wu Z. An overview of 3D printed metal implants in orthopedic applications: present and future perspectives. Heliyon. 2023;9(7):e17718. https://doi.org/10.1016/j.heliyon.2023.e17718. PMID: 37456029; PMCID: PMC10344715.

Zhang J, Zhang R, Ren G, et al. A method for using solid modeling CAD software to create an implant library for the fabrication of a custom abutment. J Prosthet Dent. 2017;117(2):209–13. https://doi.org/10.1016/j.prosdent.2016.05.018.

Swarm Intelligence in Psychiatry: Navigating Collective Wisdom for Mental Health

15

Otilia Gudana

15.1 The Basic Nature of Swarm Intelligence

At the base of swarm intelligence behaviour lies an automatic work model that allows all individuals to achieve a target without needing supervision, so it is autonomous.

Considering the well-known biological models and deducting the valuable insights from insects, mammals, ants, bees, and other social insects, we already know that individually they have limited intelligence sources (REF). However, when considered as a group, they build architectural wonders and are able to maintain optimal temperature and sufficient levels of oxygen and carbon dioxide, even as the nest grows. For social insects, teamwork is largely self-organised, coordinated primarily through the interactions of individual colony members. Together they can solve difficult problems (e.g., choosing the shortest route to a food or water source from myriad possible pathways) even though each interaction might be very simple (one ant merely following the trail left by another). The collective behaviour emerging from such groups has been defined as "swarm intelligence."

As these individual efforts get added, it creates an emerging group behaviour presenting the following characteristics [1]:

- Flexibility: the group can adapt to a changing environment.
- Robustness: even when one or more individuals fail, the group can still perform its tasks.
- Autonomy: activities are neither centrally controlled nor locally supervised.

This chapter has been independently curated and developed personally by the without any affiliation or support from any organisation.

O. Gudana (✉)
Munich, Bavaria, Germany

P. Plugmann, D. Portius (eds.), *Innovations in Healthcare and Outcome Measurement*, https://doi.org/10.1007/978-3-031-77302-0_15

The majority of current business executives and leaders models identify with the first two rules, nonetheless are hesitant to the third attribute of *autonomy*, which is, without doubt, the most intriguing and, simultaneously, the most effective of all [2]. To a greater extent, flexibility and robustness result from autonomy. To grasp the effectiveness of self-organisation (autonomy), we should first consider looking into some general rules of collective intelligence.

15.2 Collective Intelligence Rules

15.2.1 Social Dynamics

Swarm intelligence draws parallels between social insect colonies, and human societies. Just as ants communicate through chemical signals called pheromones, and bees perform elaborate dances to convey information, humans communicate through verbal and nonverbal cues expressing a specific group dynamics.

Let's take the following simple sentence and consider what it exactly means.

It's hot in here.

My co-workers would simply take this as a statement and imply that I feel warm and do not regard any other implications. On the other hand, my friend would annotate another meaning to it. They would consider the context, the tone of my voice, body language, facial expressions, and the emphasis of words within the statement and understand that I was transmitting genuine emotions.

The statement could simply mean that the temperatures are at an uncomfortable level. But it could mean that I lack fresh air or could act as an indirect invitation to open the windows. When considering it in a social context, it could be understood that based on the social atmosphere, I might be uncomfortable discussing a special topic or even being present in a specific group setting. It could also be understood positively as a statement coming from someone after battling a long winter with low temperatures.

The key takeaway is that simple words or actions might differ in their meaning depending on the contextual situation.

Based on one of the scientific behavioural analysis approaches, the "Iceberg Model" (Fig. 15.1) helps decipher and understand the meaning of (non)verbal cues, which are given by the words, thoughts, emotions, values, and beliefs of the one communicating a message.

Considering these insights, we can better determine group dynamics autonomy by individually interpreting one person's verbal to nonverbal cues, taking them as an *autonomous entity*, and then analysing their meaning based on the context this person brings to a specific "swarm".

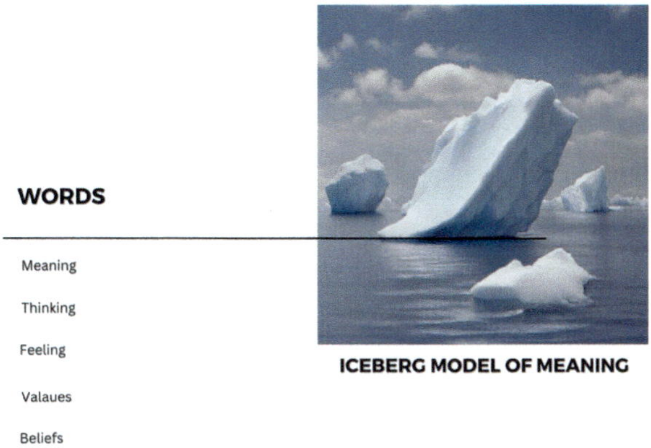

Fig. 15.1 Iceberg Model of Meaning created by Emotional Intelligence Academy

15.2.2 Crowdsourced Data and Diagnosis

The rise of the digital era of the last twenty years and the developments of social media platforms brought opportunities for young people in the sense that they are engaging with one another. In addition to that, it serves as a medium for maintaining friendships, chatting, tracking each other's activities, exchanging experiences, and even forming new connections. On the other hand, it poses significant risks for people discounting age, sex, or race. For healthcare professionals, digital platforms provide a unique advantage as they offer a vast amount of data through social media, forums, and online communities.

A study by Kim et al. [3] collected from X (formerly known as Twitter) posts of users who reportedly had been diagnosed with depression analysed the linguistic and emotional characteristics of the collected posts using the Linguistic Inquiry and Word Count (LIWC) and tracked their social engagement changes on Twitter. He was able to determine that depressed people use a specific "depression lexicon" with rather negative connotations (e.g., insomnia, imbalance, sadness, fatigue, nervousness, disturbed, isolation, moody, stressed) [3]. These insights can be detrimental to prompt diagnosis and therapeutic care for all healthcare professionals, families, and even peer groups.

Reece et al. [4] used Instagram image data to detect depression cues of users on social network services. After collecting the Instagram photos uploaded by users, he used both face detection and colourimetric analysis methods. His findings (Fig. 15.2) showed that Instagram photos posted by depressed individuals in the left photo have high saturation values (HSV), compared with photos posted by healthy individuals (right photo).

Another study attempted to predict users of postpartum depression on Facebook, based on their posts and comments and used specialised psychometric instruments to evaluate the level of postpartum depression between pre-and postnatal periods [5].

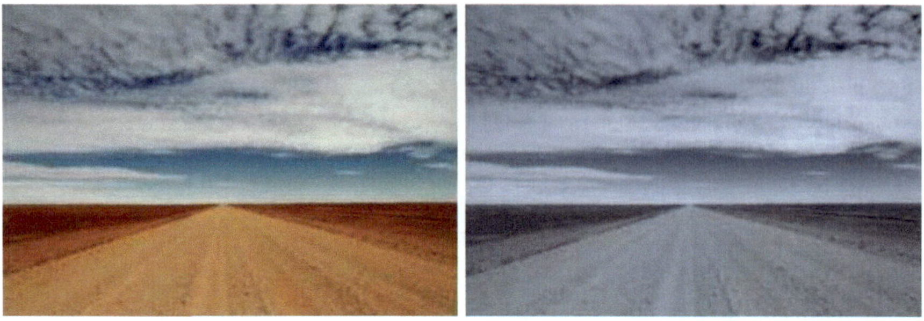

Fig. 15.2 Instagram Photos detecting cues of depression. From Reece and Danforth EPJ Data Science [4]. https://link.springer.com/content/pdf/10.1140/epjds/s13688-017-0110-z.pdf, licensed under CC-BY 4.0

It has been proven that increased social isolation and lowered availability of social capital on Facebook are the best predictors of postpartum depression in mothers.

Furthermore, Shen and Rudzicz [6] have demonstrated, based on collected user data from Reddit, that there are direct correlations between anxiety disorder and specific LDA (Linear Discriminant Analysis) topics such as school and alcohol (and drug) consumption [7].

By collecting available mental health data and analysing using swarm intelligence algorithms can identify patterns related to mental health trends, early symptom detection, and even assist in diagnosing certain disorders. Several previous studies revealed that social media is a place for users to express their feelings [8, 9]. Additionally, it can provide us with data that can be useful in observing or detecting users' emotions or potential mental problems [10].

15.3 Swarm Intelligence Algorithms in Psychiatry

15.3.1 Ant Colony Optimisation (ACO)

Algorithms are inspired by the foraging behaviour of ants. In psychiatry ACO can be used to optimise treatment plans, helping clinicians navigate the complex landscape of available interventions and personalise treatments for individual patients.

One example of a specific use case of the ACO algorithm in psychiatry is the creation of a treatment plan with the highest efficacy for a patient suffering from mild depression [11]. The leading physician, being in charge of implementing the ACO algorithm first forges by conducting an extended anamnesis, considering all biopsychosocial factors of the patients and finding the optimal, most efficient individualised treatment for patients.

Following the rules of autonomy, however, the case manager - or in this case, the leading physician — remains in the role of assessing the patient, following the algorithm protocols, and supplying holistically option plans (e.g., cognitive behavioural therapy, sleep optimisation, exercise, and various antidepressant medication) and adjacent therapies. Based on the third swarm intelligence rule of autonomy, the physician would act solely as a liaison and won't take over with supervision of complementary therapies.

Ultimately, when and if a certain number of criteria have been met and disabilities have been ruled out, the termination of the ACO algorithm and further monitoring must be taken as a last step into consideration (see Fig. 15.3).

15.3.2 Particle Swarm Optimisation (PSO) Algorithms

This is a well-known and multifaceted global optimisation method based on the social behaviour of bird flocks or fish schools.

The basic variant of the PSO algorithm works by having a population (swarm) of possible solutions (particles). These particles are moved around in the search space and are guided by their own best-known position in the search space, as well as the entire swarm's best-known position [12]. When improved positions are being discovered, these will then come to guide the movements of the swarm (see Fig. 15.4). The process is repeated, and by doing so it is hoped, but not guaranteed, that a satisfactory solution will eventually be discovered.

In mental health, particle swarm optimisation (PSO) can be applied to optimise medication dosages, behavioural therapies, or a combination of interventions, ensuring a balanced and effective treatment regimen.

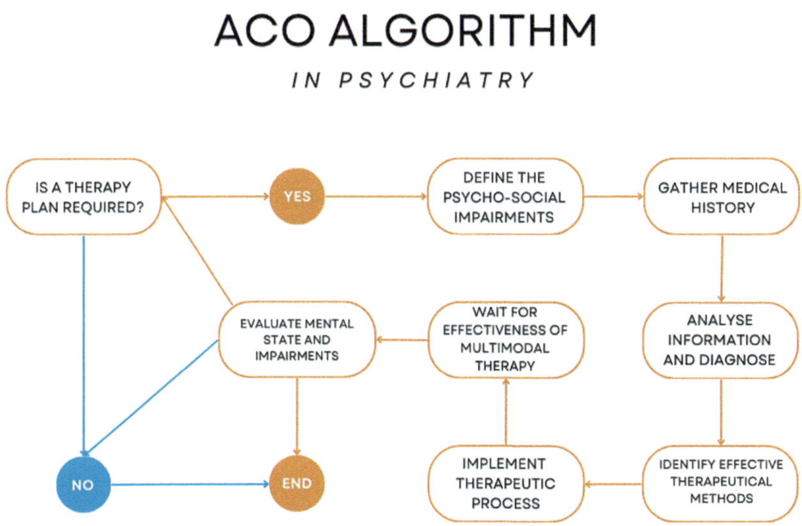

Fig. 15.3 ACO Algorithm in Psychiatry (Algorithm developed by the author)

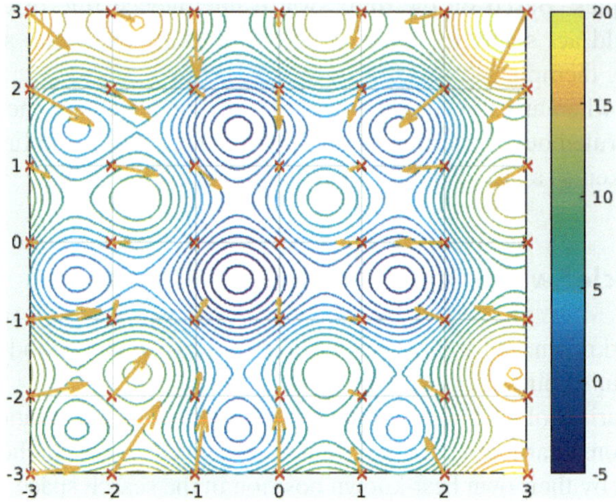

Fig. 15.4 A particle swarm searching for the global minimum of a function (Source: Photo by Ephramac. https://towardsdatascience.com/the-cartepole-problem-competitive-performance-with-particle-swarm-optimization-672f018ede3c, licensed under CC-BY 4.0)

Psychiatric disorders frequently necessitate pharmacological intervention, where finding the correct dosage, ensuring tolerability, and promoting patient compliance are paramount for achieving therapeutic success. The primary objective would be to swiftly implement pharmaceutical therapy for individuals grappling with severe mental health disorders, thereby mitigating the risk of these conditions progressing to chronic states. In many instances, however, finding the right dosage requires a prolonged time and fine-tuning of physicians based on side dosage profile, agreement, and response sensitivity.

15.3.3 Bee Algorithms

Bee Algorithms are modelled after the foraging behaviour of bees. This algorithm can be used to optimise human resource allocation in mental health care settings. It can help efficiently distribute resources, such as therapists, to areas with higher demand, ensuring more equitable access to care and therefore, reducing the possible number of psychiatric emergencies (e.g. violent outbursts).

While considering that swarm intelligence, as part of artificial intelligence, in psychiatry is still being explored and it is viewed as a black box due to its lack of transparency, there are some needs that artificial intelligence can help us quickly fill.

In 2024, one of the biggest challenges is the lack of representation of mental healthcare professionals [13]. The scarcity in rural areas is even higher. Swarm intelligence could balance multiple deficiencies: putting in place electronic health records, surveys, brain scans, social media, and sensor-based tracking systems.

Mental illness	Monitoring technique	Key findings
Schizophrenia	Electrocardiography (ECG)	- Cardiovascular mortality rates are significantly higher in individuals with schizophrenia - Changes in autonomic dysfunction during acute psychosis can predict sudden cardiac death - Non-linear complexity measures can aid in the early identification of high-risk patients
Bipolar disorder	Digital footprints	- One-minute writing sessions have a prediction accuracy of 90.31% - Passively sensed data, such as calls, SMS, activity, speech, and location, can be used to identify patients in stable or unstable states - The Social Rhythms Metric (SRM) is a clinically reliable marker for rhythmicity and stability
Depression and suicidal risk	Speech analysis	- Vocal jitter and glottal flow slope can predict near-suicidal patients - Changes in voice tone, reduced prosody, and a "lifeless" speech pattern have been observed in depressed patients - Fundamental frequency (voice pitch) is the main cue for emotion recognition, with diagnostic accuracy rates of around 70%

Fig. 15.5 Artificial intelligence monitoring techniques for mental health (Photo from Springermedizin.com, licensed under CC-BY 4.0.)

Current swarm intelligence algorithms could not only help professionals in planning treatment but also provide programs created to foresee mental illnesses, depression, and psychosis or even the chances of someone attempting suicide, just as the one presented in Fig. 15.5 [14, 15].

15.4 Swarm Intelligence and Psychotherapy

Applying the known swarm intelligence principles and following the rules of collective intelligence in group therapy sessions can enhance the collective healing process. By leading the group with the basic rules (flexibility, self--autonomy, robustness) and fostering an environment where participants can share experiences, and have the authority to self-organise or autonomously dictate, the therapeutic process can tap into the collective wisdom of the group to facilitate personal growth and a faster recovery.

Most psychiatric and/or psychosomatic illnesses do allow groups a self-reliant processes [16]. For example, dialectic behavioural therapy (DBT), which was created by Linehan in the 1970's, was created following two major concepts. One of these was that to achieve meaningful and happy lives, people must learn to accept things as they are. The other was that change is necessary for growth and happiness. Originally DBT was created as a behavioral therapeutic tool for patients suffering from borderline personality disorder (BPD), which is characterised by suicidal behaviour [17]. Along with the treatment of borderline personality disorder, DBT has also been used to treat different eating and substance abuse disorders [18]. Moreover, it was adapted to the field of forensic psychiatry in Germany in the treatment of antisocial behavioural personality to reduce aggression rates, now being called DBT-F [19].

DBT welcomes unsupervised peer-conducted self-help groups, as they provide a unique way to enable and fortify the autonomy of patients and strengthen the reliance on collective intelligence. Even though the concept of autonomy in a psychiatric context is not distant and is fully embraced, there are some severe cases where the therapeutic processes are predominantly determined by the healthcare professional (e.g. non-compliant patients or treatment-resistant schizophrenia with acute florid psychotic symptoms) [20].

Even so, the present therapeutic guidelines welcome a shared decision-making policy in psychiatric settings to improve treatment adherence, enhance patient satisfaction, and not ultimately reduce decisional conflicts.

A study demonstrated that computerised interactive multimedia cognitive-behavioural techniques conducted under minimal clinical supervision brought significant improvements in the therapy efficiency of depression and anxiety, as well as in work and social-related impairments [21].

Another possible way for patients to emulate collective intelligence is with the help of online platforms, forums, and digital communities focused on mental health support which rely on swarm intelligence principles. Unsupervised forums can facilitate discussions, harnessing the collective knowledge and experience of the community to provide valuable insights and emotional support to individuals in need [22]. As already discussed, these online platforms and digital health data are still an open faucet available for healthcare which is still not fully exploited.

Even though the dissemination of artificial intelligence in psychiatry and conducted research provide a strong evidence base regarding diagnosis, therapeutic plans, and pharmaceutical optimisation, the practical application in the healthcare field is complex.

The implementation of technological resources and available swarm intelligence algorithms in the field of psychiatry is still an ongoing process. However, with the fast-paced changes, further research is necessary before evolution will make it indispensable.

15.5 Ethical Considerations and Challenges

As with any application of data-driven technologies, ensuring the privacy and security of sensitive mental health information is paramount for the execution of swarm intelligence protocols.

Strict, multi-layered protocols and regulations must be established to protect the anonymity and confidentiality of individuals participating in swarm intelligence-based approaches. Currently, the increased stigma levels around mental health conditions represent one of the significant constraints in this technological implementation in real-life practices [23].

We must give attention to the matter of accountability of outcomes and responsibility when using artificial intelligence systems in the medical field.

Another crucial aspect of implementing swarm intelligence algorithms is inspecting potential biases in the data used to train these algorithms. Ensuring a diverse representation in the data set can help prevent the perpetuation of existing disparities in mental health care.

15.6 Conclusion

Swarm intelligence in the field of psychiatry represents an exciting frontier in mental health research and treatment. By harnessing the collective wisdom of individuals, it offers a fresh perspective on understanding and addressing mental health disorders. However, ethical considerations, along with ongoing research, regulatory clearance, and refinement of swarm intelligence algorithms, are critical for the responsible and effective implementation of this approach. As technology advances and our understanding of mental health deepens, swarm intelligence may play an increasingly significant role in shaping the future of psychiatry.

Financial Support and Sponsorship Nil.

Conflicts of Interest There are no conflicts of interest.

References

1. Bonabeu E, Meyer C. Swarm intelligence: a whole new way to think about business. Harv Bus Rev. 2001;79:106. https://hbr.org/2001/05/swarm-intelligence-a-whole-new-way-to-think-about-business
2. Krockert M, et al. Suitability of self-Organization for Different Types of production. Proc Manufac. 2021;54(2021):124–9. https://doi.org/10.1016/j.promfg.2021.07.020.
3. Kim J, et al. A deep learning model for detecting mental illness from user content on social media. Sci Rep. 2020;10:11846. https://doi.org/10.1038/s41598-020-68764-y.
4. Reece AG, Danforth CM. Instagram photos reveal predictive markers of depression. EPJ Data Sci. 2017;6:15. https://doi.org/10.1140/epjds/s13688-017-0110-z.
5. Gamon, Michael & Choudhury, Munmun & Counts, Scott & Horvitz, Eric. (2013). Predicting Depression via Social Media. Association for the Advancement of Artificial Intelligence. https://www.researchgate.net/publication/259948193_Predicting_Depression_via_Social_Media.
6. Shen J, Rudzicz F. detecting anxiety through reddit. In: Proceedings of the fourth workshop on computational linguistics and clinical psychology—from linguistic signal to clinical reality. Vancouver: Association for Computational Linguistics; 2017. p. 58–65.
7. Yoo M, et al. Semantic network analysis for understanding user experiences of bipolar and depressive disorders on Reddit. Inf Process Manag. 2019;56(4):1565–75.
8. Al-Saggaf Y, Nielsen S. Self-disclosure on Facebook among female users and its relationship to feelings of loneliness. Comput Hum Behav. 2014;36:460. https://doi.org/10.1016/j.chb.2014.04.014.
9. Valenzuela S, Park N, Kee KF. Is there social capital in a social network site?: Facebook use and college students' life satisfaction, trust, and participation. J Comput-Med Commun. 2009;14:875–901.
10. Rude S, Pennebaker J. Language use of depressed and depression-vulnerable college students. Cognit Emot. 2004;18(8):1121–33. https://doi.org/10.1080/02699930441000030.
11. Siniscalchi KA, Broome ME, Fish J, et al. Depression screening and measurement-based care in primary care. J Prim Care Community Health. 2020;11:2150132720931261. https://doi.org/10.1177/2150132720931261.

12. Zhang Y, et al. A comprehensive survey on particle swarm optimization algorithm and its applications. Artif Intell Appl. 2014;2015:1. https://doi.org/10.1155/2015/931256.
13. Mongelli F, Georgakopoulos P, Pato MT. Challenges and opportunities to meet the mental health needs of underserved and disenfranchised populations in the United States. Focus (American Psychiatric Publishing). 2020;18(1):16–24. https://doi.org/10.1176/appi.focus.20190028.
14. Avula V, et al. Artificial intelligence in psychiatry, present trends, and challenges: an updated review. Archives of Mental Health. 2023;25:1. https://doi.org/10.4103/amh.amh_167_23.
15. Terra M, et al. Opportunities, applications, challenges and ethical implications of artificial intelligence in psychiatry: a narrative review. Egypt J Neurol Psychiatry Neurosurg. 2023;59:1. https://www.springermedizin.de/opportunities-applications-challenges-and-ethical-implications-o/25672428
16. Markowitz FE. Involvement in mental health self-help groups and recovery. Health Sociol Rev. 2015;24(2):199–212. https://doi.org/10.1080/14461242.2015.1015149.
17. Chapman AL. Dialectical behavior therapy: current indications and unique elements. Psychiatry (Edgmont). 2006a;3:62.
18. Dimeff LA, Linehan MM. Dialectical behavior therapy for substance abusers. Addict Sci Clin Pract. 2008;4(2):39–47. https://doi.org/10.1151/ascp084239.
19. Wettermann A, Völlm B, Schläfke D. Highly structured treatment programs for addicted offenders: comparing the effects of the reasoning & rehabilitation program and DBT-F. Front Psychiatry. 2020;11:499241. Published 2020 Nov 13. https://doi.org/10.3389/fpsyt.2020.499241.
20. Légaré F, Adekpedjou R, Stacey D, et al. Interventions for increasing the use of shared decision making by healthcare professionals. Cochrane Database Syst Rev. 2018;7:CD006732. https://doi.org/10.1002/14651858.CD006732.pub4.
21. Proudfoot J, et al. Computerized, interactive, multimedia cognitive-behavioural program for anxiety and depression in general practice. Psychol Med. 2003;33(2):217–27. https://doi.org/10.1017/S0033291702007225.
22. Mamkyna L, Nakikj D, Elhadad. Collective Sensemaking in online health Formus. In proceedings of the 33rd annual ACM conference on human factors in computing systems (CHI '15). New York, NY: Association for Computing Machinery; 2015. p. 3217–26. https://doi.org/10.1145/2702123.2702566.
23. Wainberg ML, et al. Challenges and Opportunities in Global Mental Health: a Research-to-Practice Perspective. Current psychiatry reports. 2017;19(5):28. https://doi.org/10.1007/s11920-017-0780-z.

Correction to: Futuristic Dentistry: Towards Medical–Dental Integration and Minimalistic Approaches

Andrea Lorena Basualdo Allende

Correction to:
Chapter 8 in: P. Plugmann, D. Portius (eds.),
Innovations in Healthcare and Outcome Measurement,
https://doi.org/10.1007/978-3-031-77302-0_8

The original version of the chapter "Futuristic Dentistry: Towards Medical–Dental Integration and Minimalistic Approaches" was inadvertently published with an incorrect author affiliation. The correct affiliation details have been updated in the chapter.

The updated version of this chapter can be found at
https://doi.org/10.1007/978-3-031-77302-0_8

P. Plugmann, D. Portius (eds.), *Innovations in Healthcare and Outcome Measurement*, https://doi.org/10.1007/978-3-031-77302-0_16

GPSR Compliance

The European Union's (EU) General Product Safety Regulation (GPSR) is a set of rules that requires consumer products to be safe and our obligations to ensure this.

If you have any concerns about our products, you can contact us on ProductSafety@springernature.com

In case Publisher is established outside the EU, the EU authorized representative is:

Springer Nature Customer Service Center GmbH
Europaplatz 3
69115 Heidelberg, Germany

Batch number: 10732044

Printed by Printforce, the Netherlands